PROCEDURES and MONITORING for the CRITICALLY ILL

W9-BZX-175

THE DONKEY SANCTUARY
OF HEREFORD
SLAD, ...

PROCEDURES and MONITORING for the CRITICALLY ILL

William C. Shoemaker, MD, FCCM
Professor of Anesthesia and Surgery
University of Southern California, Keck School of Medicine
Los Angeles, California

George C. Velmahos, MD, FACS, FRCS
Associate Professor of Surgery
University of Southern California, Keck School of Medicine
Attending Surgeon
Division of Trauma and Critical Care
Los Angeles County and University of Southern California Medical Center
Los Angeles, California

Demetrios Demetriades, MD, PhD, FACS
Professor of Surgery
University of Southern California, Keck School of Medicine
Attending Surgeon and Chief
Division of Trauma and Critical Care
Los Angeles County and University of Southern California Medical Center
Los Angeles, California

Peggy Firth, Medical Illustrator

W.B. SAUNDERS COMPANY
A Harcourt Health Sciences Company
Philadelphia   London   New York   St. Louis   Sydney   Toronto

THE RICHARD STOCKTON COLLEGE
OF NEW JERSEY LIBRARY
POMONA, NEW JERSEY 08240-0195

W.B. SAUNDERS COMPANY
A Harcourt Health Sciences Company

The Curtis Center
Independence Square West
Philadelphia, Pennsylvania 19106

Library of Congress Cataloging-in-Publication Data

Procedures and monitoring for the critically ill/
[edited by] William C. Shoemaker, George C. Velmahos, Demetrios Demetriades;
Peggy Firth, medical illustrator.

p.   cm.

Includes bibliographical references.

ISBN 0–7216–8758–X

1. Critical care medicine.   2. Patient monitoring.   I. Shoemaker, William C.
II. Velmahos, George C.   III. Demetriades, Demetrios.
[DNLM: 1. Critical Illness—therapy.   2. Critical Care—methods.
3. Monitoring, Physiologic.   WX 218 P9625 2002]

RC86.7 P755 2002   616′.028–dc21   2001020319

Editor-in-Chief: Richard Lampert
Acquisitions Editor: Allan Ross
Project Manager: Mary Anne Folcher
Manuscript Editor: Linda Van Pelt
Production Manager: Frank Morales
Illustration Specialist: Peg Shaw
Book Designer: Matt Andrews

PROCEDURES AND MONITORING FOR THE CRITICALLY ILL   ISBN 0–7216–8758–X

Copyright © 2002 by W.B. Saunders Company.

All rights reserved. No part of this publication may be reproduced or transmitted in any form or by
any means, electronic or mechanical, including photocopy, recording, or any information storage and
retrieval system, without permission in writing from the publisher.

Printed in the United States of America.

Last digit is the print number: 9   8   7   6   5   4   3   2   1

RC 86.7 .P755 2002
OCLC: 45951596
Procedures and monitoring
for the critically ill

THE RICHARD STOCKTON COLLEGE
OF NEW JERSEY LIBRARY
POMONA, NEW JERSEY 08240-0195

CONTRIBUTORS

JUAN A. ASENSIO, MD, FACS
Associate Professor, University of Southern California, Keck School of Medicine, Division of Trauma and Critical Care, Department of Surgery; Attending Surgeon, Los Angeles County and University of Southern California Medical Center, Los Angeles, California
Intra-abdominal Pressure Monitoring

HOWARD BELZBERG, MD, FCCM
Assistant Professor of Surgery, University of Southern California, Keck School of Medicine; Associate Director, Division of Trauma and Critical Care, Los Angeles County and University of Southern California Medical Center, Los Angeles, California
Renal Function and Support

SUSAN I. BRUNDAGE, MD, MPH
Assistant Professor, Michael E. DeBakey Department of Surgery, Baylor College of Medicine; Director, Surgical Emergency Center Service, Ben Taub General Hospital, Houston, Texas
Pericardiocentesis and Pericardial Window

JOSÉ CEBALLOS, MD
Research Fellow, Division of Trauma and Critical Care, Department of Surgery, Los Angeles County and University of Southern California Medical Center, Los Angeles, California
Intra-abdominal Pressure Monitoring

J. COLOMBO, PhD
Adjunct Professor, Science and Technology, Bucks County Community College, Newtown, Pennsylvania; Executive Vice President, Ansar, Inc., Philadelphia, Pennsylvania
Noninvasive Autonomic Nervous System Monitoring in Critical Care

EDWARD E. CORNWELL III, MD
Associate Professor of Surgery, Johns Hopkins University; Chief of Adult Trauma, Johns Hopkins Medical Institutions, Baltimore, Maryland
Cricothyroidotomy

WILLIAM M. COSTIGAN, MD
Clinical Instructor in Orthopaedic Surgery, Los Angeles County and University of Southern California Medical Center, Los Angeles, California
Bedside Spinal Immobilization

PETER CROOKES, MD
Assistant Professor of Surgery, University of Southern California, Keck School of Medicine; Attending Surgeon, University of Southern California Hospital and Los Angeles County and University of Southern California Medical Center, Los Angeles, California
Percutaneous Feeding Catheters

JULIO CRUZ, MD, PhD
Postgraduate Professor, Escola Paulista de Medicina, Federal University of São Paulo; Director, The Comprehensive International Center for Neuroemergencies, São Paulo, Brazil
Jugular Bulb Oximetry

DEMETRIOS DEMETRIADES, MD, PhD, FACS
Professor of Surgery and Director of Trauma and Surgical Intensive Care Unit, University of Southern California, Keck School of Medicine; Chief of Trauma/Surgical Intensive Care Unit, Los Angeles County and University of Southern California Medical Center, Los Angeles, California
Tube Thoracostomy

GORDON L. ENGLER, MD
Professor of Clinical Orthopaedic and Neurologic Surgery, University of Southern California, Keck School of Medicine; Director, Scoliosis and Spinal Surgery, Los Angeles County and University of Southern California Medical Center, Los Angeles, California
Bedside Spinal Immobilization

DEBRA H. FISER, MD
Professor and Chairman, Department of Pediatrics, University of Arkansas for Medical Sciences; Chief of Pediatrics, Arkansas Children's Hospital, Little Rock, Arkansas
Intraosseous Infusion

WALTER FORNO, MD
Research Fellow, Division of Trauma and Critical Care, Department of Surgery, Los Angeles County and University of Southern California Medical Center, Los Angeles, California
Intra-abdominal Pressure Monitoring

DOUGLAS B. HOOD, MD, FACS
Assistant Professor of Surgery, Department of Surgery, Division of Vascular Surgery, University of Southern California, Keck School of Medicine, Los Angeles, California
Inferior Vena Caval Filter Placement

RIYAD KARMY-JONES, MD
Assistant Professor, Department of Surgery, Division of Cardiothoracic Surgery, University of Washington; Chief of Cardiothoracic Surgery, Harborview Medical Center, University of Washington, Seattle, Washington
Pericardiocentesis and Pericardial Window

v

LARRY KHOO, MD
Clinical Instructor, Department of Neurosurgery, University of Southern California, Keck School of Medicine, Los Angeles, California
Intracranial Pressure Monitoring

JAMES A. MURRAY, MD
Assistant Professor of Surgery, University of Southern California, Keck School of Medicine; Attending Surgeon, Los Angeles County and University of Southern California Medical Center, Los Angeles, California
Arterial Catheterization; Renal Function and Support

KATHY JEAN M. NAKANO, MD
Chief Surgical Resident, Santa Barbara Cottage Hospital, Santa Barbara, California
Pulmonary Artery Catheterization

ISMAEL N. NUÑO, MD
Assistant Professor of Surgery, University of Southern California, Keck School of Medicine; Chief, Cardiac Surgery Service, Los Angeles County and University of Southern California Medical Center, Los Angeles, California
Cardiac Pacemaker Placement

JOHN M. PORTER, MD, FACS
Associate Professor of Surgery, Northeastern Ohio Universities College of Medicine, Rootstown, Ohio; Director of Trauma/Critical Care Services, St. Elizabeth Health Center, Youngstown, Ohio
Gastric Tonometry

MARCUS L. QUEK, MD
Resident in Urology, University of Southern California, Keck School of Medicine and Los Angeles County and University of Southern California Medical Center, Los Angeles, California
Suprapubic Urinary Tube Placement

LINDA REVER, MD
Codirector of Pain Management Services, Department of Anesthesiology, Los Angeles County and University of Southern California Medical Center, Los Angeles, California
Epidural Analgesia

VINCENT L. ROWE, MD
Assistant Professor of Surgery, Department of Surgery, Division of Vascular Surgery, University of Southern California, Keck School of Medicine, Los Angeles, California
Inferior Vena Caval Filter Placement

ALI SALIM, MD
Clinical Instructor, Department of Surgery, University of Southern California, Keck School of Medicine, Los Angeles, California
Intracranial Pressure Monitoring

JACK SAVA, MD
Assistant Unit Chief, Division of Trauma and Critical Care, Department of Surgery, Los Angeles County and University of Southern California Medical Center, Los Angeles, California
Intra-abdominal Pressure Monitoring

STEPHEN M. SCHEXNAYDER, MD
Associate Professor, Pediatrics and Internal Medicine, University of Arkansas for Medical Sciences; Medical Director, Pediatric Intensive Care Unit, Arkansas Children's Hospital, Little Rock, Arkansas
Intraosseous Infusion

BRADFORD G. SCOTT, MD
Assistant Professor of Surgery, Michael E. DeBakey Department of Surgery, Baylor College of Medicine; Director of Minimally Invasive Surgery and Director of Trauma Registry, Ben Taub General Hospital, Houston, Texas
Pericardiocentesis and Pericardial Window

WILLIAM C. SHOEMAKER, MD, FCCM
Professor of Anesthesia and Surgery, University of Southern California, Keck School of Medicine; Attending Surgeon, Los Angeles County and University of Southern California Medical Center, Los Angeles, California
Routine Clinical Monitoring in Acute Illnesses; Invasive Hemodynamic Monitoring; Noninvasive Cardiac Output Monitoring: Bioimpedance and Partial CO_2 Rebreathing Methods; Noninvasive Autonomic Nervous System Monitoring in Critical Care; Physiology of Shock and Acute Circulatory Failure; Hemodynamic Therapy for Circulatory Dysfunction

MERVYN SINGER, M.D.
Reader in Intensive Care Medicine, University College London, Rayne Institute, London, England
Transesophageal Doppler Monitoring

JOHN P. STEIN, MD
Assistant Professor of Urology, University of Southern California, Norris Comprehensive Cancer Center; Attending Physician, Los Angeles County and University of Southern California Medical Center, Los Angeles, California
Suprapubic Urinary Tube Placement

MICHAEL J. SULLIVAN, MD
Assistant Professor of Anesthesiology, University of Southern California, Keck School of Medicine, Los Angeles, California
Assisted Ventilation and Intubation

GAIL T. TOMINAGA, MD
Associate Professor of Surgery, John A. Burns School of Medicine; Director, Trauma Services, The Queen's Medical Center, Honolulu, Hawaii
Flexible Bronchoscopy

GEORGE C. VELMAHOS, MD, PhD

Associate Professor of Surgery, University of Southern California, Keck School of Medicine; Attending Surgeon, Division of Trauma and Critical Care, Los Angeles County and University of Southern California Medical Center, Los Angeles, California
Central Venous Catheterization; Bedside Tracheostomy; Diagnostic Abdominal Paracentesis and Peritoneal Lavage

KENNETH WAXMAN, MD

Director of Trauma and Surgical Education, Santa Barbara Cottage Hospital, Santa Barbara, California
Pulmonary Artery Catheterization

CHARLES C.J. WO, BS

Research Associate, University of Southern California and Los Angeles County and University of Southern California Medical Center, Los Angeles, California
Invasive Hemodynamic Monitoring; Noninvasive Cardiac Output Monitoring: Bioimpedance and Partial CO_2 Rebreathing Methods; Physiology of Shock and Acute Circulatory Failure

To my father, Konstantinos, and mother, Elpida, to whom I owe everything I am or have done.
G.C.V.

To my parents.
D.D.

To doctors and nurses who wish more exposure to critical care methods and concepts to improve the care of their ICU patients.
W.C.S., G.C.V., D.D.

PREFACE

Bedside procedures are an integral part of the care delivered to our critically ill patients. Whether performed for diagnostic, monitoring, or therapeutic purposes, bedside procedures are used at a frequency that does not allow inadequate knowledge of the related technique, indications, and complications. Under the pressure of more effective utilization of operating rooms, bedside procedures in the intensive care unit are increasingly in demand. As the concept of intensive care is expanding beyond the narrow confines of the ICU, bedside procedures are increasingly more likely to be performed in several other monitored areas within the hospital. For this reason, such procedures constitute an essential part of the practice of physicians treating critically ill patients.

This book is intended to provide a comprehensive review of the most commonly used bedside procedures. Description of these procedures is usually squeezed in among information on other and more complex operations in a variety of general surgery, urology, and neurosurgery textbooks. In comparison to glorified surgical techniques, bedside procedures have little appeal. Although one can brag about performing a pancreatoduodenectomy, this opportunity is seldom given after percutaneous gastrostomy. Many of us might remember that bedside tracheostomy was not always as easy as thought, however. Definitely, all of us would agree that an emergent cricothyroidotomy can save a life in a much more effective way than most complex cancer operations.

Bedside procedures are closely associated with monitoring. What is the use of knowing how to place a pulmonary artery catheter if one cannot interpret the findings derived by it? For this reason, we decided also to include a monitoring section. Although this book is not designed to describe in detail all monitoring techniques, it became obvious that we could not exclude the monitoring methods that are related directly to bedside procedures. The Editors have provided important cross-references between the techniques and monitoring chapters.

As health care costs are spiraling and resources are dwindling, expectations of both patients and physicians have increased. These pressures constantly call into question the traditional practices of physicians taking care of critically ill patients. Assigning a task to another specialist and ignoring the details associated with it is an outdated and dangerous practice. Although the value of consulting physicians is undisputed, the patient's own doctor should synthesize all different parameters and orchestrate the optimal care for the patient. The modern intensivist, whether surgeon, pulmonologist, cardiologist, or anesthesiologist, needs to have a complete understanding of all bedside procedures and be competent to perform many of them. We hope that this book will help our colleagues obtain a better understanding of these often understated but frequently life-saving, technically challenging, and very important bedside procedures.

WILLIAM C. SHOEMAKER
GEORGE C. VELMAHOS
DEMETRIOS DEMETRIADES

NOTICE

Critical care medicine is an ever-changing field. Standard safety precautions must be followed, but as new research and clinical experience broaden our knowledge, changes in treatment and drug therapy may become necessary or appropriate. Readers are advised to check the most current product information provided by the manufacturer of each drug to be administered to verify the recommended dose, the method and duration of administration, and contraindications. It is the responsibility of the treating physician, relying on experience and knowledge of the patient, to determine dosages and the best treatment for each individual patient. Neither the Publisher nor the editor assumes any liability for any injury and/or damage to persons or property arising from this publication.

THE PUBLISHER

CONTENTS

Part
I

PROCEDURES

1 Central Venous Catheterization

George C. Velmahos

The placement of central venous catheters is an important task and one of the most frequent bedside procedures. Like any other procedure, central venous catheterization (CVC) can be associated with significant complications. Patients requiring these catheters are frail, and the related complications, although easily managed in healthy individuals, can be catastrophic in critically ill patients. For this reason, attention to technical details and knowledge of all possible pitfalls will minimize the risk of CVC.

Indications and Contraindications

The main indications are (1) rapid resuscitation via infusion of fluids or blood; (2) hemodynamic monitoring (to measure central venous pressures) or pulmonary artery catheterization; (3) long-term administration of medication, as for cancer patients on chemotherapy; (4) inability to access peripheral veins; and (5) hemodialysis, plasmapheresis, or transvenous pacemaker placement.

The main contraindications are (1) infection, (2) trauma, and (3) venous thrombosis at the selected site.

Selection of Insertion Site

Three sites are frequently used: the subclavian, the internal jugular, and the femoral vein. No site is good for all patients. Each site is associated with advantages and disadvantages and should be selected according to the individual circumstances.

The Subclavian Route. The subclavian vein is probably the most frequently used site because it is convenient for the patient and for nursing care. It is associated with the highest rate of complications, however, mainly owing to injuries to the apex of the lung (pneumothorax and hemothorax). It is the ideal site for patients who already have a chest tube in place. The subclavian route should not be used in patients with coagulopathy; in case of accidental puncture of the subclavian artery, effective manual compression cannot be maintained owing to the location of the artery under the clavicle.

The Jugular Route. The jugular route is uncomfortable for the patient, and nursing care is more difficult. It cannot be used safely in patients who need cervical spine precautions or who have tracheostomies. The

rate of complications is low, however. Lung puncture is unusual, and inadvertent injury to nearby vascular structures can be easily managed with direct pressure.

The Femoral Route. The femoral route is definitely the most uncomfortable site for the patient and therefore cannot be used for long periods of time. Because of the ease of catheter insertion at this site, it is a great choice during acute resuscitation. It is associated with a high incidence of infection, however, because it is difficult to maintain aseptic conditions at the groin; this is an additional reason precluding its prolonged use. The femoral route should not be used when trauma to the inferior vena cava or the iliac veins (as in major pelvic fractures) is suspected.

Selection of Catheter

Although there are a wide variety of catheters on the market, two types are used most frequently: the triple-lumen catheter and the Cordis catheter.

Triple-Lumen Catheter. The triple-lumen catheter has three lumina, which can be used for infusion of different kinds of fluids and medication and for monitoring central venous pressures after connection to a pressure transducer. It does not allow the insertion of a pulmonary artery catheter (Fig. 1–1).

The Cordis Catheter. The Cordis catheter has only one wide lumen with two ports. One port can be connected to a line for infusion of fluids and medication, and the other can be used for insertion of a pulmonary artery catheter. The Cordis catheter should be chosen over the triple-lumen catheter whenever massive resuscitation is required in patients who may need pulmonary artery catheterization. (The wide single lumen allows rapid infusion of fluids.) When aggressive resuscitation or pulmonary artery catheterization is no longer needed, Cordis catheters are better switched over to triple-lumen catheters, which allow connection to multiple infusion or monitoring lines (Fig. 1–2).

The Seldinger Technique

The Seldinger technique is the standard method of insertion regardless of catheter type, although there are some small variations, as described later. The entire

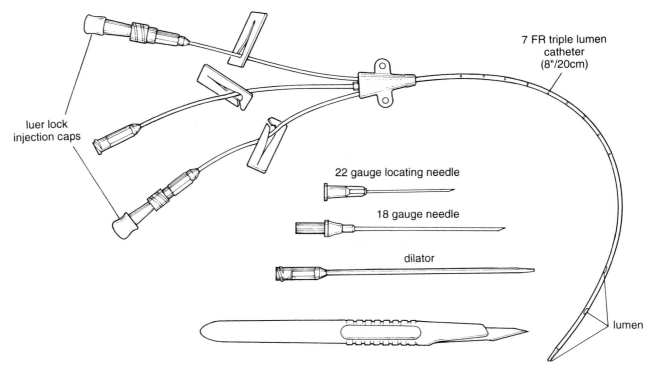

luer lock
injection caps

7 FR triple lumen
catheter
(8"/20cm)

22 gauge locating needle

18 gauge needle

dilator

lumen

FIGURE 1–1. Triple-lumen catheter set.

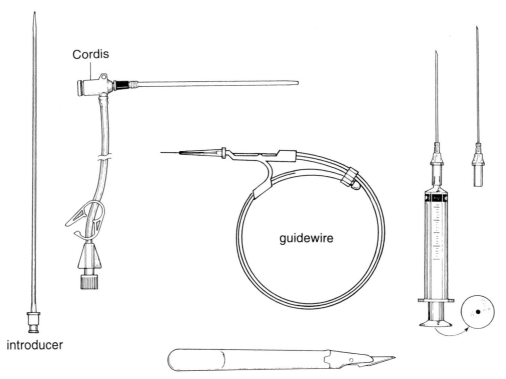

Cordis

guidewire

introducer

FIGURE 1–2. Cordis catheter set.

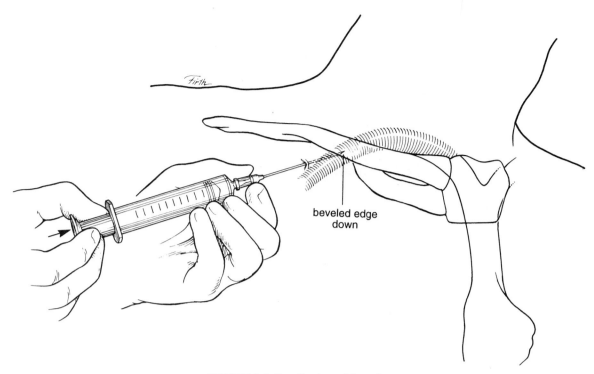

FIGURE 1–3. Localization of the vein.

procedure should be done under sterile conditions. Gown, mask, gloves, towels, and meticulous preparation of the area are mandatory. A step-by-step description of the insertion technique follows.

- The needle is inserted slowly at the appropriate landmark for the selected access site while gentle and constant suction is applied to the syringe connected to the needle (Fig. 1–3).
- When the vein has been entered, blood is aspirated into the syringe.
- For Cordis catheters, a guidewire is inserted through an opening on the plunger of the syringe (Fig. 1–4); for triple-lumen catheters, a guidewire is inserted through the needle after it has been disconnected from the syringe (Fig. 1–5). The guidewire should not be inserted more deeply than 20 cm from the skin. There is a wide mark on the guidewire to indicate approximately this distance.
- The syringe and the needle (for Cordis catheters) or the needle (for triple-lumen catheters) is withdrawn, and the guidewire is left in place (Fig. 1–6).
- The skin insertion site is incised with a No. 11–blade knife to create a skin opening of about 0.5 to 1 cm around the guidewire (Fig. 1–7).
- A dilator is introduced over the guidewire to dilate the tract and is then withdrawn. This step applies only to triple-lumen catheters.
- The catheter is introduced over the guidewire into the vein. In the case of Cordis catheters, the entire complex of introducer/dilator and catheter is inserted over the guidewire (Fig. 1–8). The introducer/dilator is then withdrawn.

- Blood is aspirated from all ports, which are flushed with saline or heparin solution, and all the port sites that are not intended for immediate use are sealed. A port should never be left open to air during insertion because air embolism may occur.
- The catheter is secured in place by suturing it onto the skin, and the entire area is covered to keep it sterile (Fig. 1–9).
- Postprocedural radiography is performed to document catheter tip position. Although a radiograph is not necessary for femoral catheters, it is mandatory for subclavian or jugular catheters.

Landmarks for Access

Subclavian Venous Catheterization. For subclavian vein catheterization, the patient is placed in reverse Trendelenburg position to distend the vein for easier access and to prevent air embolism. The most commonly used technique is the infraclavicular approach. The needle is inserted into the skin 2 cm under the middle of the clavicle. With the bevel oriented caudally, the needle is directed toward the sternal notch (Fig. 1–10). It is imperative for the needle to abut the clavicle and to pass immediately underneath it to avoid entrance into the pleural cavity and injury to the apex of the lung (Fig. 1–11). Rarely, the supraclavicular approach is used. In this approach, the needle is inserted just lateral to the tubercle marking the attachment of the anterior scalene muscle to the first rib and is directed toward the underside of the manubrium.

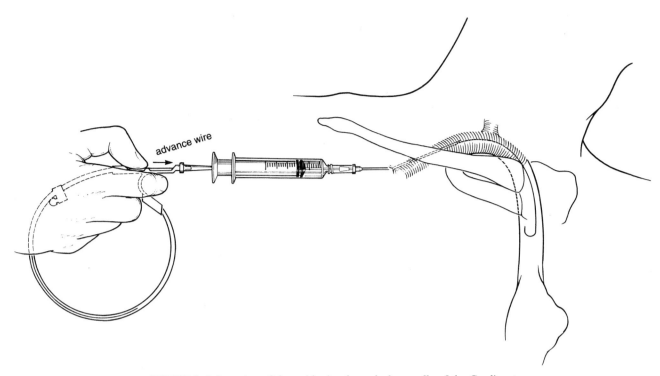

FIGURE 1–4. Insertion of the guidewire through the needle of the Cordis set.

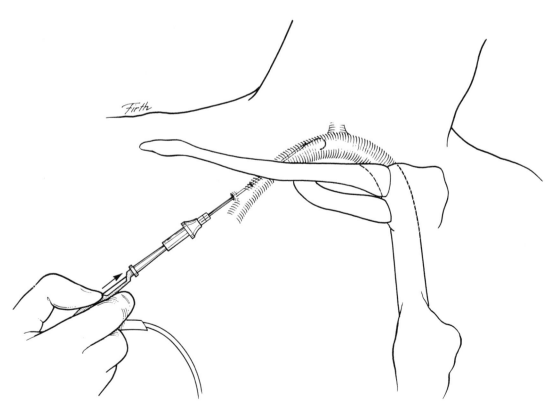

FIGURE 1–5. Insertion of the guidewire through the needle of the triple-lumen catheter set.

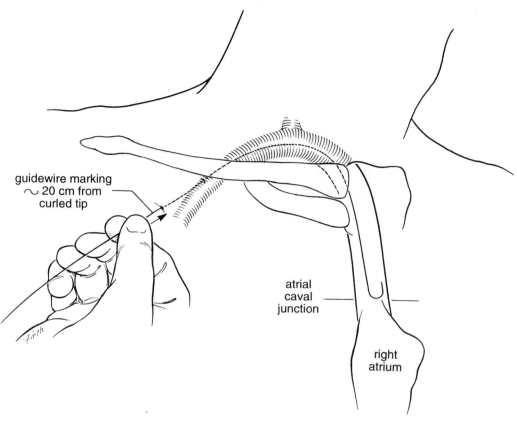

FIGURE 1–6. Guidewire in place. Needle is withdrawn.

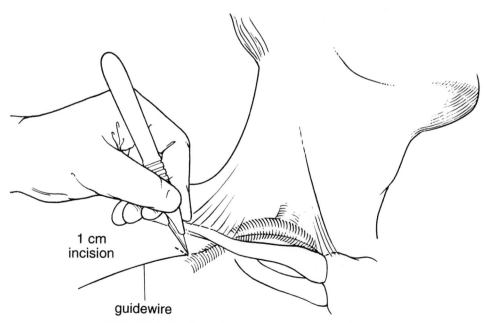

FIGURE 1–7. Small skin incision at guidewire insertion site.

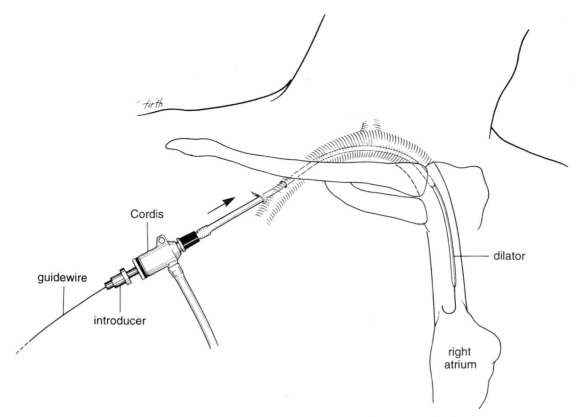

FIGURE 1–8. Insertion of Cordis catheter and introducer over guidewire.

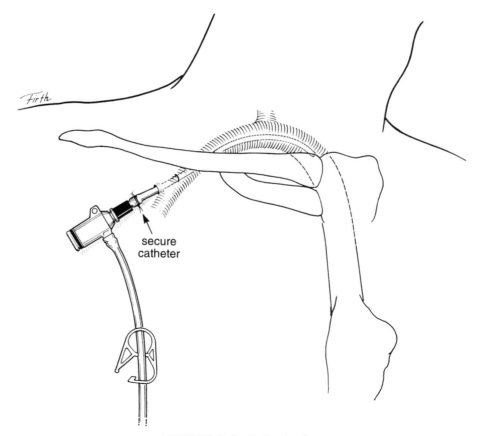

FIGURE 1–9. Cordis line in place.

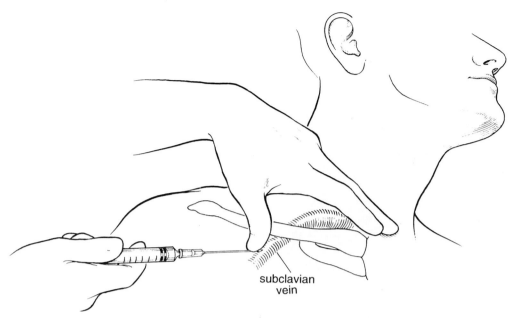

FIGURE 1–10. Position of hands during subclavian line placement.

subclavian
vein

Internal Jugular Venous Catheterization. For internal jugular vein catheterization, the patient is placed in reverse Trendelenburg position. A roll may be placed under the patient's shoulders to hyperextend the neck if spinal precautions are not required. There are three methods to access the internal jugular vein (Fig. 1–12). In the anterior approach, the skin is punctured at the anterior border of the sternocleidomastoid muscle and at mid-distance between the angle of the mandible and the sternoclavicular junction. The needle is directed at a 30- to 45-degree angle to the skin medial to the ipsilateral nipple (Fig. 1–13). In the middle approach, the needle is inserted at the junction of the sternal and the clavicular heads of the sternocleidomastoid muscle and is headed at a 30- to 45-degree angle to the skin medially to the ipsilateral nipple. These two approaches are best done with the patient's head turned away from the site of insertion, but they can also be done without moving the head. The posterior approach is my preferred method but usually requires rotation of the head to the contralateral side, a movement that is not allowed if spinal precautions are necessary. The needle is inserted at the posterior border of the sternocleidomastoid muscle, mid-distance between the angle of the mandible and the clavicle at a 30-degree angle to the skin, and is directed toward the

FIGURE 1–11. Correct orientation of needle during subclavian line placement to avoid injury to the lung. art., artery.

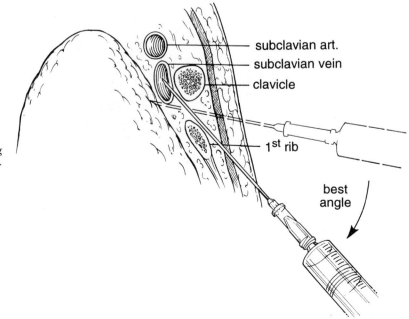

subclavian art.
subclavian vein
clavicle
1st rib
best angle

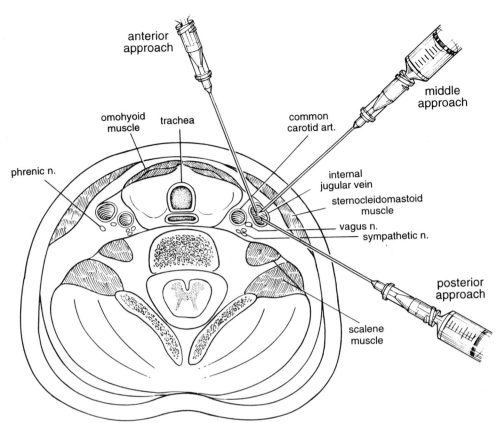

anterior approach

middle approach

omohyoid muscle

trachea

common carotid art.

phrenic n.

internal jugular vein

sternocleidomastoid muscle

vagus n.

sympathetic n.

posterior approach

scalene muscle

FIGURE 1–12. The three approaches (anterior, middle, posterior) to jugular vein catheterization. art., artery; n., nerve.

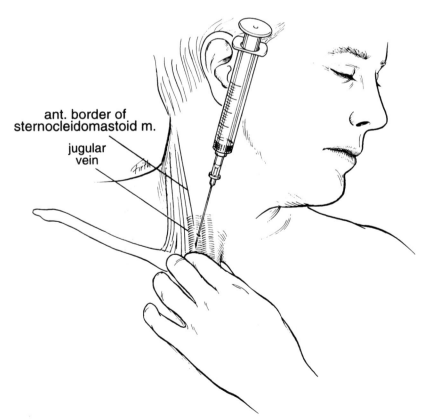

ant. border of sternocleidomastoid m.

jugular vein

FIGURE 1–13. Anterior (ant.) approach to jugular vein catheterization. m., muscle.

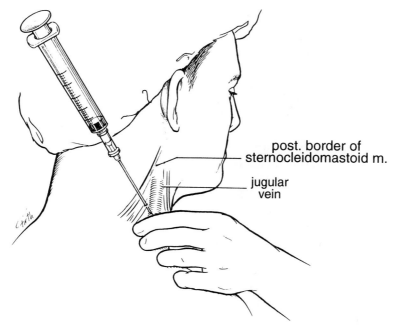

FIGURE 1–14. Posterior (post.) approach to jugular vein catheterization. m., muscle.

sternal notch (Fig. 1–14). Because the internal jugular vein crosses the posterior border of the muscle in a more superficial position than the carotid artery, the posterior approach makes localization of the vein easy.

Femoral Venous Catheterization. For femoral vein catheterization, the patient is flat, preferably with the thigh abducted. The pulse of the artery is palpated, and the needle is inserted medial to the pulsation. If pulses are absent, the needle should be inserted at the junction of the middle and the distal third of the distance between the pubic tubercle and the anterior superior iliac spine. The direction of the needle should be toward the umbilicus at a 30- to 45-degree angle to the skin (Fig. 1–15).

Complications

Pneumothorax and Hemothorax. The incidence of pneumothorax and hemothorax is 2% to 10% with subclavian vein catheterization and 1% to 2% with internal jugular vein catheterization. Aspiration of air during insertion of the syringe is pathognomonic and is associated with multiple attempts due to difficult access, overdistended lungs (as in emphysema), anatomic variants, and inexperience of the operator. To avoid air aspiration, the needle should be in immediate contact with the lower border of the clavicle while being advanced toward the vein. Ultrasound guidance during insertion may decrease the rate of inadvertent lung injury. Auscultation and urgent chest radiography after the procedure are paramount. Patients undergoing positive pressure ventilation should be closely followed even in the absence of initial symptoms. A chest

tube is the treatment of choice for pneumothoraces greater than 20% or for those of any size in patients undergoing positive pressure ventilation. The remaining patients could be managed without a chest tube if kept under close surveillance.

Inadvertent Arterial Puncture. Inadvertent arterial puncture is usually recognized when bright red pulsating blood drains from the needle. The needle should be withdrawn, and digital compression should be applied for 5 to 10 minutes. In the absence of coagulopa-

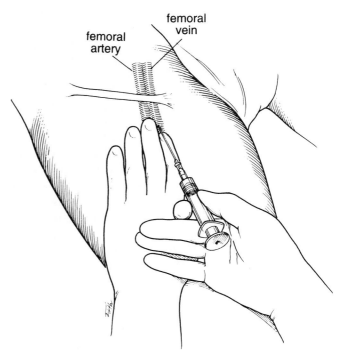

FIGURE 1–15. Femoral vein catheterization.

thy, the bleeding almost always stops. Subclavian artery injury is more difficult to control because digital compression is not adequate owing to the course of the artery behind the clavicle. Even with subclavian artery needle injuries, however, the bleeding is usually self-contained by the surrounding tissues. In patients with coagulopathy, subclavian artery catheterization should be avoided.

Worse injury to the adjacent artery occurs if the injury is not recognized early and the catheter is advanced into the artery. In this event, the catheter should be removed, and digital compression should be applied. The possibility of arterial dissection, intimal flap creation, or pseudoaneurysm should be excluded by means of duplex scanning, particularly if the carotid arteries are involved.

Tracheal Puncture. Tracheal puncture is characterized by aspiration of air. It requires only withdrawal of the needle and is invariably of no further concern.

Lymphatic Drainage. Lymphatic drainage may occur with inadvertent injury to the major thoracic duct during left subclavian or internal jugular venous catheterization. It can be in the form of a chyle fistula, a chyloma, or a chylothorax. It almost always responds to conservative treatment with drainage, a low-fat diet, or, if needed, total parenteral nutrition.

Air Embolism. Air embolism is a potentially lethal complication. It may occur if air is aspirated from the environment into the venous system during insertion of the catheter. A disconnected line or ports that are not sealed properly are common causes. Hypotensive patients who have negative venous pressure are more at risk. Although hemodynamically significant air embolism is caused by entrance of approximately 100 mL of air, smaller quantities can be deleterious in patients with limited physiologic reserve. To avoid air embolism, the patient should be placed in reverse Trendelenburg position during insertion. In this way, the pressure into the venous system increases at the site of venous puncture (for jugular and subclavian catheterization) and does not easily allow entrance of air. Additionally, if air does enter, it is captured at the apex of the heart rather than entering the pulmonary circulation. The manifestations of air embolism range from new onset of cough to cardiac arrest. Desaturation is the most common significant symptom. The treatment is quick evaluation of all lines and connections, placement of the patient in reverse Trendelenburg position, and cardiorespiratory support.

Venous or Cardiac Perforation. Venous or cardiac perforation is an unusual complication but is potentially lethal. Atrial perforations occurred with older and more rigid catheter designs. The new catheters are softer and do not irritate the endocardium. Postplacement radiography should always confirm that the tip of the catheter is lying above the superior vena caval–atrial junction (Fig. 1–16). Cardiac perforation,

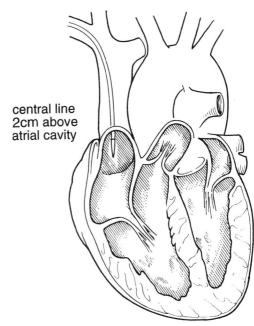

FIGURE 1–16. Correct position of the central line tip (i.e., slightly above the vena cava and the right atrial junction).

manifested by signs of cardiac tamponade, requires emergent surgical intervention. Perforation of the vein can result if a false tract is made by the dilator or the guidewire. The catheter is then placed outside the vein and, on rare occasions, hangs free in the pleural cavity. This could be extremely dangerous because fluid flow in the line is unobstructed and gives a false sense of security that the line has no problems. At the same time, all the resuscitation fluid is running into the chest. The complication is avoided by aspirating blood on insertion of the catheter.

Cardiac Arrhythmias. Arrhythmias occur if the guidewire or the catheter is irritating the endocardium. They are usually self-limited on withdrawal of the irritating device and only infrequently require antiarrhythmic medication. The guidewire should not be inserted more than 20 cm during catheter placement, and the position of the tip of the catheter should always be evaluated radiographically to ensure that it lies above the heart.

Catheter-Related Venous Thrombosis. The incidence of venous thrombosis around the catheter is unknown but is suggested to be up to 40% depending on the site, the duration of placement, the technique, the type of infusate, and the general condition of the patient. Furthermore, the percentage of catheter-related deep venous thromboses that progress to complete venous obstruction or pulmonary embolism is unknown. At this point, although routine venous duplex screening is not considered a standard of care, it is advisable to use duplex screening for certain subpopulations at risk.

Catheter-Related Infections. The breakdown of the

skin barrier will unavoidably lead to bacteremia. The incidence decreases if strict sterile techniques are maintained. Bacteremia is usually caused by gram-positive bacteria, although gram-negative bacteria and fungi are not unlikely. A rate of catheter-related bacteremia of 5% is acceptable. Antibiotic-coated catheters are manufactured to decrease the infection rates. There are many studies concluding that they do succeed, and others claim that they do not. A meta-analysis shows that the benefit is not substantial. These catheters are also very expensive. The diagnosis can be confirmed if the same pathogen is retrieved from blood cultures and from cultures of the catheter tip. Antibiotic administration or withdrawal of the catheter is appropriate according to individual circumstances.

Common Mistakes

Multiple Attempts at the Same Site. After three unsuccessful attempts, the site should be changed, or more senior help should be sought. The risk of inadvertent injury to adjacent structures increases with multiple attempts. The hematoma that forms as a result of multiple punctures compresses the vein and makes insertion even more difficult. Ultrasonographic guidance may resolve this problem.

Reluctance to Use Upper Veins Because of a Collar. Central venous catheterization may be a lifesaving intervention. Although femoral vein catheterization is preferred in the presence of a cervical collar, there will be occasions when the femoral vein cannot be used. Removal of the collar does not mean that all spinal precautions have to be aborted. Rather, sandbags, pharmaceutical paralysis, forehead taping, and manual stabilization are all adequate alternative spinal precautions that free the upper torso and the neck area for central venous catheterization.

Use of a Site Distal to an Injury. Always keep in mind that if there is a potential injury to the vein at a more proximal site than the site of catheterization, all the resuscitation fluid may extravasate through the injury. For this reason, subclavian catheterization is not a good idea in the presence of an upper presternal penetrating injury, nor is femoral catheterization a good idea in the presence of severe ipsilateral pelvic fractures or a suspected inferior vena caval injury (Fig. 1–17).

Pushing the Guidewire or the Dilator against Resistance. The insertion should be smooth. If there is resistance, a false passage is most probably created. Withdraw and repeat the procedure.

Pulling the Guidewire or the Catheter against Resistance. If the guidewire or the catheter cannot be withdrawn, one of two things has occurred: Either they are entangled by another intravenous device (a line on the other side or a vena caval filter), or there is a knot. In either case, do not try to withdraw forcefully. Stop the procedure and obtain adequate radiographs. Surgery may be necessary.

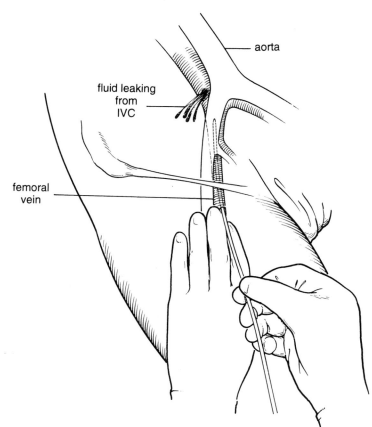

FIGURE 1–17. The femoral vein is not the site of choice for central line placement if proximal injury is suspected. IVC, inferior vena cava.

Suggested Readings

1. Collier PE, Goodman GB: Cardiac tamponade caused by central venous catheter perforation of the heart: A preventable complication. J Am Coll Surg 1995;181:459–463.
2. Parsa MH, Parsa CJ, Sampath AC: Intravenous and intra-arterial access. In Shoemaker WC, Ayres S, Grenvik A, Holbrook PR (eds): Textbook of Critical Care, 4th ed. Philadelphia, WB Saunders, 2000, pp 59–74.
3. Puri VK, Carlson RW, Bander JJ, et al: Complications of vascular catheterization in the critically ill. Crit Care Med 1980;8:495–499.
4. Raad II, Luna M, Khalil SA, et al: The relationship between the thrombotic and infectious complications of central venous catheters. JAMA 1994;271:1014–1016.
5. Trottier SJ, Veremakis C, O'Brien J, et al: Femoral deep vein thrombosis associated with central venous catheterization: Results from a prospective randomized trial. Crit Care Med 1995;23:52–59.

2 Arterial Catheterization

James A. Murray

Arterial catheters are indicated whenever a need for continuous blood pressure monitoring or frequent sampling of arterial blood gases is present. Invasive monitoring allows for the acquisition of information concerning the patient's cardiopulmonary function and the effects of therapy. Precise and continuous blood pressure monitoring is warranted in patients with shock or in patients requiring high levels of respiratory support, which may compromise cardiac function.

Although placement of arterial catheters is relatively safe and inexpensive, the need for them should be evaluated on an individual basis. Some relative contraindications to arterial catheterization include coagulation abnormalities and anticoagulation therapy. Arterial catheters should not be placed in sites with evidence of infection or trauma, through a vascular prosthesis, or in a situation in which distal ischemia is a concern (e.g., in patients with occlusive arterial disease).

Arteries from either the upper or the lower extremities may be used for invasive blood pressure monitoring. The radial artery is the most commonly used vessel. Alternative sites include the dorsalis pedis, the posterior tibial artery, and the femoral arteries of the lower extremity. The ulnar, the brachial, and the axillary arteries of the upper extremity are used very infrequently.

The ulnar artery is the dominant artery in the hand. It is connected to the radial artery through the palmar arch in 95% of patients. To ensure adequate blood supply to the hand, the Allen test is performed before a radial arterial line is placed. This test consists of occlusion of the radial artery by means of digital pressure to ensure that the ulnar artery has a pulse and that the hand is perfused adequately.

Technique

To place an arterial catheter, the patient must be able to cooperate or must be adequately sedated to prevent movement during the procedure. Local anesthetic, 1% lidocaine without epinephrine, should be used to anesthetize the skin at the site of insertion. The use of an anesthetic agent containing epinephrine can make the artery difficult to palpate owing to vasospasm.

Protective pads or towels are placed under the extremity at the site of insertion. When the wrist is the insertion site, slight extension may facilitate placement of the catheter. This maneuver makes the radial artery less tortuous and easier to cannulate, but excessive extension can make introduction of the catheter more difficult as the artery is stretched and compressed. Sterile technique should be used during placement of arterial catheters.

Except for femoral artery catheterization, a 20-gauge catheter is generally used. Smaller catheters should be used in pediatric patients and may be necessary in smaller adults. Cannulation can be achieved by directly threading an angiocatheter into the artery or by using a modified Seldinger technique. The direct techniques can be done by cannulating the artery with an angiocatheter or by using transfixation. The modified Seldinger technique can be done using catheters with a built-in guidewire or using a separate guidewire. The artery is palpated between two fingers approximately 1 cm apart. The catheter should be directed between the two palpating fingers at a 30- to 45-degree angle to the skin (Fig. 2–1).

Direct Insertion Method

In the direct insertion technique without a guidewire, an angiocatheter is inserted into the artery, maintaining the 30- to 45-degree angle. Once a flash of blood is obtained through the catheter, both the catheter and the needle are advanced 1 to 2 mm into the lumen of the artery (Fig. 2–2A). This is done to ensure that the tip of the cannula is within the artery, not just the tip of the needle. If the catheter is correctly positioned, blood will continue to return through it. Once the cannula is within the lumen of the artery, the angle is reduced to 15 degrees to facilitate advancement of the catheter. The needle portion is held steady as the catheter is advanced over the needle. Gentle twisting of the catheter may make advancement easier. As the catheter advances and the needle is withdrawn, pulsatile blood appears from the catheter (Fig. 2–2B). If resistance is met or blood is not returned, the catheter should not be advanced. The needle should be withdrawn slightly until blood return is present; then an attempt should be made to advance the catheter

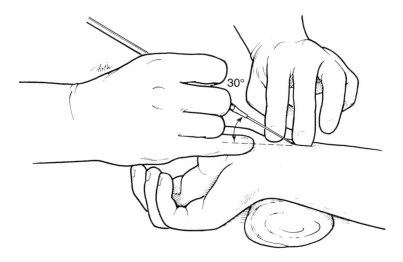

FIGURE 2–1. Catheterization of the radial artery. The catheter is inserted at a 30- to 45-degree angle to the skin. Slight wrist extension by means of a roll under the wrist facilitates placement.

again. If the attempt is unsuccessful, the needle should be removed, and the pressure should be held until bleeding stops before another attempt is made.

Transfixation Technique

An alternative method, the transfixation technique, is shown in Figure 2–3. All the initial steps remain the same. With this method, both the anterior and the posterior walls of the artery are penetrated (Fig. 2–3A). The inner needle is then withdrawn completely (Fig. 2–3B). The plastic cannula is gradually pulled back until blood flows freely from the end of the catheter (Fig. 2–3C). At this point, the angle of the cannula is reduced to 15 degrees. If blood continues to return freely at this point, the cannula may be gently advanced into the arterial lumen (Fig. 2–3D). Gentle

twisting may facilitate advancement of the catheter. If this is unsuccessful, the cannula should be removed, the pressure should be held until bleeding stops, and another try with a new catheter should be made. Because of the high failure rate, I do not advise using this technique.

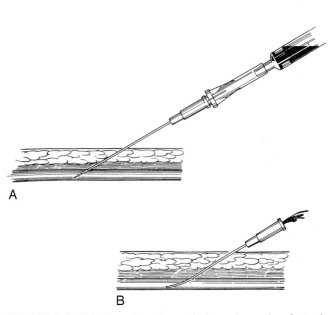

FIGURE 2–2. The direct insertion technique. An angiocatheter is advanced toward the artery. Once the needle is within the lumen (A), the cannula is advanced into the vessel (B).

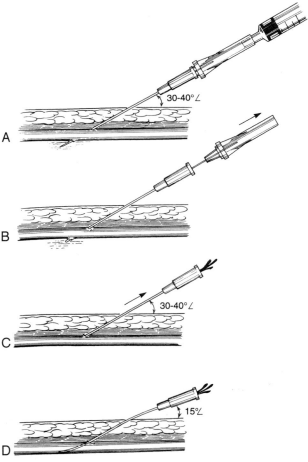

FIGURE 2–3. The transfixation technique. The needle and the cannula are guided through both the anterior and the posterior walls of the artery (A). The needle is withdrawn completely (B). The cannula is gradually pulled back until blood returns (C), and the cannula is then advanced within the lumen (D).

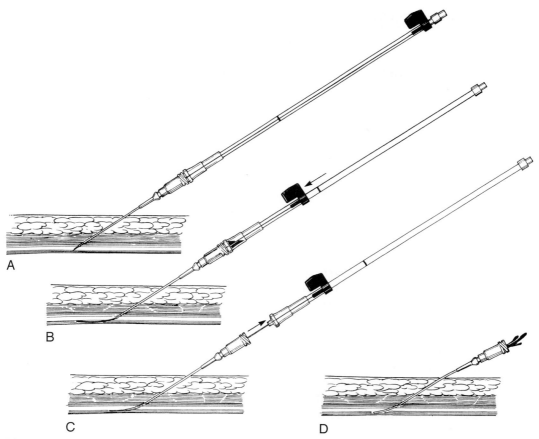

FIGURE 2–4. The Seldinger technique using a catheter with a built-in wire. The plastic sheath covering the guidewire is marked to identify the point at which the wire will exit the needle. Once the needle enters the artery, blood fills the plastic chamber (*A*). The guidewire is threaded into the vessel (*B*). The guidewire must be fully advanced to ensure that it is in the lumen. The plastic cannula is advanced over the wire, and the needle and the wire are withdrawn (*C*). Correct positioning of the wire is marked by free blood return from the cannula (*D*).

Modified Seldinger Technique

The modified Seldinger technique uses a guidewire, which is threaded into the artery after the vessel is punctured. Some catheters have built-in wires that thread through the catheter. Alternatively, a guidewire can be placed through a needle before the cannula is inserted. The basic steps remain the same.

In the Seldinger technique with a built-in guidewire, the entire needle-guidewire complex is inserted (Fig. 2–4A). Once the needle returns blood from the artery, the guidewire is advanced (Fig. 2–4B). A mark on the clear plastic cover indicates when the wire has exited the tip of the needle (see Fig. 2–4A). The wire should be advanced fully. Should resistance be felt, the wire is withdrawn, the needle is advanced 1 to 2 mm, and an attempt to pass the wire is made again. Once the wire has been inserted into the artery, the cannula is advanced over the wire, and the device is removed (Fig. 2–4C). Pulsatile blood flow should be noted from the cannula (Fig. 2–4D).

If a kit with a built-in wire is not available, the modified Seldinger technique can be performed with a separate guidewire. The needle is inserted into the artery. (The lumen of the needle should be checked

first to ensure that it accommodates the guidewire.) Once blood returns through the needle, the angle is reduced slightly, and the guidewire is inserted (Fig. 2–5A). This should advance without resistance. Then the needle is withdrawn, leaving the guidewire in place (Fig. 2–5B). A small nick in the skin may be necessary to allow passage of the cannula over the guidewire. The cannula is inserted over the guidewire, and the guidewire is withdrawn.

Once the arterial catheter is in correct position, pulsatile arterial blood flow should continue to return. The thumb is placed over the hub to prevent ongoing bleeding until the tubing can be connected. The catheter is secured with sutures, and a sterile dressing is placed. A summary of the basic equipment is outlined in Table 2–1. The general steps for placing an arterial catheter are outlined in Table 2–2. For all commonly used arteries, these steps are similar. Table 2–3 outlines small differences relevant to catheterization of the femoral artery.

Complications

The major complications associated with use of arterial catheters are related to diminished blood flow to the

TABLE 2–1. General Equipment for Arterial Catheterization

Medication for sedation (if necessary)
Local anesthetic (1% lidocaine)
Sterile gloves, drapes, gown, mask, cap, eye protection
Betadine solution or swabs
Angiocatheter
Guidewire*
Central line kit†
Pressure transducer, tubing, pressure monitor
2-0 or 3-0 nylon suture on cutting needle
Sterile gauze 4 × 4

*Individually wrapped sterile guidewires are available if the Seldinger technique is preferred and catheters with built-in wires are not available.
†A kit for central lines can be used for femoral arterial catheterization.

TABLE 2–2. Technique for Radial Artery Catheterization

1. Perform the Allen test.
2. Position the patient supine with the arm abducted. Place a small towel roll under the wrist.
3. Use aseptic technique (prepare field; use gloves, mask, cap, eye protection).
4. Identify landmarks; palpate a pulse.
5. Infiltrate with anesthetic (small volume).
6. Advance needle at 30- to 45-degree angle until arterial blood returns.
7. Advance the wire if using the Seldinger technique, then advance the catheter over the wire.
8. Remove the needle and the guidewire.
9. If using an angiocatheter, advance the catheter to the hub over the needle with a rotating motion, and remove the needle.
10. Connect tubing to the catheter.
11. Secure the catheter by suturing to the skin, and apply sterile dressing.

extremity and include local and systemic infection. Multiple prospective series have been published on the complications associated with arterial catheters. Many of these procedures were done in selected patients undergoing elective cardiac or vascular surgery. Additionally, the types of catheters and their management were different from current models.

Even catheters placed under elective conditions are associated with a significant incidence of radial artery thrombosis, reported to be around 25%. Rarely is this associated with ischemia or necrosis of the hand, however. Catheters in place for less than 24 hours very rarely cause thrombosis. Of 131 patients in one study, two (1.5%) required operative intervention for ischemia of the hand.

Infectious complications are not uncommon in patients with arterial catheters. One study evaluated the incidence of infections, both local and systemic, in patients in surgical and medical intensive care units.

The radial artery was the most common site of insertion in this group (in 72%). Local infections of the insertion site were found in 18% of all arterial lines. Four percent (5 of 130) of these catheters were felt to be responsible for systemic septicemia as well as local infection. Determined by univariate analysis, the factors associated with an increased risk of local and systemic infection were placement by means of a cutdown technique and duration of greater than 4 days.

Special Considerations

When the radial artery is used, catheterization attempts should be made first on the nondominant hand. If the axillary artery is chosen, cannulation

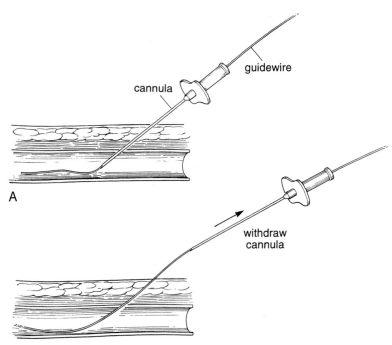

FIGURE 2–5. The Seldinger technique using a catheter without a built-in wire. Once the needle is within the artery, the guidewire is advanced into the lumen (*A*). The needle is then withdrawn (*B*). A cannula can be passed over the guidewire into the vessel.

TABLE 2–3. Technique for Femoral Artery Catheterization

1. Use aseptic technique.
2. Palpate the femoral artery.
3. Infiltrate with local anesthetic.
4. Introduce the needle into the skin over the femoral artery approximately 1 to 2 cm below the inguinal ligament.
5. Advance the needle at approximately a 45-degree angle to the skin until arterial blood returns.
6. Immobilize the needle with the free hand.
7. Advance the guidewire through the needle.
8. Remove the needle leaving the guidewire in place.
9. Make a 0.5-cm incision in the skin at the guidewire's insertion site with a No. 11–blade knife.
10. Pass the arterial catheter over the guidewire.
11. Remove the guidewire.
12. Connect tubing to the catheter.
13. Secure the catheter by suturing to the skin, and apply sterile dressing.

should be as high as possible. Risk of distal ischemia is less with the axillary artery than with the brachial artery because of the greater collateral circulation in the axillary artery. Owing to the higher incidence of brachial artery complications, this site is used the least frequently. The dorsalis pedis artery offers one of the best alternatives when the radial artery is unable to be accessed. It may be smaller and more difficult to cannulate at times. A palpable posterior tibial pulse should be present. The pressure in the dorsalis pedis artery may differ significantly from that in the more central arteries.

Suggested Readings

1. Band JD, Maki DG: Infections caused by arterial catheters used in hemodynamic monitoring. Am J Med 1979;67:735–741.
2. Bedford RF: Radial artery function following percutaneous cannulation with 18- and 20-gauge catheters. Anesthesiology 1977;47:37–39.
3. Gardner RM, Schwartz R, Wong HC, Burke JP: Percutaneous indwelling radial-artery catheters for monitoring cardiovascular function. N Engl J Med 1974;290:1227–1231.
4. Mandel MA, Dauchot PJ: Radial artery cannulation in 1000 patients: Precautions and complications. J Hand Surg 1977;6:482–485.
5. Puri VK, Carlson RW, Bander JJ, Weil MH: Complications of vascular catheterization in critically ill patients. Crit Care Med 1980;8:495–499.
6. Slogoff S, Keats AS, Arlund C: On the safety of radial artery cannulation. Anesthesiology 1983;59:42–47.
7. Weiss BM, Gattiker RI: Complications during and following radial artery cannulation: A prospective study. Intensive Care Med 1986;12:424–428.
8. Wilkins RG: Radial artery cannulation and ischaemic damage: A review. Anesthesia 1985;40:896–899.

3 Pulmonary Artery Catheterization

Kathy Jean M. Nakano and Kenneth Waxman

Since their introduction to clinical medicine in the early 1970s by Swan and Ganz, pulmonary artery (PA) catheters have significantly improved the ability to assess the cardiac function and the intravascular volume of critically ill patients. Because there was debate in the 1990s regarding the benefits of PA catheters, a panel of experts convened to review the issues surrounding their use. This panel published a consensus statement as a result of that conference. The final recommendations of the conference are listed in Table 3–1.

Indications

There are several accepted indications for the use of PA catheters (Table 3–2). Patients with severe underlying cardiopulmonary disease are candidates for PA catheters so that detailed monitoring of their cardiopulmonary status can be done. Patients who are undergoing extensive surgery (e.g., aortic surgery) with anticipated significant blood loss and fluid shifts benefit from the use of PA catheters. In patients with sepsis and shock who are unresponsive to fluid resuscitation, a PA catheter will allow more specific evaluation of intravascular fluid status, cardiac output and oxygen delivery, and oxygen use. PA catheters provide specific and important information about intravascular volume status in patients who have multiple underlying medical conditions that require fluid restriction. Patients sustaining severe polytrauma who suffer significant blood loss and direct organ injury may need a PA catheter to aid in resuscitation and monitoring, especially if they are at risk for or develop multisystem organ dysfunction.

Technique

Technique is extremely important when inserting a PA catheter. As described in Chapter 1, central venous access is obtained by means of a flexible introducer inserted using sterile technique, usually into the internal jugular or the subclavian veins. In selected situations, the femoral veins may be used.

By following these steps, one should minimize the incidence of major complications resulting from catheter insertion.

1. Flush all lines, and test the balloon with 1.0 to 1.5 mL of air (Fig. 3–1).
2. Remember that it is vitally important that pressure transduction be carried out via the *distal* port.
3. Test the adequacy of transduction by jiggling the catheter tip to confirm variance of the waveform on the monitor.
4. Place the sheath over the catheter to maintain sterility and to allow catheter manipulation in the future (Fig. 3–2).
5. With the balloon deflated, place the catheter through the introducer.
6. Advance the catheter until the tip reaches the level of the right atrium (Fig. 3–3A). From the internal jugular or the subclavian vein, the distance to the right atrium is approximately 15 to 20 cm.
7. Inflate the balloon (Fig. 3–3B).
8. Gently advance the catheter, constantly monitoring the pressure tracings. Entry into the right ven-

TABLE 3–1. Pulmonary Artery Catheter Consensus Conference

1. There is no basis for an FDA moratorium on PA catheter use at this time.
2. Clinicians should continue to weigh carefully the risks and the benefits of the PA catheter, and patients or surrogates should be fully informed before use.
3. Criteria for the appropriate use of the PA catheter in specific clinical situations should be developed.
4. Clinician knowledge about use of the PA catheter and its complications should be improved.
5. Current training, credentialing, and continuing quality improvement issues related to the PA catheter should be re-evaluated.
6. The indications and the contraindications for PA catheter use when clinical equipoise is lacking should be determined.
7. Clinical trials for indications when clinical equipoise exists should be performed.
8. Financial support for the above projects should be obtained from funding agencies and industry.

FDA, Food and Drug Administration; PA, pulmonary artery.
Data derived from Pulmonary Artery Catheter Consensus Conference: consensus statement. Crit Care Med 1997; 25:910–925.

TABLE 3–2. Indications for Pulmonary Artery Catheterization

Severe cardiopulmonary disease
Major elective surgery with anticipated blood loss
Sepsis and septic shock
Preexisting illness complicating fluid administration

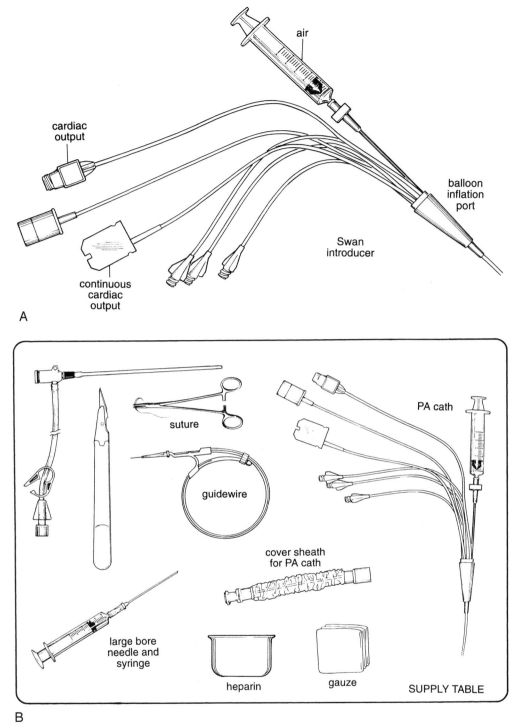

FIGURE 3–1. *A*, The Swan-Ganz catheter (newest version with continuous cardiac output capability); *B*, the entire insertion set. cath, catheter; PA, pulmonary artery.

tricle will produce higher systolic pressures than entry into the right atrium (see Fig. 3–3*B*).

9. Continue to advance the catheter, and carefully watch for development of arrhythmias.

10. Keep in mind that entry into the PA will produce a sloping diastolic curve with a higher mean diastolic pressure than will entry into the right ventricle (Fig. 3–3*C*). The distance from the right ventri-

cle to the pulmonary artery should be less than 10 cm.

11. Advance the catheter to allow the balloon tip to float into the wedge position, which appears as a dampening of the pressure tracing (Fig. 3–3*D*).

12. Note that deflation of the balloon at this point should reproduce a PA waveform.

13. Slowly reinflate the balloon to obtain a wedge

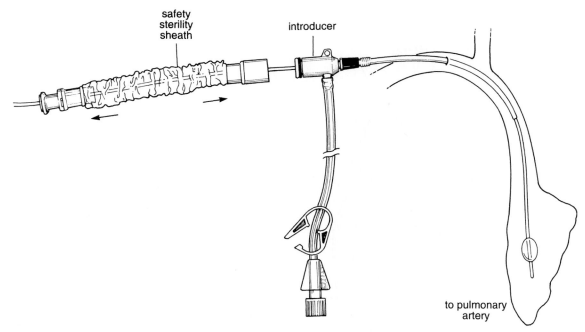

safety
sterility
sheath

introducer

to pulmonary
artery

FIGURE 3–2. The Swan-Ganz catheter inserted through the Cordis catheter via a plastic sterility sheath.

pressure and to ensure that the catheter does not wedge with less than 1.0 to 1.5 mL of air in the balloon.

14. Obtain a chest radiograph to confirm catheter position.

In general, the waveform follows the sequence shown in Figure 3–4 as the catheter is advanced.

Complications of Pulmonary Artery Catheters

Aside from the complications associated with central venous access in general, PA catheter use has additional complications. These include arrhythmias, catheter knotting, pulmonary infarction, PA rupture, right ventricular puncture, and valvular damage. Except for arrhythmias, these complications are rare and can usually be avoided with attention to proper technique.

Arrhythmias may occur during catheter insertion, especially when the catheter tip is in the right ventricle. Both atrial and ventricular dysrhythmias may occur. Most often, the arrhythmias are self-limited and cease with passage of the catheter into the PA. Occasionally, patients with excitable myocardium from preexisting arrhythmias or recent myocardial infarction may require antiarrhythmic treatment. Patients with electrolyte disturbances, particularly hypokalemia and hypomagnesemia, are also at risk. Patients with left bundle branch block are at particular risk of developing complete heart block. Careful selection of these patients for PA catheter placement is indicated. Transvenous pacemakers should be readily available during insertion.

On occasion, the catheter may curl in the right ventricle instead of passing into the PA. Rarely, the intertwining of the catheter produces a knot (Fig. 3–5A). If this occurs, fluoroscopically assisted untying or surgical removal is necessary on rare occasions.

Infarction of a pulmonary segment may occur when the PA catheter is permanently wedged, thereby occluding blood flow to the segment distal to the balloon (Figure 3–5B). Radiographically, the infarction may appear as a wedge-shaped opacity extending peripherally from the tip of the PA catheter, but it may not be apparent on routine chest x-ray. Surveillance for loss of the PA waveform with appearance of a permanent wedge pressure tracing will help circumvent the occurrence of this complication.

Hemoptysis in a patient with a PA catheter should alert one to the possibility of PA rupture (Figure 3–5C). This often-fatal complication may occur during catheter insertion or wedge pressure measurement. Patients who have sepsis, pulmonary hypertension, an overwedged PA catheter, or any condition associated with friable pulmonary vasculature are at higher risk of PA rupture. Avoidance of this complication necessitates close monitoring of catheter tip position by means of chest x-ray, monitoring of the PA waveform, and ensuring that the wedge pressure is not obtained with less than 1.0 to 1.5 mL of air in the balloon.

Knowledge of catheter tip location during insertion is imperative. One should see clear, sequential progression of the waveforms from the right atrium to the right ventricle to the PA to the wedge (see Fig. 3–4). Any deviation from this sequence generally indicates that the catheter is in the wrong position. Occasionally, the catheter may pass directly into the inferior vena

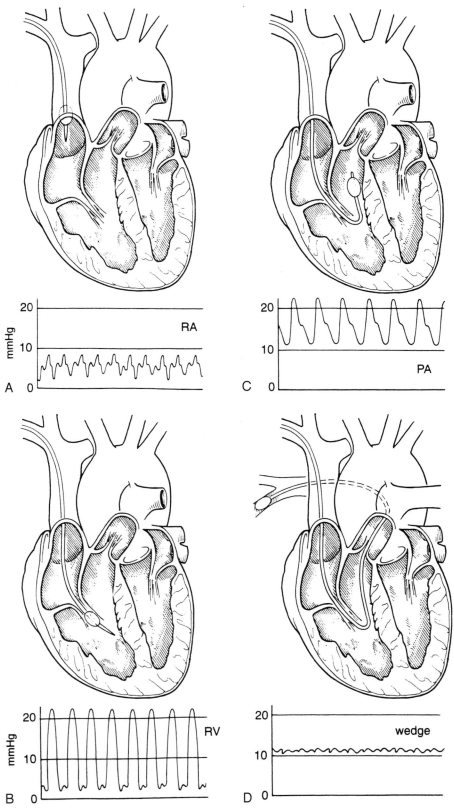

FIGURE 3–3. *A* to *D*, Advancement of the Swan-Ganz catheter through the cardiac chambers and respective waveforms. PA, pulmonary artery; RA, right atrium; RV, right ventricle.

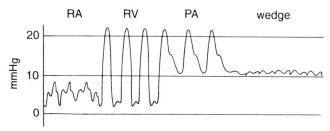

FIGURE 3–4. The waveform sequence as the catheter is advanced. PA, pulmonary artery; RA, right atrium; RV, right ventricle.

cava. More common, however, is progression from the right atrium to the right ventricle, then directly to an apparent wedge position. This may occur when the catheter tip has lodged in a trabecula of the right ventricle. Continued advancement of the catheter may lead to puncture of the right ventricle and subsequent risk of cardiac tamponade.

Valvular damage (tricuspid or pulmonic) may occur as a result of long-term use of a PA catheter that traverses the valves. Damage may also occur if the balloon is inflated during catheter removal. Thus, it is important always to know if the balloon is inflated or deflated and never to withdraw the catheter while the balloon is up.

Applications of Pulmonary Artery Catheters

Valuable data are obtained from the PA catheter. Some of the information is measured directly, and some is calculated. Important measured values obtained from the PA catheter include cardiac output, PA wedge pressure, mixed venous oxygen saturation, PA pressures, and right heart pressures. Cardiac output is a function of the stroke volume multiplied by the heart rate. The technique used to monitor cardiac output is thermodilution. The PA wedge pressure is used as an estimation

of left ventricular end-diastolic pressure, which reflects left ventricular filling pressure. As the balloon on the PA catheter floats forward and occludes the pulmonary arteriole or capillary, the wedge pressure measured at the distal end of the catheter will reflect the back pressure from the left atrium, which is equivalent to the end-diastolic pressure of the left ventricle (assuming that there is no mitral valvular disease). The wedge pressure is also referred to as the PA occlusion pressure. To provide further information, the mixed venous oxygen saturation can be measured by either (1) direct oximetry with continuous fiberoptic light transmission at the catheter tip or (2) removal of a sample of mixed venous blood from the distal port of the PA catheter and measurement of its saturation. In removing a mixed venous sample from the PA catheter, it is important to remember that there should be slow, steady withdrawal of blood after it has been removed from the catheter itself. If the blood is drawn back too quickly, there will be "contamination" of the sample with oxygenated blood from the postcapillary circulation. Direct measurement of the PA systolic and diastolic pressures provides valuable information about the resistance within the pulmonary vasculature. With normal pulmonary vascular resistance, the PA diastolic pressure should approximate the PA wedge pressure.

There are also calculated values that can be derived (Table 3–3). The four most important values are cardiac index, oxygen delivery, oxygen consumption, and systemic vascular resistance. The cardiac index establishes cardiac output based on body surface area to normalize the value across all body sizes. Oxygen delivery is a function of arterial oxygen saturation, hemoglobin concentration, and cardiac output. Oxygen consumption is a function of hemoglobin concentration, cardiac output, and the difference between arterial oxygen saturation and mixed venous oxygen saturation. Monitoring oxygen consumption as it relates to oxygen delivery allows one to determine if enough

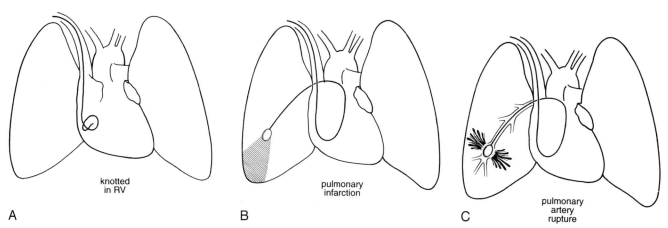

FIGURE 3–5. *A,* Knotting of catheter in right ventricle (RV). *B,* Pulmonary infarction due to inappropriate advancement. *C,* Pulmonary artery branch rupture.

TABLE 3-3. Variables and Important Equations

Variable	Equation	Normal Value
Cardiac output: CO (L/min)	$= SV \times HR$	5.0 ± 0.5
Cardiac index: CI (L/min/m²)	$= CI/BSA$	3.2 ± 0.2
Oxygen delivery index: DO_2 (mL/min/m²)	$= CO \times CaO_2 \times 10$	520 ± 16
Oxygen consumption index: VO_2	$= CI(CaO_2 - CvO_2) \times 10$	131 ± 2
Arterial oxygen content: CaO_2 (mL/dL)	$= (Hgb \times 1.36 \times SaO_2) + (PaO_2 \times 0.0031)$*	19 ± 1
Mixed venous oxygen content: CvO_2 (mL/dL)	$= (Hgb \times 1.36 \times SvO_2) + (PaO_2 \times 0.0031)$*	14 ± 1
Oxygen extraction: O_2 ext (%)	$= DO_2/VO_2$	26 ± 1
HR: heart rate		
Hgb: hemoglobin		
Systemic vascular resistance index: SVRI (dyne.5/cm⁵.m²)	$= 79.2 (MAP - CVP)/CI$	2180 ± 210
Pulmonary vascular resistance index: PVRI (dyne.5/cm⁵.m²)	$= 79.92(MPAP - WP)/CI$	270 ± 15
Stroke index: SI (mL/m²)	$= CI/HR$	46 ± 5
Left ventricular stroke work: LVSW (g.m/m²)	$= SI \times MAP \times 0.144$	56 ± 6
Right ventricular stroke work: RVSW (g.m/m²)	$= SI \times MPAP \times 0.144$	9 ± 0.9

*In the estimation of CaO_2 and CvO_2, only the first part of the equation is used because the second part is negligible.
79.92 and 0.144 are conversion values.
BSA, body surface area; CVP, central venous pressure; MAP, mean arterial pressure; MPAP, mean pulmonary arterial pressure; PaO_2, partial pressure of arterial oxygen; SaO_2, arterial oxygen saturation; SV, stroke volume; SvO_2, mixed venous oxygen saturation; WP, wedge pressure.

oxygen is being provided to supply the needs of the tissue.

Suggested Readings

1. Connors AF Jr, Speroff T, Dawson NV, et al: The effectiveness of right heart catheterization in the initial care of critically ill patients. JAMA 1996;276:899–907.
2. Gattinoni L, Brazzi L, Pelosi P, et al: A trial of goal-oriented hemodynamic therapy in critically ill patients. SvO2 Collaborative Group. N Engl J Med 1995;333:1025–1032.
3. Nelson LD: The new pulmonary arterial catheters: Continuous venous oximetry, right ventricular ejection fraction, and continuous cardiac output. New Horiz 1997;5:251–258.
4. Pulmonary Artery Catheter Consensus Conference: consensus statement. Crit Care Med 1997;25:910–925.
5. Shoemaker WC, Parsa MH: Invasive and noninvasive monitoring. In Gronvik A, Ayres SM, Holbrook PR, Shoemaker WC (eds): Textbook of Critical Care, 4th ed. Philadelphia, WB Saunders, 2000, pp 74–91.
6. Swan HJC, Ganz W, Forrester JS, et al: Catheterization of the heart in man with use of a flow-directed balloon-tipped catheter. N Engl J Med 1970;283:447–451.

4 Intraosseous Infusion

Stephen M. Schexnayder and Debra H. Fiser

Intraosseous infusion (IOI) has been used to provide rapid vascular access for critically ill infants and children. Originally described in the 1940s, this procedure fell out of favor as vascular access devices such as the butterfly (scalp vein) needle and the plastic intravascular catheter were developed. With advances in pediatric life support, the technique has regained popularity, and it can be a lifesaving means to deliver both resuscitation fluids and medications to critically ill pediatric patients.

Intraosseous infusion takes advantage of the rich vascular network in the intramedullary cavity of long bones in children (Fig. 4–1). Blood flows from venous sinusoids into a central venous canal in long bones. This central canal empties into nutrient and emissary veins, which drain into central veins. The time needed to deliver drugs to the central circulation is essentially equivalent to that seen with peripheral intravenous devices, although some studies have shown slightly more rapid absorption. As children age, the red marrow found in young children is replaced by a less vascular yellow marrow, which may cause slower absorption in children older than 5 years of age. Although 6 years of age is frequently cited as the upper limit for this technique, IOI has been used in adults; however, volume resuscitation is somewhat limited by the resistance to flow.

Indications

Intraosseous infusion is indicated when rapid vascular access is required in children and cannot be readily established in peripheral veins. In critically ill children, attempts at peripheral intravenous access should be limited to three (or 90 seconds), as recommended in the American Heart Association's Pediatric Advanced Life Support course. The most frequently encountered clinical scenarios requiring this procedure are cardiopulmonary arrest, shock, status epilepticus, and severe burns. Nearly all medications can be given by this route, although some antibiotics may need to be given in larger doses to achieve similar therapeutic levels. It is also possible to send aspirated marrow for blood chemistry studies, pH analysis, typing and crossmatching, and blood culture. Absolute contraindications to the procedure are osteogenesis imperfecta and os-

teopetrosis. Relative contraindications are ipsilateral fracture, local infection, and major trauma proximal to the potential site of placement. It may not always be possible in patients with severe multiple trauma to avoid such placement, however. Failure of intraosseous placement in a bone precludes further attempts in that bone because subsequent attempts may increase the risk of compartment syndrome.

Technique

A number of needles are commercially available for IOI, although plain hypodermic, butterfly (scalp vein),

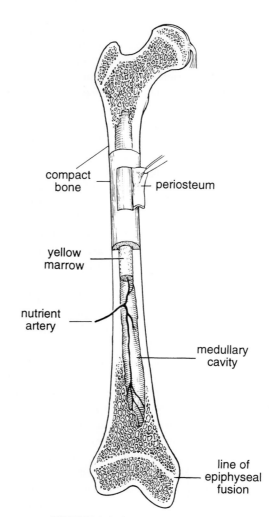

FIGURE 4–1. Anatomy of long bones.

compact bone

periosteum

yellow marrow

nutrient artery

medullary cavity

line of epiphyseal fusion

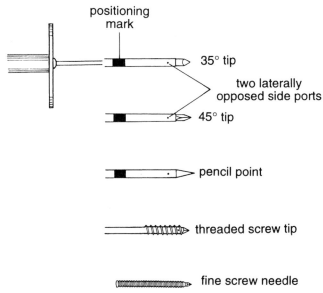

FIGURE 4–2. Various needle types for intraosseous infusion. *Top three,* Dieckmann modifications. *Fourth from top,* Sur-Fast needle. *Bottom,* Sussmane-Raszynski needle.

and spinal needles may be used. Because regular hypodermic needles lack a stylet, they may become clogged with bone or other tissues during insertion. Spinal needles are more difficult to use because of their propensity to bend. Jamshidi bone marrow aspiration needles are frequently used, and a number of modifications have been made to facilitate easier insertion (e.g., Cook, Dieckmann, and Sussmane-Raszynski needles). Some needles are threaded in an attempt to make them more secure. Various needle designs are shown in Figure 4–2. A study comparing the Jamshidi with the Cook needle found the Jamshidi needle more user friendly in a laboratory model. A novel automatic bone-injection gun has been employed in adults, but this device is not commercially available.

The site should be prepared with alcohol or povidone-iodine solution. Local anesthesia is rarely required because of the altered mental status accompanying critical illness. In alert patients, however, a local anesthetic such as lidocaine can be infiltrated into the skin, the subcutaneous tissue, and the periosteum to reduce the amount of pain associated with this procedure.

The most frequently used site for IOI is the proximal tibia, as demonstrated in Figure 4–3. Other sites for consideration include the distal tibia, the distal femur, and the anterior superior iliac spine. The humerus has been used in experimental animals, and both the calcaneus and the clavicle have been used in adults. The precise location for placement is described in Table 4–1. Needles should be inserted using a twisting motion with firm pressure, as shown in Figure 4–4, because the rotary motion will reduce the chance of bending the needle. Care should be taken to stabilize

the extremity with firm pressure, but one should avoid placing the hand posterior to the insertion site. Owing to extreme pressure, the needle might penetrate both cortices of the bone and the posterior soft tissues, injuring the operator's hand.

When the needle penetrates the marrow cavity, a sudden decrease in resistance ("give") is frequently felt. The needle should stand upright without support. Confirmation of correct placement is made by aspirating marrow after removal of the stylet. If no marrow can be obtained, inject a small volume of isotonic saline solution and reattempt aspiration. Blood-tinged fluid should be aspirated if the needle is properly placed. The site should be frequently observed for swelling, which might indicate extravasation, and distal pulses should be monitored frequently.

A number of different methods of stabilization of the needle have been used. Gauze dressings may be placed on the sides of the needle to stabilize it, with a tape bridge to the needle. The gauze dressings should then be firmly secured to the leg with tape. Alternatively, a hemostat may be applied to the needle immediately past the point where the needle exits the skin. The hemostat is then secured with tape to the skin. The needle should be removed as soon as more permanent vascular access has been obtained.

Pitfalls

A number of procedure-related complications have been described, including soft tissue and bone infection. Infection is rarely a problem when needles are left in place for less than 12 hours. Compartment syndrome has been reported and should be suspected when swelling or tension develops. Fracture of the bone may occur, although the clinical significance of this is uncertain. Animal studies have shown no changes in developmental and histologic studies 6 months after IOI. Leg length discrepancy following IOI is extremely unlikely. Fat embolism is also a theoretical concern, although laboratory studies have not found this to be a significant risk.

TABLE 4–1. Locations for Intraosseous Needle Placement

Proximal tibia	Anterior tibial surface on the medial flat surface of the tibia 1–2 cm below the tibial tuberosity; direct needle away from the epiphysis (60–90 degrees); in young infants, use the tibial tuberosity
Distal tibia	Just proximal to the medial malleolus and posterior to the saphenous vein at a 90-degree angle
Distal femur	2–3 cm proximal to the external condyle in the midline, directed superiorly 75–80 degrees
Anterior superior iliac spine	Insert needle perpendicular to the long axis of the body

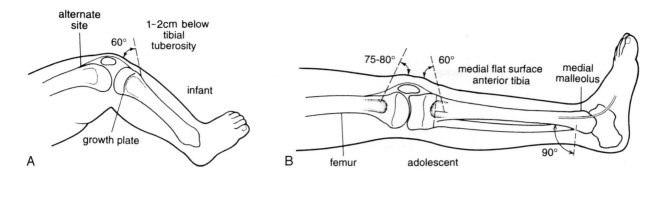

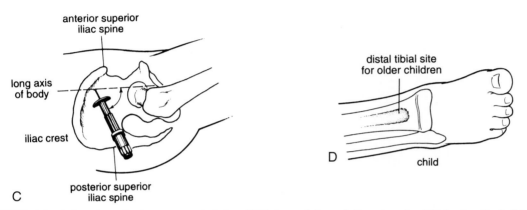

FIGURE 4–3. *A*, Locations for intraosseous infusion (IOI) in an infant. *B*, Locations for IOI in the distal tibia and the femur in older children. *C*, Location for IOI in the iliac crest. *D*, Location for IOI in the distal tibia.

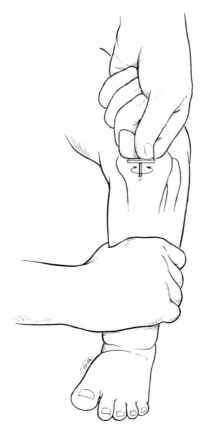

FIGURE 4–4. Technique for insertion of intraosseous infusion needle.

Suggested Readings

1. Brickman K, Rega P, Schoolfield L, et al: Investigation of bone development and histopathologic changes from intraosseous infusion. Ann Emerg Med 1996;28:430–435.
2. Fiser D: Intraosseous infusion. N Engl J Med 1990;322:1579–1591.
3. Fiser R, Walker WM, Siebert JJ, et al: Tibial length following intraosseous infusion: A prospective, radiographic analysis. Pediatr Emerg Care 1997;13:186–188.
4. Glaeser P, Hellmich TR, Szewczuga D, et al: Five-year experience in prehospital intraosseous infusion in children and adults. Ann Emerg Med 1993;22:1119–1124.
5. Halm B, Yamamoto LG: Comparing ease of intraosseous needle placement: Jamshidi versus Cook. Am J Emerg Med 1998;16:420–422.
6. Orlowski J, Julius CJ, Petras RE, et al: The safety of intraosseous infusion: Risks of fat and bone marrow emboli to the lungs. Ann Emerg Med 1989;18:1062–1067.
7. Simmons C, Johnson NE, Perkin RM, et al: Intraosseous extravasation complication reports. Ann Emerg Med 1994;23:363–366.
8. Vidal R, Kissoon N, Gayle M: Compartment syndrome following intraosseous infusion. Pediatrics 1993;91:1201–1202.

5 Bedside Tracheostomy

George C. Velmahos

Bedside tracheostomy is increasingly being used because of growing concerns regarding health care costs and effective use of operating room time. Although perceived as a relatively easy procedure, it is associated with considerable intra- and postoperative morbidity. Some of the complications, such as loss of the airway, can be catastrophic, and the damage caused can be nonreversible. Therefore, performance of a tracheostomy by the bedside of an intensive care unit (ICU) patient should not be undertaken lightly. The operating room is undisputedly the safest place for any surgical procedure; however, the trip to the operating room may be dangerous for critically ill patients. Additionally, operating rooms are not immediately available, and often "simple" and nonemergent procedures (e.g., tracheostomy) are postponed in favor of other more complex operative cases.

The ability to perform this procedure at the bedside should not result in relaxation of the measures and the techniques that would have otherwise been followed in the operating room. Many studies have shown that bedside tracheostomy is safe only if done under proper conditions. Sterile technique, adequate illumination, and instrument availability are prerequisites of success. In other words, the need to perform a tracheostomy by the ICU bedside should serve as an impetus to convert the ICU room to a mini–operating room rather than as an excuse to perform a surgical procedure under suboptimal conditions.

The advances in percutaneous tracheostomy, a technique that has existed a long time but that was recently refined to become easier and safer, have revolutionized the way in which clinicians are performing tracheostomy. There is a documented increase in the number of bedside tracheostomies—up to 100% in some studies, compared with historical controls—presumably because percutaneous tracheostomy is easily done by the bedside and there is no dependence on operating room availability. It is possible, however, as with many minimally invasive techniques, that the increase in incidence occurs owing to relaxation of the indications. Unfortunately, the indications for tracheostomy are widely debated and cannot be clearly defined.

In this chapter, I describe open and percutaneous bedside tracheostomy. There are numerous modifications of each technique. This chapter covers the most frequently used and safest methods, according to the experience of the author.

Indications

Tracheostomy is mandatory in two situations and is advisable in another.

- Protection of the airway (mandatory), as with a nonemergent need for a surgical airway and an inability to establish oro- or nasotracheal intubation. Major facial injuries would be a typical scenario for this indication. Remember, if an emergent surgical airway is required, a cricothyroidotomy—not a tracheostomy—should be performed.
- Permanent tracheostomy (mandatory), as for major resectional surgery of the upper airway due to cancer or high spinal cord injury resulting in ventilator dependence.
- Temporary tracheostomy in critically ill patients (advisable).

Patients in the ICU who require prolonged mechanical ventilation are better managed by means of tracheostomy. The duration of time that should be considered prolonged is still unknown, however. Several studies have shown that the rate of endotracheal complications (e.g., granuloma, subglottic stenosis) increases after the 10th day of oro- or nasotracheal intubation. Other studies place this time point as early as the 7th day or as late as the 21st day. Whatever the duration may be, it is important to perform tracheostomy earlier rather than later. The worst time to perform tracheostomy is many days after oro- or nasotracheal intubation of an inflamed and injured trachea. It makes much better sense to perform tracheostomy early after identification of the patients who have a high likelihood of requiring prolonged mechanical ventilation.

Unfortunately, prolonged ventilation has been used in the presence of many risk factors with moderate sensitivity and specificity. In our trauma ICU, we use the following as indicators at 48 hours after admission that the patient will require more than 7 days of mechanical ventilation: a high injury severity score (>20), a low partial arterial oxygen tension to fractional inspired oxygen ratio (<250), an increased need for fluid resuscitation (positive fluid balance of more than 2 L), and a need for a pulmonary artery catheter. In such patients, we consider early tracheostomy on a case-by-case basis. In a wider sense, tracheostomy should also be thought of as a weaning tool in patients with prolonged ventilatory dependence because it facilitates bronchial toilet, decreases dead space, and makes disconnection from the ventilator safer in the presence of a secure airway.

Considerations before the Procedure

As emphasized earlier, the potential technical challenge of bedside tracheostomy should not be understated. Although the majority of these procedures proceed uneventfully, technical difficulties on certain occasions produce major discomfort to even the most experienced surgeons. For this reason, adequate preparation is imperative. Illumination is probably the most important and the least optimal aspect of a bedside procedure. If you cannot see, you cannot operate. If portable lights do not resolve the problem, headlights are the best solution. Adequate equipment is the second most important aspect. Do not try to do a tracheostomy with a scalpel and a forceps. Have a complete surgical tray open or at least on standby. On the other hand, unnecessary instruments will only flood the operative field and will make selection of the appropriate tools—in the absence of a scrub nurse—almost impossible. It is advisable to design a special bedside tracheostomy tray with all the necessary instruments. Although the ICU room does not accommodate multiple helpers, it is my recommendation that there always be four persons involved: two operators (one necessarily a surgeon), one individual who is responsible for the airway, and one circulator. The operative field should be properly sterilized; the operators should be gowned, gloved, and masked; and the entire procedure should be done under aseptic technique. Although cost considerations are understandably an issue, the patient's safety is the primary concern and can be ensured only when all the necessary precautions are taken.

In contrast to operating room procedures, the majority of bedside tracheostomies are done without an anesthesiologist, so a common mistake is to give inadequate analgesia to the patient. This should be of special concern in chemically paralyzed patients who cannot indicate pain. Local analgesia should be given. I routinely sedate heavily and give intravenous analgesia to these patients when they are already intubated. There is no point in avoiding this for the short duration of the procedure.

Technique

Open Method

A 5-cm horizontal or vertical incision is made at mid-distance between the cricoid cartilage and the sternal

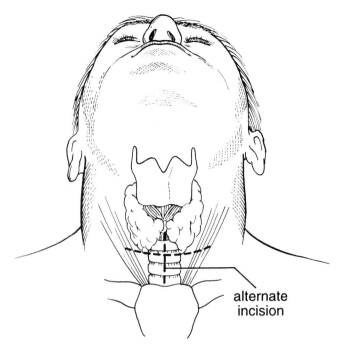

FIGURE 5–1. Skin incision for open tracheostomy.

notch (Fig. 5–1). A horizontal incision produces a more cosmetic scar, and a vertical incision avoids bleeding from the external jugular veins and can be extended along the trachea in complex cases. The subcutaneous tissue is incised by means of electrocoagulation. The anterior jugular veins run close to the midline on either side of the neck and may require ligation. The pretracheal muscles are split in the midline. Meticulous hemostasis is important to maintain a clean operative field. Take advantage of the entire length of the skin incision by opening the subcutaneous tissue and muscles up to the two edges of the skin. A common mistake is to create a progressively smaller incision as one goes deeper, resulting in "working through a hole" at the tracheal level. The thyroid isthmus is frequently in the way and can be retracted upward. On rare occasions, a large isthmus may require ligation and division over the trachea.

The pretracheal fascia is a strong layer of tissue that usually requires sharp dissection. This can be done via electrocoagulation, taking care not to burn the underlying tracheal rings. The trachea is visualized under the pretracheal fascia as a white structure. The second to fifth tracheal rings should be exposed. Two nonabsorbable (usually Prolene 2–0) stay sutures are placed on each side of the trachea (Fig. 5–2). Each suture should circle the third or the fourth tracheal ring as laterally as possible. A knot is tied at the edge of each suture. These two sutures are used to maintain traction during insertion of the tracheostomy tube and to replace a tracheostomy tube if the airway is lost postoperatively by mistake. By cutting the knot, which lies outside the wound, the suture can be pulled out when a tracheostomy tract has been firmly established

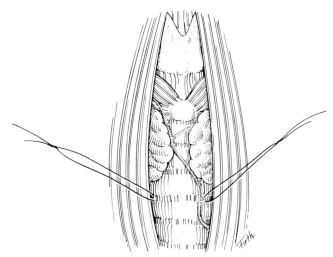

FIGURE 5–2. Stay sutures on lateral tracheal walls.

(usually around the seventh postoperative day). After identification of the tracheal rings, a hook is placed at the first ring to pull the trachea upward and forward. Traction is applied to the stay sutures to bring the trachea into the operative field. The person who handles the oro- or nasotracheal tube is then asked to cut the tapes, secure the tube to the skin, and deflate the balloon.

Following this, the trachea is incised via a No. 11–blade scalpel in one of three ways: a vertical H (with a long limb through the third and the fourth rings and two short limbs across the second and the fourth cartilage interspaces), a cross (with a long limb through the third and the fourth rings and an equal limb across the third interspace), or a trap door (with its base at the fourth interspace).

There are numerous variations, but these three are used most commonly (Fig. 5–3). I prefer the vertical H because it causes the least trauma to the trachea, and I make a second short limb only if I feel that the opening is not wide enough to accommodate the tube. It is important never to cut the trachea by means of electrocoagulation because the contact with oxygen may lead to an explosion.

Under direct vision, the endotracheal tube is withdrawn to a level immediately above the tracheal incision. At this point, a lubricated No. 8 tracheostomy tube with introducer is inserted through the opening, taking care not to invert the edges of the tracheal incision as the trachea is stabilized by the hook and the stay suture (Fig. 5–4). The introducer is then withdrawn, the balloon is inflated, and the tracheostomy tube is connected through a sterile connection to the ventilator (Fig. 5–5). Only after correct placement is confirmed by the detection of bilateral breath sounds and capnography is the endotracheal tube completely removed. This is an important precaution because if a complication arises, the oro- or nasotracheal tube can always be advanced, and the airway will never be lost. By suturing it to the skin and tying a tape loosely around the neck, the tracheostomy tube is secured on site.

Percutaneous Dilational Method

There are several kits for percutaneous tracheostomy. The two most frequently used are the Cook kit (Cook

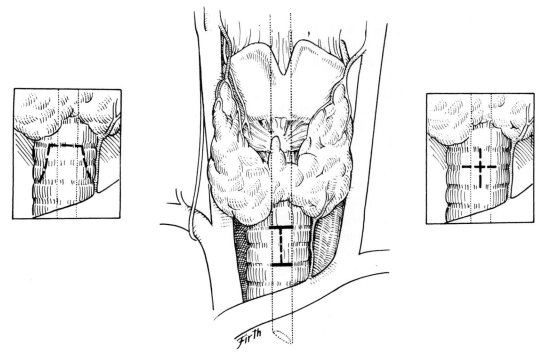

FIGURE 5–3. Tracheal incisions: trap door incision (*left*), H-incision (*middle*), cross incision (*right*).

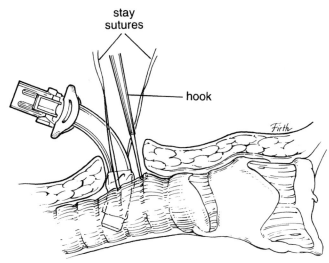

FIGURE 5–4. Hook and stay sutures pull the trachea up as the tracheostomy tube is inserted.

Critical Care, Bloomington, Ind) and the Portex kit (SIMS Portex, Keene, NH). The following description is based on use of the Cook kit and is a variation of a method known as the Ciaglia technique.

A 2-cm horizontal or vertical incision is made at mid-distance between the cricoid cartilage and the sternal notch (Fig. 5–6). The opening should be only large enough to accommodate a digit. I prefer a vertical incision because it avoids injuring the anterior jugular veins, and bleeding from these veins may be difficult to control through a small incision. The pretracheal muscles are spread gently, and the trachea is palpated by a digit inserted through the incision. It is not important to clear the trachea of any overlying tissue because this maneuver is difficult through a small incision and may cause bleeding. The balloon of the endotracheal tube is deflated, but the endotracheal tube is not moved. A needle attached to a 10-mL syringe half-filled with saline solution is inserted under digital guidance through the incision toward the midline of the trachea around the second or the third tracheal ring. Constant suction on the syringe is applied during insertion. On entrance into the trachea, air is aspirated into the syringe, noted as bubbles floating out of the saline solution. It is very important at this step to stabilize the needle with one hand while disconnecting the syringe with the other.

A guidewire is passed through the needle into the tracheal lumen. The needle is then withdrawn, and a short and stiff dilator is passed over the guidewire to dilate the existing tract slightly (Fig. 5–7). After the short dilator is withdrawn, a guiding catheter is placed over the guidewire and is inserted into the trachea (Fig. 5–8). A mark on the guiding catheter is used to indicate the length of insertion. All dilations will take place over the guidewire and guiding-catheter complex. Progressive dilations are then done, starting with

the smallest 12 Fr curved dilator up to the largest 36 Fr curved dilator (Fig. 5–9). It is important to direct the dilator at a 60-degree angle to the skin, pointing cranially. Because the trachea does not run parallel to the skin but tracks posteriorly, this orientation of the dilator will result in a vertical insertion that is 90 degrees to the trachea. If the pointed tip of the dilator is vertical to the trachea, insertion will be easy with minimal force. If, on the other hand, the dilator is advanced against the trachea at a different angle, considerably more force is required, risking either false pretracheal passage (Fig. 5–10) or injury to the trachea (Fig. 5–11).

On insertion, the dilator should be curved downward over the anterior wall of the trachea to avoid injury to the posterior membranous portion and the adjacent esophagus (Fig. 5–12). After the larger dilator is inserted and withdrawn, a digit is entered through the incision into the trachea to palpate the endotracheal tube. Up to this point, because all dilations were done next to the endotracheal tube, the operator will realize how easily the average person's trachea accommodates both the endotracheal tube and the dilators. The person handling the endotracheal tube is instructed to pull the tube out slowly and to stop when the tip of the tube lies right over the palpating digit (Fig. 5–13). The 28 Fr dilator is then inserted into a No. 8 Shiley tracheostomy tube and should fit snugly. Both are introduced over the guidewire and guiding-

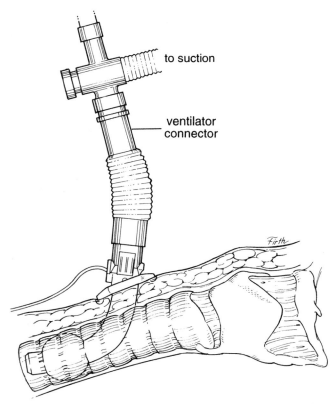

FIGURE 5–5. Tracheostomy tube in correct position.

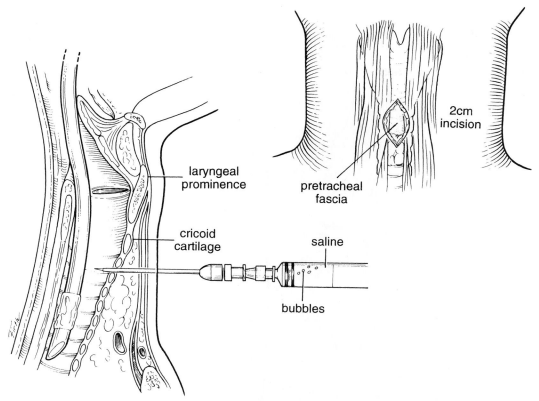

FIGURE 5–6. Small skin incision for percutaneous tracheostomy (*right*). The needle is inserted into the trachea under constant aspiration. Bubbles enter the saline solution once the trachea is punctured (*left*).

catheter complex into the trachea (Fig. 5–14). The guidewire, the guiding catheter, and the 28 Fr dilator are withdrawn, and the tracheostomy tube remains in place (Fig. 5–15). The balloon is inflated, and placement is confirmed by means of chest auscultation and capnography. Only then is the endotracheal tube completely removed.

A recent Cook kit includes only one progressively wider dilator (blue rhino). Dilation is done by insertion of this single dilator (Fig. 5–16). The Portex kit has straight dilators. Although the Portex dilator may perforate the trachea more easily, the lack of a curve risks inadvertent perforation of the posterior tracheal wall. A new Portex kit uses a specially designed clamp, through which the guidewire passes. Opening the clamp dilates the tract. No further dilations are required, and the tracheostomy tube is passed over the guidewire.

Bronchoscopy is a useful technique that makes the procedure safer, particularly during the operator's learning period. The person handling the endotracheal tube can place a bronchoscope through the tube. Then the tube is withdrawn to a level distal to the vocal cords. Needle, guidewire, and dilator insertion is done under direct bronchoscopic guidance. Eccentric insertion, bleeding, or false passage can be easily seen and corrected.

Pitfalls of Percutaneous Technique

Incorrect Placement of the Needle in Relation to the Paratracheal Structures. To avoid incorrect placement of the needle, it should be introduced under digital guidance (Figs. 5–17 and 5–18). Manual stabilization of the trachea should be accomplished by means of gentle pressure on the cricoid cartilage during needle insertion. Bronchoscopy can confirm placement of the needle in the tracheal lumen (Fig. 5–19).

Incorrect Orientation of Dilators. The dilators used for progressive tract dilation should be introduced at a 60-degree angle to the skin. Owing to the curved shape of the dilators as well as the natural course of the trachea, which distances itself from the skin as it enters the mediastinum, dilator insertion vertical to the skin may result in pretracheal dilation (see Fig. 5–10) or major damage to the anterior tracheal wall. This is caused by dilators being in contact with the wall along a wide surface rather than just a pointed tip (see Fig. 5–11).

Perforation of the Posterior Wall of the Trachea with Possible Entry into the Esophagus. Tracheal perforation may occur for two reasons (see Fig. 5–12). First, it could result from unnecessary force having been applied to the dilator to achieve entry into the trachea. If the dilator is placed at the correct angle, the pointed tip will easily perforate the anterior tra-

Text continued on page 40

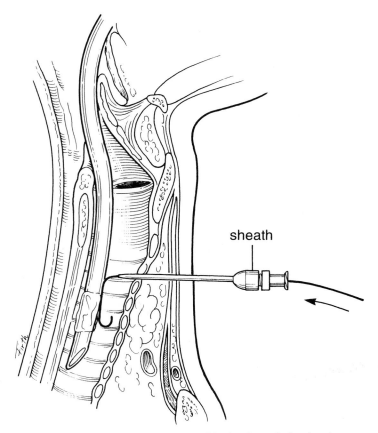

FIGURE 5–7. Introduction of a guidewire through the sheath.

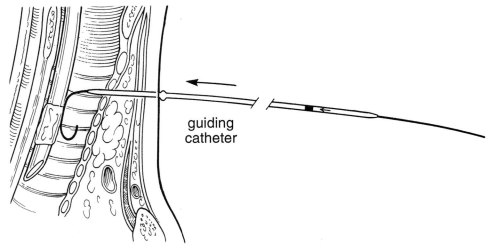

FIGURE 5–8. Introduction of a guidewire catheter over the wire.

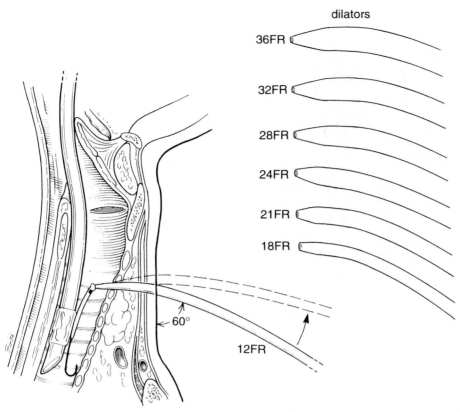

dilators

36FR

32FR

28FR

24FR

21FR

18FR

60°

12FR

FIGURE 5–9. Progressive dilatation up to 36 Fr at a 60-degree angle to the skin. The dilator is tilted caudally when the trachea is entered. Note that dilators are inserted without removing the endotracheal tube.

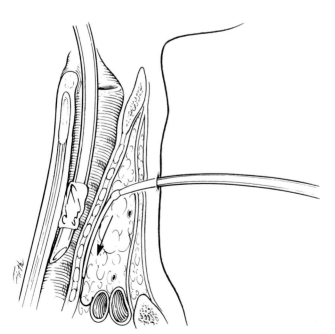

FIGURE 5–10. Inserting the dilator vertical to the skin rather than maintaining the 60-degree angle may lead to pretracheal dilation owing to the curved tip of the dilator.

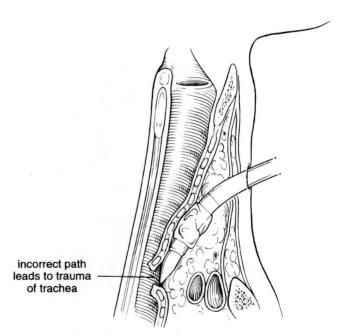

incorrect path leads to trauma of trachea

FIGURE 5–11. Damage to the trachea may also occur.

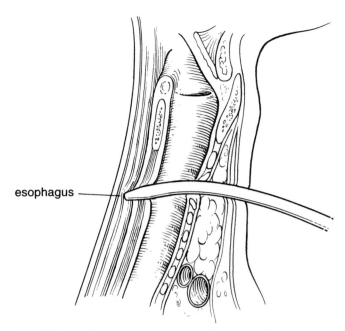

esophagus

FIGURE 5–12. Forgetting to direct the dilator caudally may lead to perforation of the posterior trachea and the esophagus.

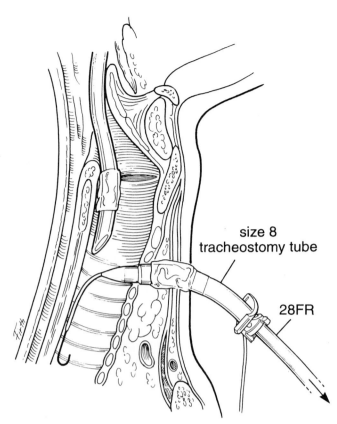

size 8
tracheostomy tube

28FR

FIGURE 5–14. Insertion of a No. 8 tracheostomy tube over a 28 Fr dilator.

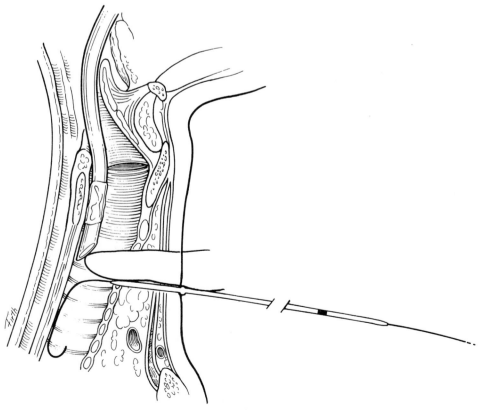

FIGURE 5–13. Withdrawal of the endotracheal tube under digital guidance.

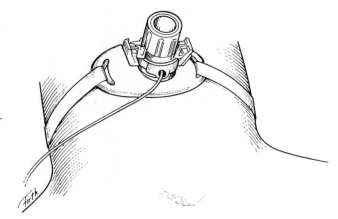

FIGURE 5–15. Tracheostomy unit in place.

38 FR

do not insert
under skin beyond
this point

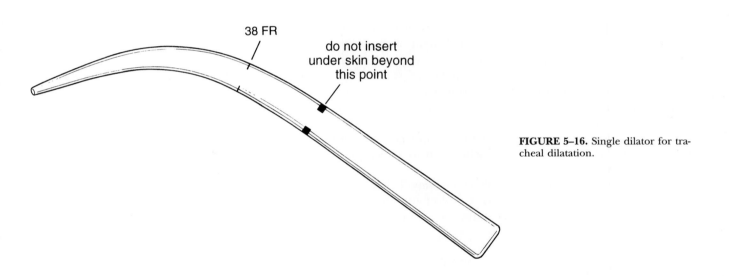

FIGURE 5–16. Single dilator for tracheal dilatation.

needle misses trachea

thyroid
gland

trachea

neurovascular
bundle

esophagus

FIGURE 5–17. Paratracheal insertion of the needle.

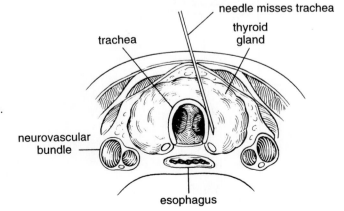

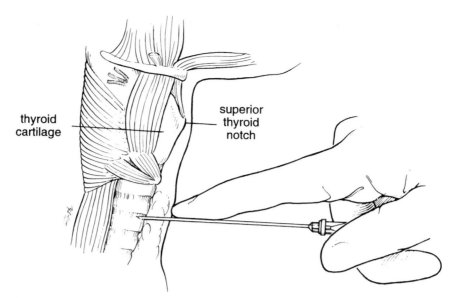

FIGURE 5–18. Digital guidance during needle insertion.

chea, and entry will be facilitated. If force is needed to insert the dilator into the trachea, placement of the dilator is incorrect. The procedure should be stopped, and the position of the dilator should be adjusted. Second, perforation of the posterior trachea is a risk if the dilator is not directed downward after a "give" is felt after insertion. The dilator should be tilted toward the mediastinum once the tip is inserted to follow the natural course of the trachea and to avoid injuring its posterior wall.

Resistance at Insertion of the Tracheostomy Tube. Resistance usually occurs owing to a discrepancy between the lumen of the tracheostomy tube and the dilator used to guide the tracheostomy tube into the tracheal lumen (Fig. 5–20). A 28 Fr dilator fits tightly into a No. 8 tracheostomy tube and eliminates this problem. Unfortunately, such an ideal fit does not exist for tracheostomy tubes of other sizes. New commercial kits, which provide specifically manufactured tracheostomy tubes for different dilator sizes, may solve this problem.

Early Removal of the Orotracheal Tube. The orotracheal tube should remain in place right above the site of percutaneous tracheal perforation until the correct position of the tracheostomy tube is confirmed. If for any reason the tracheostomy tube is not inserted into

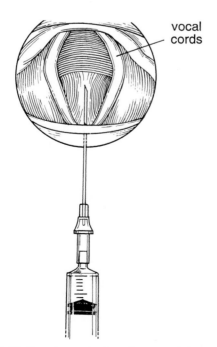

FIGURE 5–19. Bronchoscopic view of a correctly inserted needle.

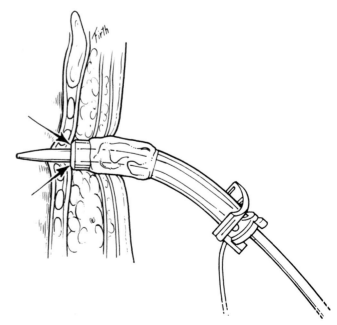

FIGURE 5–20. Discrepancy between size of dilator lumen and size of tracheostomy tube lumen, resulting in difficult insertion.

the trachea and desaturation occurs, the orotracheal tube can be advanced back into position. Intubation should never be lost with this technique.

Too High or Too Low Placement of the Tracheostomy Tube. High placement of the tracheostomy tube may cause long-term complications, such as subglottic stenosis. Low placement may cause bleeding due to direct contact with thoracic inlet vessels (Fig. 5–21). The most frequently affected vessel of this unusual but highly lethal complication is the innominate artery. A tracheoinnominate fistula may occur with catastrophic bleeding into the trachea. To avoid this complication, the skin incision should be placed approximately in the middle of the distance between the cricoid cartilage and the sternal notch. The guiding digit should direct the needle to be inserted at a point that is not close to the cricoid or the notch. If this complication occurs, direct digital pressure may be lifesaving until the patient is taken to the operating room for surgical repair (Fig. 5–22).

General Complications of Tracheostomy

Complications of tracheostomy can be intraoperative, short-term postoperative, or long-term postoperative. Bleeding, loss of airway, and injury to adjacent structures are the most common intraoperative complications. The same complications, if not recognized intraoperatively, will present shortly after the operation as external bleeding or local hematoma, desaturation, subcutaneous emphysema, pneumothorax, or tracheoesophageal fistula. Long-term complications include

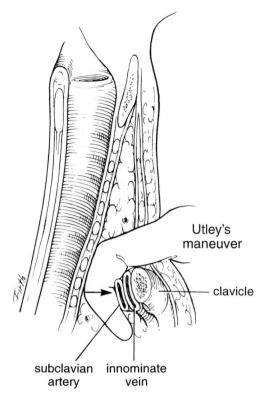

FIGURE 5–22. Digital compression of the innominate vessels in the presence of severe bleeding from a tracheoinnominate fistula.

subglottic stenosis, laryngeal nerve injury, tracheal granulomas and constriction, and alteration of phonation. Although minor complications are frequent and usually self-limited, major complications occur with a frequency of 1% to 3%. The procedure carries a mortality rate ranging from 0.1% to 1% and underscores the importance of meticulous technique and attention to detail.

Percutaneous versus Open Bedside Tracheostomy

There is ongoing debate about the safety and the cost-effectiveness of percutaneous and open bedside tracheostomy. To date, there are six prospective randomized trials and one meta-analysis comparing the two techniques. All but one of the prospective randomized trials conclude that the percutaneous technique is as safe as and possibly more cost-effective than the open technique. These trials include groups ranging from 12 to 40 patients per method, however, and therefore lack adequate power to find differences in the rates of complications of low incidence. Their conclusions should be viewed with caution. The meta-analysis, which included a variety of controlled and uncontrolled studies done over a long period of time, concluded that percutaneous tracheostomy is associated with a higher prevalence of perioperative complica-

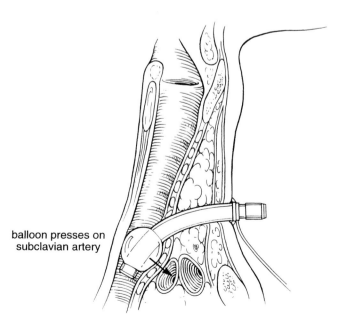

FIGURE 5–21. Low insertion of the tracheostomy tube results in balloon compression of the thoracic inlet vessels.

tions but that open tracheostomy is associated with more postoperative complications.

It is evident from these data that the question is still not settled. As is true for every technique, it is unlikely that either of the two methods can serve as a panacea for all patients. It is important for surgeons who treat critically ill patients to be familiar with both techniques and to be able to apply each one to the appropriate patient for the appropriate indications.

Suggested Readings

1. Ciaglia P, Firshing R, Syniec C, et al: Elective percutaneous dilatational tracheostomy. Chest 1985;87:15–19.
2. Dulguerov P, Gysin C, Perneger TV, Chevrolet JC: Percutaneous or surgical tracheostomy: A meta-analysis. Crit Care Med 1999; 27:1617–1625.
3. Friedman Y, Fildes J, Mizock B, et al: Comparison of percutaneous and surgical tracheostomies. Chest 1996;110:480–485.
4. Gysin C, Dulguerov P, Guyot JP, et al: Percutaneous versus surgical tracheostomy: A double-blind randomized trial. Ann Surg 1999;230:708–714.
5. Heikkinen M, Aarnio P, Hannukainen J: Percutaneous dilational tracheostomy or conventional surgical tracheostomy? Crit Care Med 2000;28:1399–1402.
6. Muttini S, Melloni G, Gemma M, et al: Percutaneous or surgical tracheotomy. Prospective, randomized comparison of the incidence of early and late complications. Minerva Anestesiol 1999;65:521–527.
7. Porter JM, Ivatury RR: Preferred route of tracheostomy—percutaneous versus open at the bedside: A randomized prospective study in the surgical intensive care unit. Am Surg 1999;65:142–146.
8. Velmahos GC, Demetriades D: Common bedside procedures in the intensive care unit. In Shoemaker WC, Ayres SM, Grenvik A, Holbrook PR (eds): Textbook of Critical Care, 4th ed. Philadelphia, WB Saunders, 2000, pp 114–119.
9. Velmahos GC, Gomez H, Boicey CM, Demetriades D: Bedside percutaneous tracheostomy is safe and easy to teach: Prospective evaluation of a modification of the current techniques on 100 patients. World J Surg 2000;24:1109–1115.

6 Cricothyroidotomy

Edward E. Cornwell III

Consider these scenarios.

1. A physician walking through an intermediate care area at 2:00 AM is summoned by nurses at the bedside of a 32-year-old female who has severe reactive asthma and who has had four tracheostomies. The patient is in obvious respiratory distress with agitation, air hunger, audible wheezing, and an oxygen saturation of 65%.
2. A brain-injured patient (Glasgow Coma Scale score of 4) is brought to the emergency department following a motor vehicle accident. Rapid-sequence intubation is attempted, but "difficult anatomy" and maxillofacial trauma render endotracheal intubation impossible.
3. A recently extubated patient in the intensive care unit experiences acute desaturation and becomes agitated, with a heart rate of 140 beats per minute. The upper airway is markedly edematous, the vocal cords cannot be visualized during attempts at endotracheal intubation, and the oxygen saturation is 65%.

These three scenarios (all actual) highlight how important it is for physicians involved in the care of critically ill or injured patients to be well versed in the technique of cricothyroidotomy. Undoubtedly one of the most underrated procedures in all of medicine, cricothyroidotomy is virtually always lifesaving if performed when truly necessary. Stated more dramatically, its failure to be performed successfully virtually ensures the demise of the patient. True estimates are difficult to come by, but survey of trauma registries at several urban trauma centers indicates that about 0.5% of all patients admitted with major trauma require an emergency surgical airway.

Indications

Surgical cricothyroidotomy is indicated in patients who require emergent intubation but have the following problems:

1. Visualization of the vocal cords is impossible owing to local edema, bleeding, or abnormal anatomy.
2. Severe maxillofacial trauma precludes use of naso- or oropharyngeal routes.
3. Strict immobilization of the cervical spine is required owing to a partial neurologic deficit at this level, which may be converted to a complete deficit if the neck is manipulated during orotracheal intubation.

Technique

Equipment

One is tempted simply to provide the standard instructions regarding the need for a tracheostomy tray that is well stocked with a tracheal spreader and various clamps. Such instruction would ignore the emotionally charged environment that typically exists whenever an emergency cricothyroidotomy becomes necessary, however. Because an emergency tray is occasionally not available when it is most needed, it is important to know the six bare necessities for performing the procedure, as follows:

1. Index finger.
2. Kelly or Crile clamp.
3. Scalpel.
4. Sterile preparation solution.
5. Surgical gloves.
6. Tracheostomy tube, size No. 6. (In its absence, an endotracheal tube will suffice, but the excitement of the moment will invariably lead to advancing the tube too far and into the right mainstem bronchus.)

Procedure

The patient should be supine with the neck in the neutral position. The most time-consuming aspect of the procedure should be identification of the cricothyroid membrane. Clinicians who work in emergency settings should make it a practice to assess this membrane on colleagues and patients under controlled circumstances. One should not spend much time on this practice in patients with thin necks and easy anatomy because these patients are easily intubated endotracheally. Even in patients with short, fat necks, however, the sternal notch and the thyroid cartilage (Adam's apple) should be quickly and easily identified.

The cricoid cartilage is the first small notch felt as the index finger ascends in the midline from the sternal notch toward the thyroid cartilage. The firm, pliable membrane between it and the thyroid cartilage is the cricothyroid membrane.

During cricothyroidotomy, it is important for the thumb and the index finger of the nondominant hand to stabilize the tracheal-laryngeal complex by firmly fixing the thyroid cartilage in place (Fig. 6–1). There is a variable amount of soft tissue compliance, which allows this complex to be easily moved away from the midline if not properly fixed. At this point, a 3- to 4-cm transverse or vertical incision should be made through the skin, the dermis, and the cricothyroid membrane. In teaching this procedure over the past 10 years, the author has observed that the novice tends to be too superficial rather than too aggressive with the incision. As soon as the cricothyroid space has been identified, it is opened transversely by means of sharp dissection with the knife. In unparalyzed patients making any respiratory effort, the bubbling gush (gush of air and blood droplets) signifies successful incision of the membrane and reminds us of the importance of protective eyewear.

At this point, the surgeon may be surprised to find that in some patients, the space between the cricoid and the thyroid cartilage is frequently narrow and may permit only part of the fifth finger to be inserted. The importance of keeping part of a finger in the membrane cannot be overemphasized. This takes on even greater importance in uncontrolled situations when one is both performing the procedure and giving directions regarding what equipment is needed. A clamp is inserted to spread the membrane wide (Fig. 6–2). With the clamp in place, the trachea is elevated by pulling the clamp up. A No. 6 tracheostomy tube is inserted under the clamp, and the clamp is removed. For some reason, tracheostomy tubes are packaged with the inner cannula inside the tube (rather than the white, blunt-tipped plastic obturator, which is needed to guide the tube into the airway). A nervous, inexperienced assistant will drop the obturator, cannula, or tracheostomy tube (or some combination thereof) unless forewarned. (More commonly, he or she may hand the surgeon the tracheostomy tube as packaged with the inner cannula in place.) Forethought regarding this scenario is invaluable.

Pitfalls and Complications

There are several potential pitfalls that should be contemplated ahead of time. Laceration of the anterior jugular veins is a potential complication, given their paramedian location. Fortunately, their superficial location makes them just as easy to control as to injure. Manual pressure and suture ligation once the airway is secure will solve this problem. If the skin incision is made vertically rather than transversely, the likelihood of injuring the anterior jugular veins is less. The aforementioned packaging of most tracheostomy tubes lends itself to delays that may occur as a result of fumbling of the obturator and the inner cannula that are packaged with the tube. It is helpful to forewarn nursing or medical personnel who are assisting the operator about the need to place the blunt-tipped obturator through the tracheostomy tube before passing it to the operator.

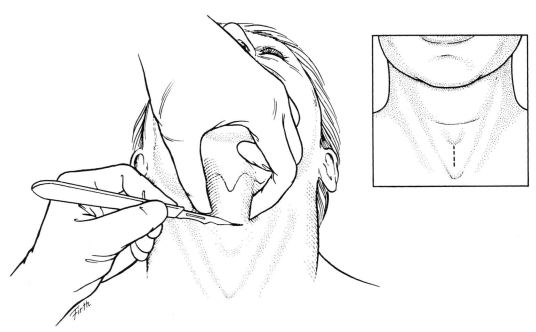

FIGURE 6–1. A transverse or a vertical incision is used at the level of the cricothyroid space. The trachea should be stabilized with the other hand. Employing a vertical incision avoids cutting the anterior jugular veins *(inset).*

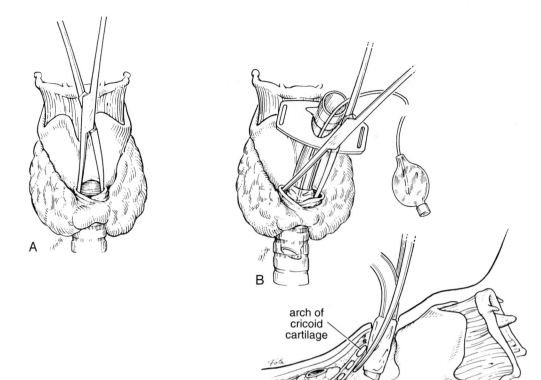

FIGURE 6–2. The cricothyroid membrane is incised and is then enlarged with a clamp *(A)*. With the clamp in place and spread, the size 6 tracheostomy tube is advanced behind the clamp *(B)* while the trachea is pulled upward by the clamp *(C)*.

A major complication is esophageal injury, which is possible if the scalpel penetrates the posterior trachea. This is avoided by controlling the incision at the level of the cricothyroid membrane and not penetrating it with anything other than the examining finger or a blunt-tipped clamp. Again, fixation of the thyroid and the cricoid cartilage by the index finger and the thumb of the nondominant hand is critical.

Mistaking the location of the cricothyroid space and cutting above rather than below the thyroid cartilage is not uncommon. An adequate skin incision allowing good visualization of the thyroid and the cricoid cartilage prevents this mishap.

Bleeding from muscular structures, local veins, or thyroid is probably the most common occurrence. There is not enough time for adequate hemostasis before the tracheostomy tube is inserted, and it is difficult to find bleeding once the tube is in place and obstructs the field. Bleeding can only be avoided by staying in the midline and identifying vital structures correctly. Although cricothyroidotomy is perceived as an easy surgical maneuver on a superficial structure, it can be complicated, and the pressure of the circum-stances can lead to failure to establish an airway expeditiously. It requires experience, calmness under strenuous circumstances, and good surgical skills.

Long-term complications include swallowing dysfunction due to posterior displacement of the epiglottis (a phenomenon that may be reversible after tube removal), as well as hoarseness and vocal cord dysfunction.

Suggested Readings

1. Goumas P, Kokkinis K, Petrocheilos J, et al: Cricothyroidotomy and the anatomy of the cricothyroid space. An autopsy study. J Laryngol Otol 1997;111:354–356.
2. Isaacs JH Jr, Pedersen AD: Emergency cricothyroidotomy. Am Surg 1997;63:346–349.
3. Jacobson LE, Gomez GA, Sobieray RJ, et al: Surgical cricothyroidotomy in trauma patients: Analysis of its use by paramedics in the field. J Trauma 1996;41:15–20.
4. Lim JW, Lerner PK, Rothstein SG: Epiglottic position after cricothyroidotomy: A comparison with tracheotomy. Ann Otol Rhinol Laryngol 1997;106:560–562.
5. Surgical cricothyroidotomy. In Chen H, Sola J, Lillemoe K (eds): Manual of Common Bedside Surgical Procedures by the Halsted Residents of the Johns Hopkins Hospital. Baltimore, Williams & Wilkins, 1996, p 20.

7 Tube Thoracostomy

Demetrios Demetriades

Chest tubes are used to drain intrathoracic air or fluid collections. As opposed to other drains, they require connection to a special system that does not allow entrance of air into the thoracic cavity when negative intrapleural pressure is generated. The monitoring of chest tube output guides clinical management. The main indications for chest tube insertion are (1) pneumothorax, (2) hemothorax, (3) thoracic operations, and (4) other fluid collections, such as chylothorax and empyema. Following trauma, acute sanguinous chest tube output of more than 1000 to 1500 mL usually requires an operation, although correlation with the hemodynamic status of the patient may place this threshold at a lower or a higher level. Pneumothoraces of less than 15% may be treated with close monitoring without a chest tube unless they cause clinical symptoms or the patient requires positive pressure ventilation. Chest tubes are generally removed when the drainage is less than 2 mL/kg in cases of blood or serosanguineous fluid, or until they stop draining completely in cases of infected collections. One must always remember that chest tubes may malfunction and therefore do not always reflect intrathoracic fluid production. Although potentially lifesaving tools, they are associated with complications. Their need should be evaluated daily and their use discontinued in the absence of solid clinical indications.

Technique

The patient is placed in the supine position with the arm abducted at 90 degrees (Figs. 7–1 and 7–2). The insertion site should be in the midaxillary line at the fourth or the fifth intercostal space. The insertion site should always be above the level of the nipple to avoid injury to the diaphragm or the intra-abdominal organs, such as the liver or the spleen. During expiration, the diaphragm easily reaches the nipple level. This insertion site is satisfactory for both hemothorax and pneumothorax. Bending the arm over the patient's head to the contralateral side pulls the latissimus dorsi muscle to the incision site (Fig. 7–3). Therefore, the arm should be abducted in a relaxed position.

Following administration of local anesthesia, a 1.5- to 2-cm transverse incision through the skin, the subcutaneous tissue, and the superficial layers of the intercostal muscles is made at the insertion site (see Fig. 7–2). The sharp dissection should be kept close to the upper edge of the rib to avoid injury to the intercostal vessels, which are located at the inferior border of each rib. Entry into the pleural cavity is made via blunt dissection using a Kelly forceps (Fig. 7–4). After the initial dissection, the Kelly forceps is forced into the pleural cavity in a controlled manner to avoid injury

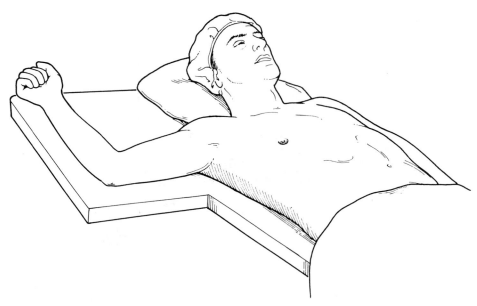

FIGURE 7–1. Position for insertion of thoracostomy tube: supine, arm abducted 90 degrees.

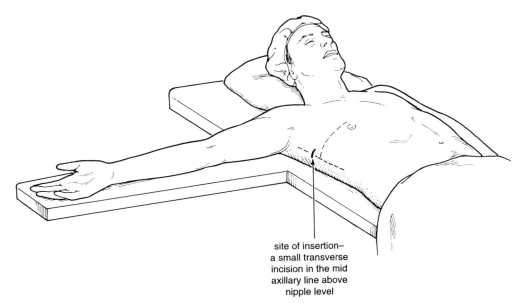

site of insertion–
a small transverse
incision in the mid
axillary line above
nipple level

FIGURE 7–2. The insertion site is in the midaxillary line at the fourth to fifth intercostal space.

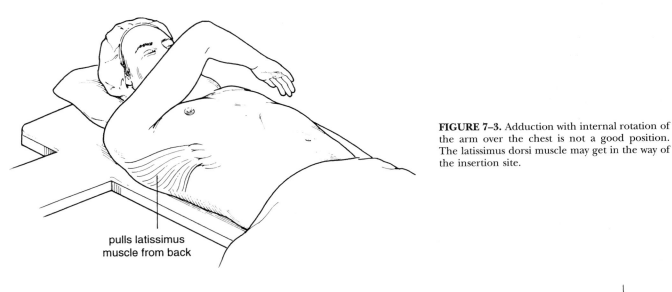

pulls latissimus
muscle from back

FIGURE 7–3. Adduction with internal rotation of the arm over the chest is not a good position. The latissimus dorsi muscle may get in the way of the insertion site.

FIGURE 7–4. The pleural cavity is entered by means of blunt dissection using a Kelly forceps. After the initial dissection, the forceps is forced into the cavity in a controlled manner.

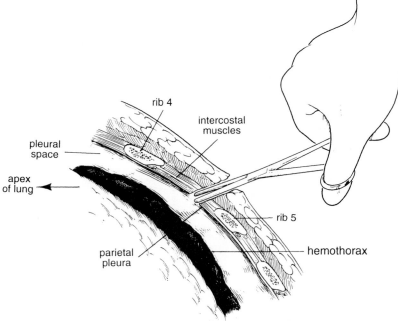

rib 4

intercostal
muscles

pleural
space

apex
of lung

parietal
pleura

rib 5

hemothorax

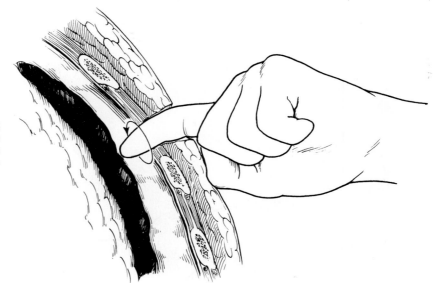

FIGURE 7–5. Digital exploration of the pleural cavity is recommended for patients with previous chest injury or infection or for intensive care unit patients with suspected pneumonia or adult respiratory distress syndrome.

to the intrathoracic organs. Subcutaneous tunneling is painful, makes the procedure more difficult, and does not have any benefits.

The next step is digital exploration of the wound and the adjacent pleural space to evaluate for intrapleural adhesions and to avoid accidental insertion of the thoracostomy tube into the lung parenchyma (Fig. 7–5). This maneuver is important in patients with previous chest injury or infection and in all intensive care unit patients with suspected pneumonia or adult respiratory distress syndrome. In these situations, the presence of adhesions or a stiff lung increases the risk of accidental intraparenchymal tube placement. In other patients, however, routine digital exploration is not necessary.

Insertion of the chest tube is next. The size of the tube depends on the nature of the material to be drained (blood, thin liquid, or air) and the age and the sex of the patient. To provide adequate drainage without excessive pressure on the adjacent ribs, which can be painful, a size 36 tube should be used for hemothorax in adult males. In adult females, a size 32 to 36 tube should be used, and in children, a size 10 to 28 tube should be used. The tube is grasped with a clamp through its distal fenestration. The proximal end of the tube is clamped with a second clamp to avoid splashing of blood. The tube is firmly forced into the pleural cavity in the direction of the apex of the lung and posteriorly (Fig. 7–6). As soon as the tube enters the pleural cavity, the clamp is released and withdrawn (Fig. 7–7) while the tube is advanced in a twisting fashion toward the apex, as described previously. When the tube is in place, it should be rotated 360 degrees to prevent inappropriate kinking. If the tube does not rotate freely, it should be pulled back slightly and rotated again. The tube is then connected to the collection system.

If the incision at the insertion site is too long, it should be closed with interrupted sutures. The tube should be anchored to the thoracic wall with a separate suture (Fig. 7–8). A horizontal mattress suture should be placed around the tube and left untied, to be used for wound closure later during tube removal. The tube is further secured to the thoracic wall with adhesive tape (Fig. 7–9).

Components of System

Collection System

The standard collection system consists of three chambers: the collection chamber, the one-way seal chamber, and the suction chamber control. Negative suction of about 20 cm H_2O is advisable immediately after thoracostomy tube insertion. Its role at later stages is not clear, and there is no evidence that it is of any benefit. Certainly, in the presence of air leaks, continuous negative pressure may cause the condition to deteriorate.

Autotransfusion System

Autotransfusion of blood from the pleural cavity is easy, safe, and cost-effective. Commercially available collection bags may be attached to the side of the standard thoracostomy collection system. The collected blood can be reinfused through a standard blood filter. Anticoagulant (100 mL of citrate for every 600 mL of blood) is advisable but not required.

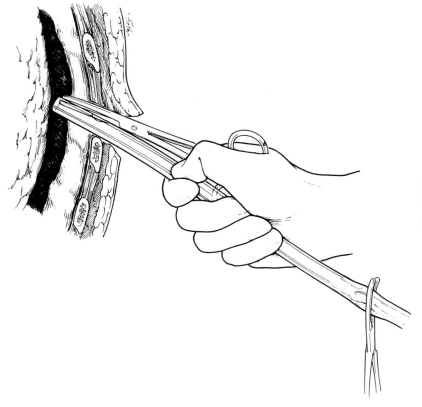

FIGURE 7–6. Insertion of the thoracostomy tube. While firm traction is maintained, the tube is grasped through its distal fenestration with a Kelly forceps and is forced into the pleural cavity.

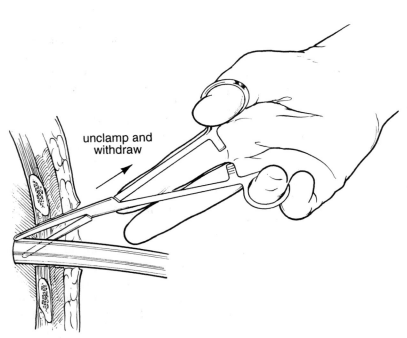

unclamp and withdraw

FIGURE 7–7. The clamp is withdrawn.

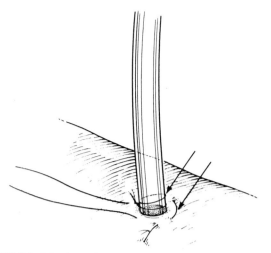

FIGURE 7–8. A horizontal mattress suture is placed around the tube and is left untied, to be used for later wound closure after removal of the tube.

Adjuvant Treatment

If the patient is awake and stable, and there is no suspicion of spinal injury, early chest physiotherapy immediately after thoracostomy tube insertion is strongly recommended. The patient should be instructed to cough vigorously while lying on his or her back, while lying on his or her side, and, later, while sitting. This simple physiotherapy maneuver encourages drainage of the hemothorax before it clots and expansion of the lung before atelectasis occurs. Prophylactic antibiotics with staphylococcal coverage are essential in preventing intrathoracic infections. A single dose is as effective as prolonged prophylaxis.

Postinsertion Care

Chest X-ray

A chest film should be obtained immediately after insertion of the tube to confirm its position, the presence of residual hemothorax, or persistent pneumothorax. The tube should be in the pleural cavity (including its last fenestration) without any kinking.

Removal of Thoracostomy Tube

The thoracostomy tube should be removed at the earliest possible time to reduce the risk of empyema. In most cases, it can be safely removed within 2 or 3 days, when any air leak stops completely and blood drainage is reduced to less than 30 to 50 mL/day. In the presence of an infected pleural collection, the tube should be left in place until it stops draining completely. Obtaining a chest x-ray after at least 6 hours of water sealing is advisable before tube removal. In the awake and alert patient, the tube can be removed in either deep inspiration or deep expiration, so long as the patient holds his or her breath at the moment of removal.

The procedure should be explained to the patient in advance. This is a two-person procedure. One person prepares the sutures, which had been placed during insertion of the tube in anticipation of wound closure. A second person removes the tube with the right hand while supporting the thoracic wall by applying firm pressure with the left hand, with the tube between the

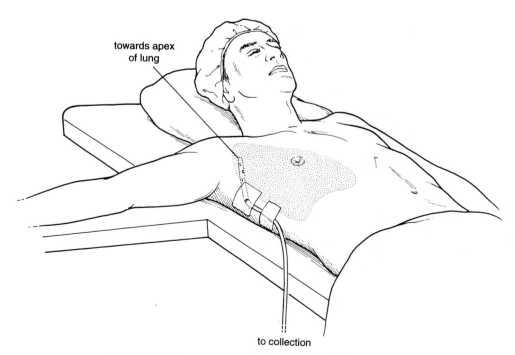

towards apex
of lung

to collection

FIGURE 7–9. Thoracostomy tube in place and taped to the skin.

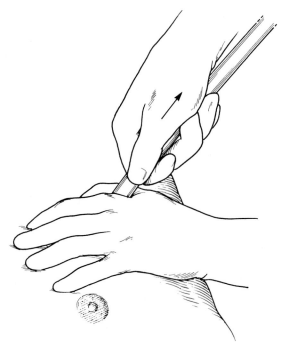

FIGURE 7–10. Removal of thoracostomy tube. The tube is pulled out with the right hand while the thoracic wall is supported with the left hand.

thumb and the index finger (Fig. 7–10). Then the assistant pulls and ties the pursestring suture (Fig. 7–11). Suturing of the entry site of the tube is not absolutely necessary. The wound can be covered with petroleum jelly–impregnated gauze during tube re-

moval and can be secured firmly with adhesive tape. This is useful to remember in case the suture breaks during tying.

In the unconscious, mechanically ventilated patient, the tube should be removed at the end of inspiration when the intrathoracic pressure is positive and the risk of accidental pneumothorax is reduced.

Routine chest films should be obtained immediately after removal of the tube.

Complications

Persistent Air Leak

Rarely does any air leak persist for more than 3 or 4 days. In such cases, the first step is to confirm the intrathoracic position of all the fenestrations of the tube. Sometimes the air leak is due to intrapulmonary insertion of the tube, especially in patients with previous chest trauma or intrathoracic infection or in patients who have been in the intensive care unit for many days and have developed a stiff lung. A computed tomographic scan may confirm the intraparenchymal position, and withdrawal of the tube usually controls the air leak. If these steps do not uncover any problems, bronchoscopy should be performed to exclude a major bronchial tear. Air leaks from pulmonary injuries are usually self-controlled, and they rarely need surgical repair. To accelerate healing, the negative suction in the thoracostomy tube should be main-

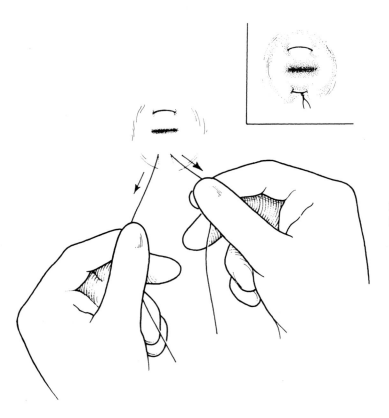

FIGURE 7–11. A second individual ties the previously placed pursestring suture. *Inset* shows completed closure.

tained at very low levels. In mechanically ventilated patients, the tidal volume should be as low as possible. High-frequency percussive ventilation or independent lung ventilation may be helpful in persistent cases.

Residual Hemothorax

In the presence of a suspected significant residual hemothorax after thoracostomy tube insertion, a computed tomographic scan of the chest should be performed within 2 or 3 days to evaluate the nature of the opacification in the chest. A plain film cannot distinguish between a clotted hemothorax and an intrapulmonary hematoma or lung atelectasis. If the computed tomographic scan confirms the presence of significant residual hemothorax, thoracoscopic evacuation should be performed within 4 or 5 days. Delayed evacuation is always more difficult, and the results are inferior to early evacuation because of organization of the clot.

Complications Related to the Thoracostomy Tube

The most common related complication is intrathoracic infection. Risk factors include poor aseptic technique during insertion of the tube, long duration of the tube in the chest, the presence of residual hemothorax, and no prophylactic antibiotics. Other tube-related complications include insertion of the tube in the lung and perforation of the diaphragm or other organs (e.g., liver, spleen, heart, or stomach).

Encysted Hemothorax or Pneumothorax

Blind insertion of a tube in an intensive care unit patient with suspected encysted hemothorax or pneumothorax is usually not effective and might be dangerous. A pigtail catheter with underwater drainage that is inserted under computed tomographic or ultrasonic guidance is the safest and most effective management tool.

Pitfalls

1. Insertion of the thoracostomy tube below the nipple level may result in diaphragmatic or intra-abdominal injury.
2. Subcutaneous tunneling at the tube insertion site is difficult and very painful and does not reduce the incidence of empyema.
3. Antibiotic prophylaxis for the duration of thoracostomy tube use does not reduce the incidence of intrathoracic infection. A single dose is as good as prolonged prophylaxis.
4. Multiple insertions of thoracostomy tubes for persistent hemothorax are rarely effective and increase the risk of empyema. Early operative evacuation should be performed (thoracoscopy or minithoracotomy).
5. Planning a surgical procedure for suspected residual hemothorax should never be done solely on the basis of chest film findings. A chest film cannot reliably distinguish between a hemothorax and an intrapulmonary hematoma or atelectasis. Computed tomographic evaluation should always be performed.

Suggested Readings

1. Dalbec DL, Krome RL: Thoracostomy. Emerg Med Clin North Am 1986;4:441–457.
2. Demetriades D, Breekon V, Breckon C, et al: Antibiotic prophylaxis in penetrating injuries of the chest. Ann R Coll Surg Engl 1991;73:348–351.
3. Quigley RL: Thoracocentesis and chest tube drainage. Crit Care Clin 1995;11:111–116.
4. Velmahos G, Demetriades D, Chan L, et al: Predicting the need for thoracoscopic evacuation of residual traumatic hemothorax: Chest radiography is insufficient. J Trauma 1999;46:65–70.

8 Pericardiocentesis and Pericardial Window

Susan I. Brundage, Bradford G. Scott, and Riyad Karmy-Jones

Anatomy of the Pericardium

Twin membranes form the pericardium. The monolayer visceral pericardium, which overlies the epicardium, is clinically indistinguishable from the epicardium. The second layer, the parietal pericardium, is formed by an inner layer of mesothelial cells and an outer layer of fibrous connective tissue. The parietal pericardium is anchored to the central portion of the diaphragm inferiorly, to the proximal portion of the aortic arch superiorly, and to the costal margin and the sternum anteriorly. Posteriorly, the pericardium lies against the pleura and the esophagus and joins the epicardium at the entrance sites of the cava and the pulmonary veins. The pulmonary arteries are extrapericardial structures that dive deep into the parietal pericardium shortly after the bifurcation of the main pulmonary trunk.

Pericardial Tamponade

The pericardial space physiologically contains less than 50 mL of serous fluid. Drainage of the pericardial space is via the lymphatics. Cardiac function can be compromised by increases in the volume of intrapericardial fluid or by obliteration of the pericardial space by fibrosis (constrictive pericarditis). Constrictive pericarditis is managed surgically, and discussion of its treatment is beyond the scope of this chapter.

The impact of a pericardial effusion is determined by a number of features: the volume, the rapidity of development, coexisting hypovolemia, and underlying cardiac function. For example, following cardiac surgery in a patient with compromised ventricular function, a small posterior loculated collection of blood can cause significant compromise in left ventricular function. On the other hand, the pericardial sac can accommodate a large slow-growing chronic effusion without significant myocardial compromise in patients with diseases of the connective tissue who have intact cardiac function.

There are a large number of causes of pericardial effusion (Table 8–1). In nonacute pericardial effusions, diagnosis may be made by means of chest radiography, which demonstrates a "water-bottle" cardiac silhouette; ultrasonography; echocardiography; or computed tomography. Although diagnosis of pericardial effusion is important, the key question is whether there is a degree of cardiac tamponade. The mechanism underlying tamponade is occlusion of the superior and the inferior vena cava, which results in decreased preload with loss of right-sided filling. Additionally, both ventricles become compressed with impaired diastolic filling and systolic outflow. Beck's triad describes the clinical signs of tamponade; it consists of (1) hypotension, (2) distended neck veins, and (3) muffled heart sounds.

An accentuated (more than 10 mm Hg) difference between the systolic pressure on expiration and the pressure on inspiration, the so-called pulsus paradoxus, indicates impaired left-sided filling secondary to increased right ventricular pressure and increased pulmonary capacitance. Shift of the septum to the left also occurs and further impairs left ventricular function. This accentuated pulsus paradoxus can be detected by noting a drop in blood pressure on the arterial waveform with inspiration. While allowing the blood pressure cuff to deflate slowly, however, one may note a level at which the blood pressure is heard intermittently (i.e., only during expiration) and then a point at a lower pressure when it is heard more constantly (i.e., during both expiration and inspiration). The difference between these points is then

TABLE 8–1. Etiology of Pericardial Effusions

Trauma	Infection
Blunt	Tuberculous
Penetrating	Viral
Malignancy	Bacterial
Lymphoma	Fungal
Lung	Aortic dissection
Breast	Postpericardiotomy syndrome
Other	Myxedema
Uremia	Radiation
Connective tissue disorder	Cardiac catheterization
	Central line placement
	Idiopathic causes

calculated. Central venous pressure higher than 15 mm Hg and readings from a pulmonary artery catheter demonstrating "equalization" of the central venous pressure, the pulmonary artery systolic pressure, and the wedge pressure should raise the suspicion of tamponade. Echocardiography reveals right ventricular collapse during diastole.

In the acute setting, because of the lack of distensibility of the pericardium, as little as 250 mL of fluid can lead to cardiogenic shock. One or more elements of Beck's triad may be absent, and the chest radiograph may demonstrate a normal cardiac silhouette. Therefore, diagnosis can be complicated, and a high index of suspicion is essential.

Effusions that develop slowly over several days or weeks, such as those caused by most malignancies or metabolic diseases, result in gradual distention of the pericardium. Secondary to increased compliance, significantly greater volumes of intrapericardial fluid may accumulate (as much as 2 L) before symptoms become apparent. Symptoms can be similar to those of acute tamponade but are often subtle, including shortness of breath, cough, and lower extremity edema. In these settings, massive enlargement of the cardiac silhouette is generally apparent on a chest radiograph.

Pericardiocentesis

Pericardiocentesis may be performed to diagnose or treat tamponade. In the stable patient, it is appropriate to perform the procedure under ultrasonographic guidance. In rare settings, computed tomography–guided pericardial drainage may be useful for loculated effusions. Coagulation parameters should be checked, especially in patients with chronic tamponade who have a concomitant degree of hepatic engorgement. In patients who are unstable, the procedure is performed "blindly." While preparing for pericardial drainage, it is critical to remember that these patients are preload dependent. Therefore, adequate volume replacement is essential, and overuse of sedation should be avoided. Induction of anesthesia with an associated increase in pleural positive pressure and a decrease in preload in the face of inadequate intravascular volume can precipitate cardiac arrest. The cause of cardiac arrest is multifactorial and includes increased positive pressure following intubation, loss of venous tone with sedation, or loss of peripheral vasoconstriction as a consequence of hyperventilation. When pericardiocentesis is done for traumatic pericardial tamponade, it is critical to remember that it is not a diagnostic tool but is a temporizing therapeutic intervention. Pericardiocentesis as a diagnostic tool in traumatic injury is associated with a prohibitively high false-negative and -positive rate as well as a risk of significant complications; therefore, it has been almost abandoned for diagnosis in traumatic injury. Patients who undergo pericardiocentesis as a temporizing measure must rapidly proceed to the operating room for a definitive procedure, usually median sternotomy.

When the procedure is being performed, the patient should lie supine if possible. Usually, unintubated patients cannot lie flat and need to be elevated. A standard pericardiocentesis kit is available, but in urgent settings, a central line kit may be used. The site should be sterilized and, if time permits, infiltrated by local anesthesia. When the procedure is being performed without radiologic or ultrasonic guidance, the preferred insertion site is 0.5 cm to the left of the xiphoid and 0.5 to 1.0 cm inferior to the costal margin. The needle is aimed at the left shoulder tip and enters the skin and the subcutaneous tissue at a 45-degree angle (Fig. 8–1). Once the needle is posterior to the costal margin (usually 1.0 to 2.5 cm deep), the angle is changed to 15 degrees (Fig. 8–2). Electrocardiographic guidance can be helpful in determining when epicardial contact has occurred. Electrocardiography is performed by connecting an alligator clip to the needle and monitoring for ST segment elevation or premature ventricular contractions. Aspiration of 50 to 100 mL of blood or fluid should result in dramatic improvement in blood pressure and narrowing of pulsus paradoxus.

After draining a nonacute pericardial effusion, most institutions currently recommend using the Seldinger technique to place an intrapericardial catheter. Use of a three-way stopcock attached to a drainage bag allows ongoing aspiration as well as measurement of intrapericardial pressures (ideally between −3 and +3 mm Hg). In nontraumatic effusions, fluid should be sent for diagnostic purposes, including cytologic examination, culturing, and chemistry analysis. In nontraumatic effusions, options include dilating the tract to 8 Fr or larger or subsequent operative interventions. Malignant or persistent effusions can be managed by means of sclerosis. A 30% recurrence rate was noted when pericardial catheter drainage alone was employed, compared with a 1% incidence of recurrence when a subxiphoid window was used. Complications of pericardiocentesis are described in Table 8–2.

TABLE 8–2. Complications of Pericardiocentesis

Cardiac puncture
Right or left anterior descending coronary artery laceration
Arrhythmia
Pneumothorax
Injury to abdominal organs
Cardiac arrest
Incomplete drainage
Infection

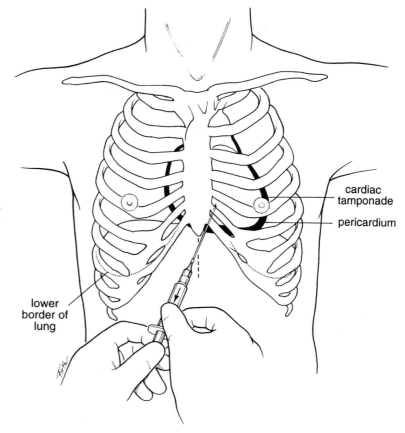

FIGURE 8–1. Insertion of needle for pericardiocentesis at the junction of the xiphoid and the left costal margin, aiming toward the left shoulder.

cardiac tamponade

pericardium

lower border of lung

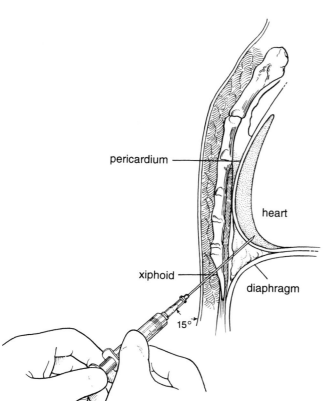

pericardium

heart

xiphoid

diaphragm

15°

FIGURE 8–2. In pericardiocentesis, the needle is inserted slowly under continuous aspiration toward the heart at a 15-degree angle to the skin.

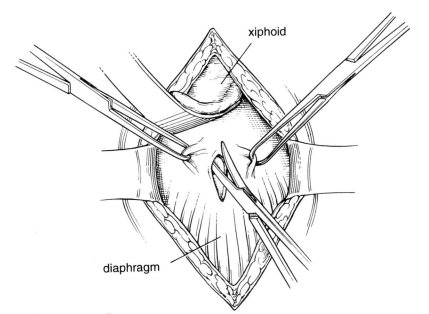

FIGURE 8–3. Pericardial window. The central diaphragm is opened by means of sharp dissection (scissors, knife, or electrocoagulation) after it has been grasped and elevated by two clamps.

Pericardial Window

Ideally, a diagnostic subxiphoid or transdiaphragmatic pericardial window is created in the operating room. If blood is noted, median sternotomy with appropriate operative intervention follows.

After sterile preparation, a longitudinal incision is made, starting at the xiphoid process and extending to approximately 3.5 cm below it. The midline fascia is opened, avoiding entry to the peritoneum. If the tip of the xiphoid is in the operative field, it may be mobilized, elevated, and resected. Blunt finger dissection beneath the xiphoid and the inferior sternum will allow access to the anterior pericardium, which usually merges with the diaphragm (Fig. 8–3). The latter structure is marked by transverse muscle fibers, whereas the

pericardium appears smooth and gray. Finger palpation identifies the cardiac pulsation. The pericardium can be very difficult to grasp. Allis clamps or Crile clamps may be useful, but often a small nick must be made using a No. 15 or 11 blade (Fig. 8–4). The incision can be enlarged to 2 cm by use of a knife or scissors to allow careful visualization of the pericardial cavity. It is very important to keep the surgical field blood free by means of careful cauterization. Otherwise, blood dripping from muscular structures may change the color of the pericardial fluid to red and give a false-positive result. In chronic conditions, a catheter (20 Fr chest tube or any other type of drain) may be placed into the pericardial sac. In traumatic injury, creation of a positive pericardial window is followed by immediate median sternotomy. Complica-

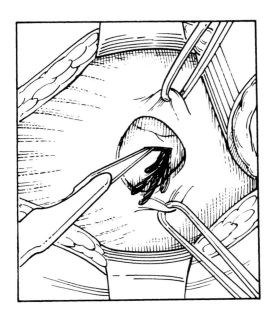

FIGURE 8–4. The underlying pericardium is incised in a similar way after careful hemostasis has been obtained.

TABLE 8–3. Complications of Pericardial Window

Right ventricular laceration	Infection
Pneumothorax	Bleeding from edges
Abdominal hernia	Incomplete drainage
Diaphragmatic laceration	

tions of pericardial window creation are described in Table 8–3.

Suggested Readings

1. Allen KB, Faber LP, Warren WH, Shaar CJ: Pericardial effusion: subxiphoid pericardiostomy versus percutaneous catheter drainage. Ann Thorac Surg 1999;67:437–440.
2. Callaham ML: Pericardiocentesis in traumatic and nontraumatic cardiac trauma. Ann Emerg Med 1984;13:924–945.
3. Duvernoy O, Magnusson A: CT-guided pericardiocentesis. Acta Radiol 1996;37:775–778.
4. Focht G, Becker RC: Pericardiocentesis. In Rippe JM, Irwin RS, Fink MP, et al (eds): Procedures and Techniques in Intensive Care Medicine. Boston, Little, Brown, 1995, pp 111–116.
5. Franco KL, Breckenridge I, Hammond GL: The pericardium. In Baue AE, Geha AS, Hammond GL, et al (eds): Glenn's Thoracic and Cardiovascular Surgery, 5th ed. Norwalk, CT, Appleton and Lange, 1991, pp 1977–1987.
6. Ivatury RR, Simon RJ, Roham M: Cardiac injuries and resuscitative thoracotomy. In Maul KI, Rodriguez A, Wiles CE III (eds): Complications in Trauma and Critical Care. Philadelphia, WB Saunders, 1996, pp 279–288.
7. Jimenez E, Martin M, Krukenkamp I, Barrett J: Subxiphoid pericardiotomy versus echocardiography: A prospective evaluation of the diagnosis of occult penetrating cardiac injury. Surgery 1990;108:676–679.
8. Shoemaker WC: Pericardial tamponade. In Webb AR, Shapiro MJ, Singer M, Suter PM (eds): Oxford Textbook of Critical Care. New York, Oxford University Press, 1999, pp 276–279.
9. Wilkes JD, Fidias P, Vaickus L, Perez RP: Malignancy-related pericardial effusion. 127 cases from the Roswell Park Cancer Institute. Cancer 1995;767:1377–1387.

9 Percutaneous Feeding Catheters

Peter Crookes

Seriously ill and injured patients are generally unable to eat. They are consequently at risk of malnutrition and all its secondary complications. In addition, failure to use the gastrointestinal (GI) tract for a prolonged period leads to atrophy of the intestinal mucosa, which may take a very long time to reverse. This may have the additional effect of reducing the barrier to bacterial translocation, a situation with the potential to exacerbate sepsis. Localized injury or malfunction of the upper GI tract, even without serious systemic illness, may be a major impediment to recovery. For these reasons, safe and ready access to the GI tract is an important component of intensive care. Nutrition can be provided either by the enteral or the parenteral (intravenous) route. This chapter concentrates on access to the GI tract for the provision of nutrition. The unique advantages of providing nutrition directly to the GI tract rather than intravenously include a reduced risk of central line sepsis, fluid overload, and mucosal atrophy of the GI tract.

Short-term enteral nutrition is often provided via a nasogastric (NG) tube. A specially designed tube with a weighted end can sometimes be made to pass into the duodenum for postpyloric feeding, but the poor gastric motility often observed in these patients demands endoscopic or fluoroscopic assistance. Although many ingenious ways have been designed to assist transpyloric placement of the NG tube (including the use of a narrow-gauge angioscope passed through the tube), NG and nasoenteric tubes are best suited for short-term use because of the high incidence of patient discomfort, accidental dislodgement, and sinusitis with prolonged use. Percutaneous cannulation of the GI tract is then preferred.

Percutaneous Techniques

The stomach is the most accessible part of the GI tract for percutaneous cannulation. The basic principle underlying all methods of access—whether with endoscopic or fluoroscopic guidance—is that the stomach should be distended with air until its anterior wall comes to lie directly beneath the peritoneum of the anterior abdominal wall without the interposition of other structures. This allows it to be safely cannulated.

Percutaneous Endoscopic Gastrostomy

Elective percutaneous endoscopic gastrostomy (PEG) is commonly performed by gastroenterologists, but in the intensive care unit (ICU), a surgeon or an intensivist with good endoscopic skills is often available. He or she also has the advantage of being familiar with other potentially important aspects of the patient's condition, such as a history of recent abdominal surgery.

Preparation. If the patient has an indwelling NG tube, ensure that the stomach is empty before commencing. It is best not to remove the NG tube until you are sure that the PEG tube can be placed. Patients without NG tubes must be kept on nothing-by-mouth status overnight. There is a high incidence of delayed gastric emptying in the ICU, and aspiration is a real risk. Patients who are not already receiving antibiotics should receive broad-spectrum antibiotic prophylaxis, particularly to guard against bacteremia. Heparin should be stopped before the procedure. If the coagulation parameters are abnormal, administer fresh frozen plasma before the procedure. Expose the upper abdomen, but do not prepare and drape the area or open the PEG kit until you are sure that the procedure is possible. PEG catheters come in several sizes, commonly 20 or 24 F. The larger size is preferable because it easily allows the passage of a jejunostomy tube.

Sedation. Conscious sedation is easy to administer and monitor in the ICU setting. In cooperative alert patients, we usually spray the throat with benzocaine (Cetacaine) before giving sedation. It is best to use a short-acting benzodiazepine such as midazolam, and most add an opiate such as meperidine (Demerol) or morphine. Both are given in small incremental doses until sedation has been achieved. Place a mouth guard between the teeth before the patient is totally sedated. Intubated patients are easier to sedate and keep comfortable, but the positioning of equipment is sometimes a nuisance, and care must be taken to ensure that access to the endotracheal tube is not impeded.

Procedure. Have suction available at the head of the bed. Turn the smaller knob of the endoscope forward to lock movement in the lateral plane. The larger knob can then be moved back and forward with the thumb to provide upward and downward curving of the scope. Introduce the scope into the back of the pharynx with

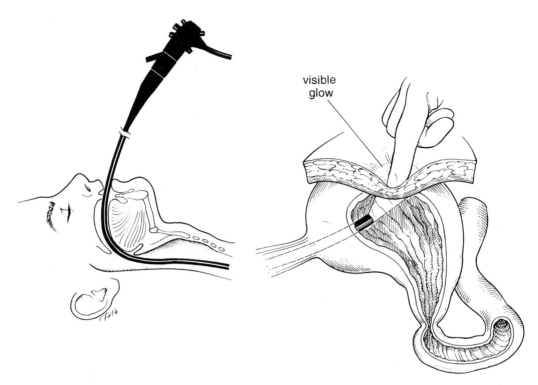

visible glow

FIGURE 9–1. Endoscopic method of identifying the optimal site for insertion of the percutaneous catheter.

a gentle flexion curvature. Follow the line of the NG tube if there is one. If the scope stays in the midline, you will be able to advance it to about 18 to 20 cm from the mouth guard without difficulty. Resistance before this usually means that you are not in the midline but are pushing into a piriform sinus. If you see the larynx, withdraw 1 cm and unflex the scope slightly so that it travels behind the epiglottis. It will then be sitting at the top of the cricopharyngeus. Have the patient swallow, and gently advance the scope into the esophagus.

In an intubated patient, the easiest way to introduce the gastroscope is to stand at the patient's head and use a laryngoscope to elevate the tongue and the endotracheal tube. Then insert the gastroscope along the posterior pharyngeal wall until it passes into the esophagus. Keep your finger on the inflate button until you see that the lumen of the esophagus is widely patent. Advance the scope down to the gastroesophageal junction, which can be recognized by the bunching up of the folds of the cardia and by the abrupt transition between the pearl-gray squamous esophageal mucosa and the salmon-pink columnar mucosa of the stomach (Z line). Pass the scope into the stomach, and inspect the body and the fundus, which are characterized by rugal folds, and the antrum, which is flat and featureless. It is important to ensure that the pylorus can be cannulated and that there is no duodenal ulcer.

With the stomach well inflated, look for a spot in the body of the stomach just proximal to the antrum. An assistant should press on the epigastrium to aid

orientation. Through the endoscope, observe where the assistant's finger can be seen indenting the stomach wall (Fig. 9–1). Darken the room, and rotate the monitor away from the field of view so that the light from the endoscope can be seen transilluminating the abdominal wall. The ideal spot is just to the left of the midline in the epigastrium and preferably at least 2 cm below the left costal margin. If the light can be clearly seen, mark the spot. A scrubbed assistant will then prepare and drape the area. Reconfirm the spot at which the indentation of the assistant's finger can be visualized endoscopically, and pass the snare down the biopsy channel until it emerges into the stomach. The assistant will then infiltrate local anesthesia into the area, making sure that the guidewire in its circular sheath is ready for use, and will push the large needle through the anesthetized skin into the stomach. When it is observed in the lumen, the central needle is removed, and the guidewire is passed down the cannula into the stomach. The endoscopist encircles the wire with a snare and tightens it (Fig. 9–2). As the assistant feeds more of the guidewire into the stomach, the endoscope is drawn back out through the mouth, keeping the snare tightly closed until the wire has been brought out through the mouth (Fig. 9–3).

There are two ways to insert the gastrostomy tube, depending on its design. In the "push" method, a gastrostomy tube is used that has a long extension tapering to a fine point. It is passed over the wire to emerge in the epigastrium. It is important to hold the guidewire straight with one hand and to advance the

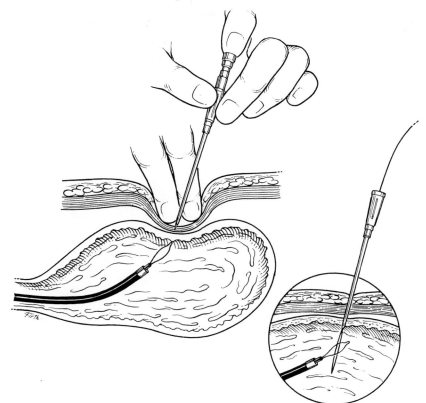

FIGURE 9–2. The guidewire is passed into the stomach through the needle and is encircled by the snare (*inset*).

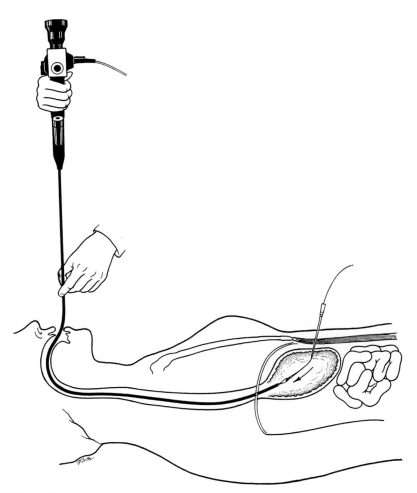

FIGURE 9–3. The endoscope is withdrawn, and the guidewire is pulled out through the mouth.

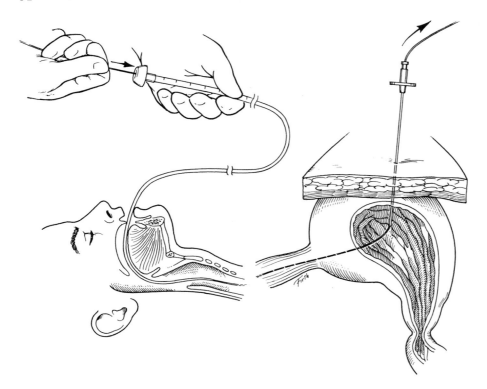

FIGURE 9–4. The percutaneous endoscopic gastrostomy catheter is passed over the guidewire and is pushed down into the stomach.

gastrostomy tube extension with the other (Fig. 9–4). At this point, the assistant cuts the site where the wire enters the skin to make an opening of about 4 mm (Fig. 9–5). Once the tapered extension emerges in the epigastrium, the whole assembly can be pulled through the oropharynx and down into the stomach. Typically, the gastrostomy tube can be pulled through until the 3-cm mark appears at the skin, depending on the amount of subcutaneous fat. This is the level at which the flange on the gastrostomy tube is snugly against

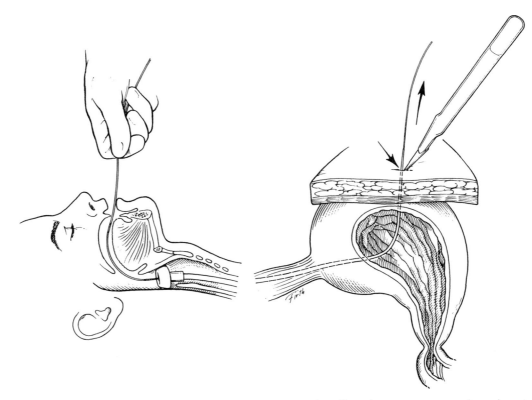

FIGURE 9–5. Enlargement of the skin opening at the site of guidewire insertion allows the percutaneous endoscopic gastrostomy catheter to exit.

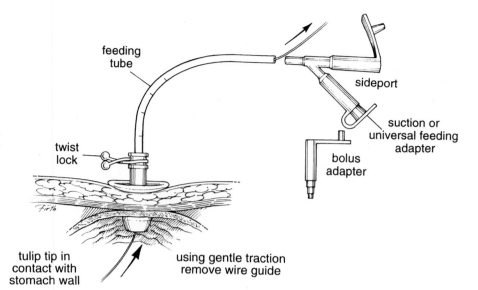

FIGURE 9–6. The percutaneous endoscopic gastrostomy unit in situ, demonstrating the methods of fixation to the skin and of attachment of the feeding ports.

the gastric wall. Pull out the guidewire; pass the Silastic retention rings over the tapered extension and down over the gastrostomy tube until flush with the skin; trim the tube to about 15 cm in length; and apply the stopcock fitting, which connects to feeding pumps or a syringe (Fig. 9–6).

The "pull" method employs a looped guidewire. When brought through the mouth by the snare, the guidewire is looped onto a loop of wire at the end of the gastrostomy tube. The wire is then pulled down,

bringing the gastrostomy tube out into the enlarged epigastric incision, as before (Fig. 9–7). The physical characteristics of both types of gastrostomy tubes are identical; they differ only in mode of insertion, and choice is a matter of personal preference.

Special Situations

What Happens When You Cannot Transilluminate?

Sometimes the reason for inability to transilluminate is trivial, such as too much subcutaneous fat or too much ambient light. The most serious reason is the

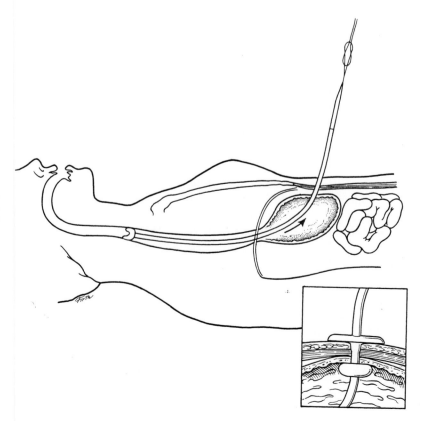

FIGURE 9–7. Looped guidewire pulling the percutaneous endoscopic gastrostomy unit through the stomach. (*Inset,* Correct position of the gastrostomy tube with flange flush against gastric wall.)

interposition of other structures between the gastric wall and the anterior abdominal wall. Transverse colon or small bowel may be stuck there, especially after previous abdominal surgery. Many ICU patients with a lot of third-space fluid retention have enlargement of the liver, which comes down well below the costal margin and can overlap the stomach. In a thin patient in a darkened room, inability to see the endoscopic light through the skin is a danger signal. If upper abdominal or chest computed tomography has been done recently, inspect the position of the stomach relative to the anterior abdominal wall before scheduling PEG insertion.

Previous Gastric Surgery

Dealing with a patient who has had previous gastric surgery is easy if the patient has had an antecolic reconstruction. The efferent limb of a Billroth II or a Roux-en-Y reconstruction is usually fairly superficial, and it can often be made to transilluminate, and to be punctured, in the same way as the stomach. Because retrocolic gastrojejunostomy makes the efferent limb less accessible, it may be necessary to pass the endoscope much further down the limb before it can be made to reach the anterior abdominal wall.

The Very Obese Patient

Very obese patients, despite their apparent overnutrition, often still require access to the GI tract when in the ICU for prolonged periods. The chief problem is the practical difficulty of getting a needle safely into the stomach. In morbidly obese patients, the needle supplied with the PEG kit is often not long enough, and a long needle (i.e., the type used to insert a central line) can be used. The needle needs to be big enough to accept the guidewire. There is a higher incidence of skin problems in obese patients, but otherwise the complications are similar.

Gastroparesis or Gastric Outlet Obstruction

If the stomach is full of fluid on endoscopy, or the volume of NG aspirate is large, suspect an outlet problem. Old duodenal ulcer scarring or a new stress ulcer may cause physical outlet obstruction. Diabetic patients and others with major sepsis may simply have a nonemptying stomach, and patients with stroke or head injury also exhibit dysfunction of the lower esophageal sphincter. In these patients, tube feedings accumulate in the stomach and create a great risk of aspiration. This is an indication for provision of feeding distal to the pylorus.

Percutaneous Endoscopic Jejunostomy

For patients who require postpyloric feeding, one simple method is to insert a jejunostomy feeding tube through the PEG and to guide it endoscopically into the duodenum. It is helpful to tie a short length of silk suture to the end of the jejunostomy tube so that it can be grasped by biopsy forceps or a snare. The scope is then carried down through the pylorus into the duodenum and is positioned as far as it will go, generally in the third portion of the duodenum. It is always frustrating to accomplish this, only to find that the jejunostomy tube backs out into the stomach as the scope is withdrawn. To prevent this, advance the snare or the biopsy forceps, grasping the jejunostomy tube as the scope is withdrawn; when it is in the stomach, apply strong suction to the jejunostomy tube. (This means connecting suction to the port marked "feeding," because the port marked "suction" applies suction to the stomach.) It is then possible to relax the snare and to advance it slightly to disengage it from the jejunostomy catheter before withdrawing it.

Fluoroscopic Nonendoscopic Procedures

In the ICU, endoscopic insertion of feeding tubes can be carried out at the bedside with minimal disruption to the routine. Sometimes it is not possible or safe to insert a PEG tube. These situations include trauma to or recent surgery of the pharynx, the neck, or the esophagus or an undilatable stricture due to caustic ingestion, previous radiation therapy, or a bulky tumor. In such circumstances, provided an NG tube can be positioned in the stomach, percutaneous gastrostomy and jejunostomy can be performed by an interventional radiologist using fluoroscopic guidance. The principle of this method is similar to that of PEG tube insertion: The stomach must be distended with air until it lies just beneath an accessible part of the abdominal wall. The advantage of fluoroscopy is that the distended stomach can be seen in the lateral projection, and its proximity to the abdominal wall can be observed. It has the further advantage that tube site infection seems to be less of a problem, because the gastrostomy tube is not dragged through the mouth and contaminated by oral flora. In practice, if the patient can be safely moved to the radiology suite, the relative advantages of PEG and fluoroscopic gastrostomy depend on local enthusiasm and expertise.

Randomized controlled trials show little advantage of one technique over the other except for a reduction in the frequency of wound site sepsis with the fluoroscopic technique. Because insertion of the gastrostomy tube could potentially displace the stomach away from the abdominal wall, one common preliminary step is to insert a needle into the stomach and to pass a T-fastener into the lumen. As the needle is withdrawn, the T-fastener, which is inserted in a straight position, assumes a T shape and is drawn upward to fix that portion of the stomach against the anterior abdominal wall. Generally, three or four such fasteners are in-

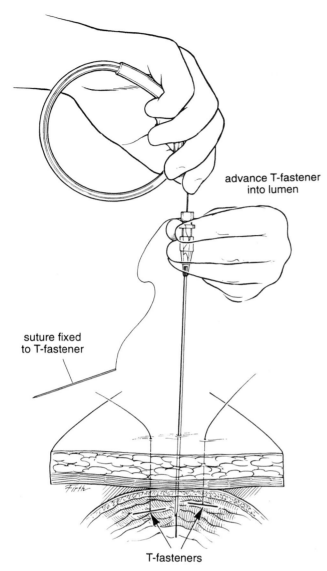

advance T-fastener into lumen

suture fixed to T-fastener

T-fasteners

FIGURE 9–8. T-fasteners keep the stomach applied to the anterior abdominal wall before placement of fluoroscopically guided gastrostomy unit.

serted to attach an area of stomach approximately 1 inch in diameter to the back of the abdominal wall (Fig. 9–8). The threads of the T-fasteners are sutured to the abdominal skin over a cotton roll. The needle and the subsequent guidewire are then easily inserted in the middle of the area outlined by the T-fasteners, and the track is dilated in a manner similar to central line insertion. The actual gastrostomy tube has a self-retaining device distally, either a pigtail curl or a small balloon. The sutures holding the T-fasteners are removed in a few days, when adherence of the stomach to the abdominal wall has occurred.

Jejunostomy Insertion

Fluoroscopic guidance can be used to position a feeding tube more distally than is usually possible endo-

scopically. This is best done with an established gastrostomy site. A mature gastrostomy tract, no matter how it was created, can be used to insert a steerable guidewire through the pylorus and beyond the ligament of Treitz into the proximal jejunum. The catheter is then passed over the guidewire under fluoroscopic control until it lies in the proximal jejunum.

Recannulation of Previous Jejunostomy Site

A patient who has undergone jejunostomy and develops recurrent disease may need repeat jejunostomy. A similar situation may develop acutely in the hospital if the jejunostomy tube is accidentally removed. If this is noticed at once (within 1 or 2 hours), the tube can simply be washed and reinserted. If the tube can be easily advanced and flushed, there is no need to confirm its position by a "tubogram." Often, the opening has closed over, however, and it is not possible to reinsert the tube blindly. The problem can be solved by using fluoroscopic guidance to position a needle in the bowel at the site of the previous jejunostomy and injecting water-soluble contrast material to identify the bowel lumen. A guidewire is then positioned well into the bowel, and a catheter is introduced over the guidewire, as previously described.

Indications

Prolonged Access to the Gastrointestinal Tract

Many patients undergoing major surgery for trauma or a major elective resection will have a jejunostomy tube inserted at the time of surgery. In the ICU setting, patients needing access to the GI tract are those who remain ill and who are unable to eat because of a major complication that develops in the process of recovery. Any type of major organ failure may cause this inability to receive oral feedings, especially failure resulting from prolonged ventilator dependency, neurologic injury, or prolonged sepsis. If the duration of this prolonged recovery period is short (1 to 2 weeks), feeding can be given by the NG tube without the need for a more invasive procedure. Longer periods of NG intubation are associated with sinusitis and perhaps an increased tendency toward reflux, aspiration, and even esophageal stricture. Percutaneous techniques are valuable in these situations.

Choice of Procedure

If there is no peroral access to the stomach via either endoscopic or NG tube, an open procedure in the operating room is usually required. If endoscopy cannot be done but an NG tube can be passed, fluoroscopic gastrostomy is the simplest solution. This may be necessary after major head and neck surgery—which may be accompanied by dense proximal scarring from radiation therapy or a large tumor mass—or after major facial or neck trauma. If there is no barrier to upper GI endoscopy, perform PEG unless the stomach is nonfunctional (owing to gastric outlet obstruction, gastroparesis, or a very large hiatal hernia causing reflux and aspiration), in which case percutaneous endoscopic jejunostomy is useful. In the special situation in which the stomach is needed for subsequent reconstruction (e.g., after esophagectomy or pharyngolaryngectomy), it is better to keep the stomach intact and to perform open jejunostomy directly, because the presence of an additional suture line in the tubularized stomach might lead to ischemia of the gastric conduit postoperatively.

Pitfalls

These procedures are safe and effective in experienced hands, as indicated by several studies with large numbers of patients. Complications are related to the initial endoscopic procedure, the actual puncturing of the stomach or the jejunum, and the administration of tube feedings.

Complications of Endoscopy

Aspiration is an important risk in all ICU patients but especially when it is associated with malfunction of the foregut. Gastroparesis, hypotonia of the lower esophageal sphincter, esophageal trauma, retention of secretions or tube feedings, and bacterial overgrowth in the acid-suppressed stomach can all contribute to the risk. It is minimized by keeping the stomach empty and taking care when introducing the endoscope.

Oversedation may result in desaturation and the need for intubation of a patient with precarious respiratory status. Narcotic medications such as meperidine may be reversed by naloxone (Narcan), and midazolam can be reversed by flumazenil. Oversedation can be prevented by giving medications in small increments and allowing enough time for them to take effect before increasing the dose.

Perforation is rare if the upper GI tract is structurally normal. A patient who cannot cooperate is at risk during the initial introduction of the endoscope, however, and there is no substitute for care and gentleness. If there is a known stricture, do not start the procedure unless a narrow-gauge or a pediatric endoscope is immediately available.

Early Complications of Puncture and Intubation

Other structures may be punctured, including the colon and the small bowel. If the stomach is distended enough to permit clear transillumination of the skin, it is rare for there to be any intervening structures. Bleeding may be due to correction of coagulopathy or damage to an omental vessel close to the greater curve.

Patients with jejunostomy tubes can sometimes develop pneumatosis intestinalis, which is usually minor but may create an alarming appearance on a computed tomographic scan of the abdomen. We have noticed it after operative jejunostomy when the needle catheter technique is used, because there is presumably a tract through which bowel gas can track within the wall. It does not have the serious significance of spontaneously occurring pneumatosis, however.

Dislodgement of the feeding tube, if it occurs early, will lead to the twin disasters of gastric perforation and infusion of nourishment and medications into the peritoneal cavity. This presents with peritonitis but is often hard to recognize in critically ill patients, who may be obtunded or have other sources of a fever that cause the complication to be disregarded.

Late Complications

Dislodgement. Dislodgement after the tract has matured is of less consequence. An agitated patient or an inattentive nurse may accidentally dislodge the tube. If this is noticed at once, a Foley catheter or a replacement gastrostomy tube with a retention device may be positioned through the same opening. Confirm that it is in the stomach by aspirating gastric juice or tube feeding material. If repositioning is necessary in the first 2 weeks, we recommend radiologic confirmation before using the replaced tube again. After this time, the stomach is usually so adherent that there is little danger of misplacing a new tube. If the tube cannot be easily repositioned through the old site, however, it should be replaced under x-ray control.

Infection of the Skin. Skin infection may develop at the site of insertion. This is a relatively common problem, which is often of concern to the patient and the nurses but rarely causes serious morbidity. A number of factors are thought to be important in reducing its incidence and its severity.

1. Aseptic technique during insertion of the gastrostomy tube.
2. Care in dressing the wound.
3. Avoidance of overtight application of the Silastic retention devices to the skin. In typical patients, the disk should be approximately at the 3-cm mark.
4. Avoidance of excessive movement of the catheter

against the skin. Tape it gently to the skin a few centimeters away.

5. Keeping the site amenable to easy inspection. Do not cover it with bulky dressings. Gently massage the skin toward the tube, looking for subcutaneous pus.

Intolerance of Tube Feedings. It is surprisingly rare, even in patients with serious sepsis and organ failure, for true intolerance to be seen. The stomach may be slow to empty, so that feedings administered to the patient 4 hours previously are still present; however, unless mechanical small bowel obstruction is present, jejunal feedings are usually well tolerated. Diarrhea may result when too great a volume of hyperosmolar material is infused into the jejunum. One should beware of attributing diarrhea to this mechanism in ICU patients, however, because other potentially disastrous causes, including *Clostridium difficile* colitis, are very common in this setting. Diarrhea can usually be controlled by adding attapulgite (Kaopectate), 30 mL to each 1-liter bag of tube feeding material. Up to 90 mL may be added. A formula containing soluble fiber is also useful.

Complications of Tube Feedings. Small bowel obstruction and ischemia have been described in several settings, in some cases associated with excessive fiber in the formula. The more seriously ill the patient, the more difficult it is to detect early abdominal signs. The development of abdominal distention or guarding should alert the physician to this possibility, particularly if there are other signs of intestinal dysfunction (e.g., cessation of bowel movements).

Tube Blockage and Malfunction. Small-caliber jejunostomy tubes are much more likely to clog than large (20 to 24 F) tubes. Inserting crushed medications into the tubes is a potent reason for blockage. Flush narrow-gauge tubes with acidic material such as coke after administering medications to prevent blockage. A blocked tube may often be cleared by flushing it with water using a small (2-mL) syringe. Larger syringes are less effective. Refractory blockage may respond to infusion of a small quantity of vinegar or other acidic substance, leaving it for 30 minutes before another attempt to clear the tube is made. If these measures fail, replace the tube.

Therapeutic Interventions

Explanation of detailed feeding regimens is not appropriate to this chapter, but some simple guidelines are offered. Percutaneously placed tubes can be used for feeding after 24 hours. Jejunal feedings cannot be given by syringe in a large bolus and require constant infusion using a pump. Most formulas produce 1 kcal/mL, making it easy to calculate requirements. A rate of 44 mL/hour delivers 1000 mL and 1000 kcal/day.

Special formulations exist for use in diabetic patients or in those with hepatic or renal insufficiency. Even a patient with a fistula can often be fed enterally if an elemental diet is administered. It is best to begin with small volumes, say 15 mL/hour, and advance the amount by 15 mL/hour every 12 hours until the goal rate is reached. Do not forget to reduce the intravenous rate as this process is advancing. There is no point in waiting for traditional signs of return of bowel function in these patients. Small bowel motor activity returns early after the stress of surgery or sepsis, before return of activity in either the stomach or the colon.

Gastrostomy feedings are usually given by administering a bolus of 200 to 250 mL (equivalent to one can of tube feeding material) by syringe. Feedings are given every 4 hours, and the amount is increased until the nutritional goal is met. Before administering each feeding, aspirate the gastrostomy tube to measure the residual volume. A large or an increasing residual volume is an indication to consider providing a jejunostomy tube through the pylorus.

Suggested Readings

1. Dewald CL, Hiette PO, Sewall LE, et al: Percutaneous gastrostomy and gastrojejunostomy with gastropexy: experience in 701 procedures. Radiology 1999;211:651–656.
2. Gossner L, Keymling J, Hahn EG, Ell C: Antibiotic prophylaxis in percutaneous endoscopic gastrostomy (PEG): A prospective randomized clinical trial. Endoscopy 1999;31:119–124.
3. Grathwohl KW, Gibbons RV, Dillard TA, et al: Bedside videoscopic placement of feeding tubes: Development of fiberoptics through the tube. Crit Care Med 1997;25:629–634.
4. Hoffer EK, Cosgrove JM, Levin DQ, et al: Radiologic gastrojejunostomy and percutaneous endoscopic gastrostomy: A prospective randomized comparison. J Vasc Interv Radiol 1999;10:413–420.
5. Kudsk KA, Croce MA, Fabian TC, et al: Enteral versus parenteral feeding: Effects on septic morbidity after blunt and penetrating abdominal trauma. Ann Surg 1992;215:503–511.
6. Larson DE, Burton DD, Schroeder KW, DiMagno EP: Percutaneous endoscopic gastrostomy. Indications, success, complications, and mortality in 314 consecutive patients. Gastroenterology 1987;3:48–52.
7. Lo CW, Walker WA: Changes in the gastrointestinal tract during enteral or parenteral feeding. Nutr Rev 1989;47:193–198.
8. Lowe JB, Page CP, Schwesinger WH, et al: Percutaneous endoscopic gastrostomy tube placement in a surgical training program. Am J Surg 1997;174:624–628.
9. Lucas CE, Yu P, Vlahos A, Ledgerwood A: Lower esophageal sphincter dysfunction often precludes safe gastric feeding in stroke patients. Arch Surg 1999;134:55–58.
10. Miller RE, Castlemain B, Lacqua FJ, Kotler DP: Percutaneous endoscopic gastrostomy. Results in 316 patients and review of literature. Surg Endosc 1989;3:186–190.
11. Moore FA, Feliciano DV, Andrassy RJ, et al: Early enteral feeding compared with parenteral reduces postoperative septic complications: The results of a meta-analysis. Ann Surg 1992;216:172–183.
12. Ponsky JL, Gauderer MWL: Percutaneous endoscopic gastrostomy: A nonoperative technique for feeding gastrostomy. Gastrointest Endosc 1981;27:9–11.
13. Scaife CL, Saffle JR, Morris SE: Intestinal obstruction secondary to enteral feedings in burn trauma patients. J Trauma 1999;47:859–863.
14. Schachter P, Finkelstein A, Cohen O: Bizarre early and late complications of percutaneous endoscopic gastrostomy. J Clin Gastroenterol 1999;29:102.

10 Diagnostic Abdominal Paracentesis and Peritoneal Lavage

George C. Velmahos

Diagnostic peritoneal lavage (DPL) continues to provide useful information 35 years after its original description. Its major use is in trauma cases when there is a question about intra-abdominal injuries. DPL includes insertion of a catheter into the peritoneal cavity, aspiration through the catheter to identify the presence of gross blood, infusion of 1 L of fluid in the absence of bloody aspirate, and microscopic examination of the returned fluid for a variety of factors. Abdominal paracentesis is also used in nontraumatic conditions (e.g., ascites). The principles of the two techniques are the same. The only difference is that abdominal paracentesis for drainage of ascites is often done through the lateral abdominal wall, whereas DPL is almost exclusively done in the midline.

Indications and Contraindications

Diagnostic peritoneal lavage is used in hemodynamically unstable patients with traumatic injuries in whom clinical examination of the abdomen is unreliable owing to intoxication or injuries to the head, the spinal cord, or multiple associated sites. Because of increasingly easier access to computed tomography (CT), which has higher specificity, hemodynamically stable patients in whom clinical examination is unreliable are better evaluated by means of abdominal CT. A potential scenario for the use of DPL in hemodynamically stable patients with traumatic injury is after emergent transport to the operating room for neurosurgical intervention. These patients are usually not able to be evaluated clinically, a condition that will continue for many hours intraoperatively and postoperatively. Because CT is not an option in many of these cases, intraoperative DPL performed in parallel with the neurosurgical intervention would be appropriate to evaluate the abdominal cavity.

Abdominal paracentesis is used for tense ascites to relieve symptoms of compression. The threshold that should be maintained before draining ascites is debatable. The benefits of the procedure should be balanced against the risks of contaminating a sterile collection and allowing the development of more ascitic fluid as a result of the release of intra-abdominal pressure.

Contraindications include the presence of abdominal scars from previous surgery; pelvic fractures with suspected large pelvic hematomas, which may extend beyond the boundaries of the pelvis and interfere with the DPL insertion site; and advanced pregnancy. All the problems associated with these conditions can be bypassed if DPL is really needed, however, by selecting alternative abdominal sites or techniques and exercising particular caution when entering the abdominal cavity.

Criteria and Reliability

The results of DPL are considered positive if any of the following are found in the effluent: (1) more than 100,000 red blood cells per milliliter; (2) more than 500 white blood cells per milliliter; (3) amylase, urea, or bilirubin levels higher than serum levels; (4) food particle, feces, or high bacterial counts. These criteria were developed for patients with blunt trauma. In the majority of cases, only the red blood cell count is measured. For patients with penetrating trauma, the red blood cell count associated with positive DPL results is unknown; in various studies, the value has been set at 1000, 5000, 10,000, and 50,000/mL. Although I rarely, if ever, use DPL for penetrating abdominal trauma, I favor the use of a threshold of positivity of 1000 red blood cells per milliliter, simply because no red blood cells should be in the abdominal cavity in the absence of peritoneal penetration.

The count of 100,000 red blood cells per milliliter in the DPL effluent may be produced by as little as 50 mL of blood in the abdominal cavity. This explains why DPL is very sensitive (close to 99%) in detecting intra-abdominal injuries but is not specific in distinguishing between those who need operative intervention and those who can be managed nonoperatively.

In almost 90% of patients with active intraperitoneal bleeding, gross blood will be aspirated immediately on insertion of the catheter, and infusion of fluid will become obsolete. It is not necessary to return the entire infusate for microscopic examination because this is time-consuming and at times impossible. A return of 250 mL is considered sufficient to produce reliable cell counts.

Although DPL is used mostly in the emergency department, it is occasionally required in the intensive care unit to rule out initially undiagnosed injury in a patient who cannot be transported to the CT suite and who has an unknown source of sepsis shortly after admission. Under these circumstances, the threshold of white blood cells or bacterial count in the effluent that would characterize a positive DPL result is unknown. Using the same criteria as for acute patients will probably not affect the sensitivity but will decrease the specificity of the procedure even further.

Technique

There are two techniques: open and closed. A peritoneal dialysis catheter is used for either technique. Additionally, there is a percutaneous DPL set that can be used only for the closed technique.

Open Technique

A 3- to 5-cm vertical skin incision is created under the umbilicus. In pregnant patients or those with pelvic fractures, the incision can be made over the umbilicus (Fig. 10–1). The subcutaneous fat is dissected, and the fascia is grasped with a Kocher clamp and is lifted toward the skin (Fig. 10–2). Two stay sutures (2–0 nylon) are placed on either side of the Kocher clamp, and the clamp is released. The fascia is incised with the knife between the two sutures (Fig. 10–3). The underlying muscle and the peritoneum can be incised via knife or scissors until the abdominal cavity has been entered. Then the DPL catheter, which has multiple side holes to avoid obstruction by clots or viscera, is inserted under direct visualization toward the pelvis. Aspiration via the catheter follows to examine for gross blood. If 5 to 10 mL of blood is aspirated, the DPL result is considered positive. If no blood is aspirated, 1 L of sterile fluid is instilled from an intravenous bag into the abdominal cavity. Unobstructed flow of the fluid confirms good position of the catheter. Then the intravenous bag is lowered below the level of the patient to act as a siphon for fluid return (Fig. 10–4). When effluent flow stops, the intravenous bag is disconnected to terminate suction, and a specimen is sent for laboratory testing. The DPL catheter is removed, and the stay sutures are tied together to close the fascial opening.

Closed Technique

A 0.5-cm incision is made in the skin at the abovementioned site. In the trocar method (Fig. 10–5), which uses a peritoneal dialysis catheter, a trocar is fed into

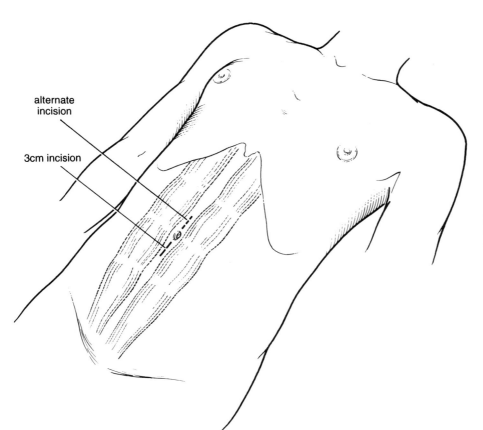

alternate incision

3cm incision

FIGURE 10–1. Incision over or under the umbilicus for open diagnostic peritoneal lavage.

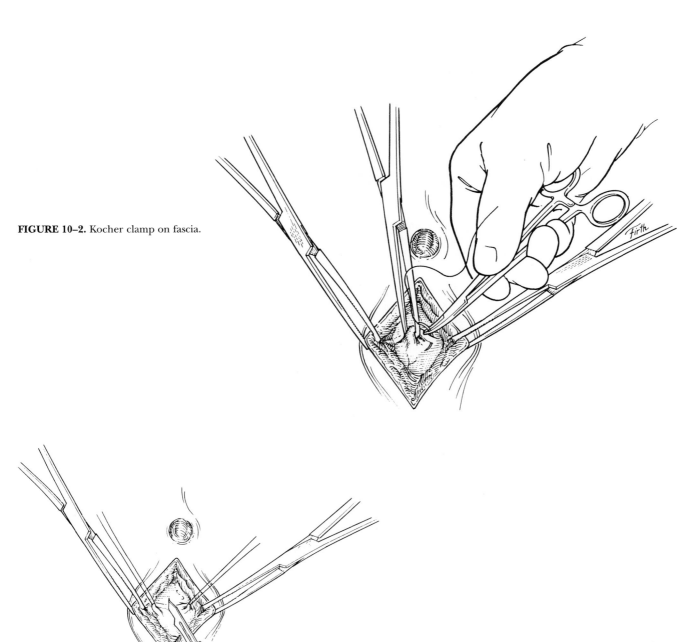

FIGURE 10–2. Kocher clamp on fascia.

FIGURE 10–3. Stay sutures in place and opening of the fascia.

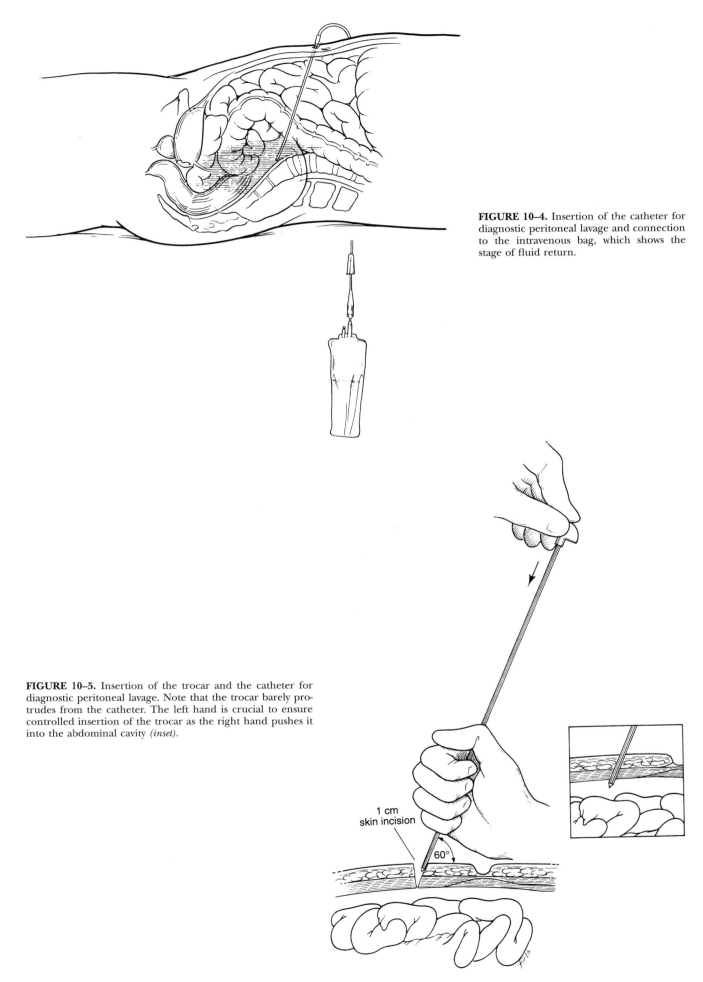

FIGURE 10–4. Insertion of the catheter for diagnostic peritoneal lavage and connection to the intravenous bag, which shows the stage of fluid return.

FIGURE 10–5. Insertion of the trocar and the catheter for diagnostic peritoneal lavage. Note that the trocar barely protrudes from the catheter. The left hand is crucial to ensure controlled insertion of the trocar as the right hand pushes it into the abdominal cavity *(inset)*.

1 cm
skin incision

60°

the catheter until the trocar barely protrudes from the end of the catheter. Then the trocar and the catheter are advanced through the skin incision toward the pelvis. It is important for the left hand of the operator to control the trocar as the right hand pushes it to prevent abrupt insertion into the abdominal cavity. Two "gives" are felt as the catheter passes through the anterior and the posterior abdominal fascia. If insertion is being done with properly controlled movements, after the second "give," the catheter will be just barely in the peritoneal cavity. At this point, the trocar is withdrawn, and the catheter is advanced toward the pelvis (Fig. 10–6). Some operators use an assistant to elevate the skin during insertion of the trocar. Although this is advisable for the novice operator, I do not consider it necessary as experience builds.

In the percutaneous Seldinger method, a preset kit (Arrow International, Inc., Reading, PA) is used. The needle connected to the syringe, which is half-filled with water, is inserted slowly at the same site as mentioned previously. On insertion into the abdominal cavity, the water flows easily (Fig. 10–7). The needle remains in place, a J-wire is fed through the needle, and the needle is withdrawn (Fig. 10–8). A small skin

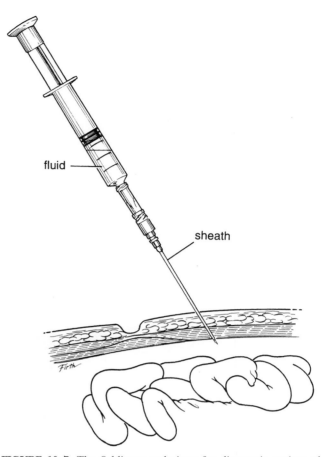

FIGURE 10–7. The Seldinger technique for diagnostic peritoneal lavage. The needle is advanced until the water in the syringe flows easily.

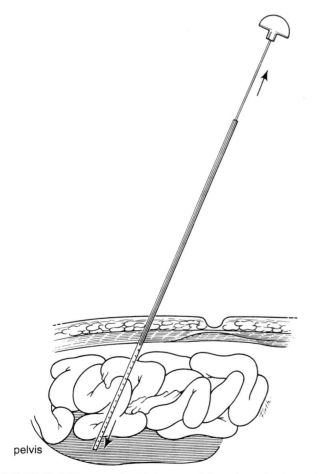

FIGURE 10–6. The trocar is withdrawn, and the catheter is advanced toward the pelvis.

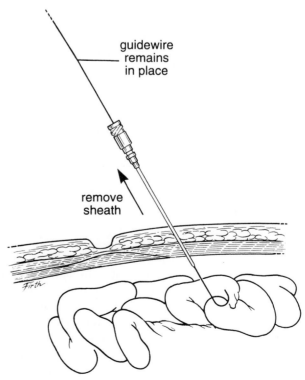

FIGURE 10–8. A J-wire is inserted through the needle.

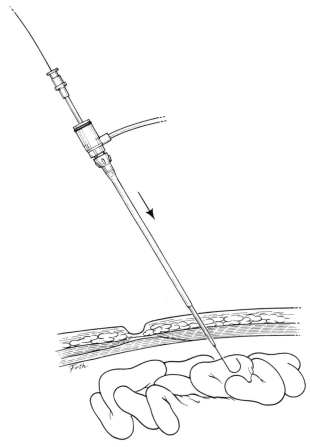

FIGURE 10–9. After a skin incision has been made at the site of J-wire insertion and the tract has been dilated, the catheter for diagnostic peritoneal lavage, guided by a dilator, is advanced over the J-wire.

incision is made around the wire, and a dilator is used to enlarge the tract. Then a percutaneous DPL catheter combined with a dilator is advanced over the guidewire (Fig. 10–9). The J-wire and the dilator are removed, leaving the catheter in place (Fig. 10–10).

Pitfalls and Complications

The most worrisome complication is injury to underlying viscera during insertion of the trocar, the needle, or the catheter. Although the incidence is low (1% to 2%), there are reports of injuries to almost every possible abdominal structure, including the aorta and the inferior vena cava. Open DPL was associated with fewer such complications in some studies, although other studies did not find any difference in complication rates between the open and the closed techniques. I prefer the closed technique under emergent conditions. In this era of unrestricted access to CT for hemodynamically stable patients, DPL is reserved for patients who are hemodynamically unstable and who require a fast procedure to evaluate the abdominal cavity as the potential source of bleeding. Open DPL is

considerably slower than closed DPL. In a prospective comparative study of the two techniques, we recorded an average time of 11 minutes for the open technique versus 2 minutes for the closed technique. On the other hand, if DPL is done under nonemergent conditions (e.g., in a patient taken to the operating room for neurosurgical intervention or in an intensive care unit patient with sepsis of unknown origin), I prefer to do open DPL and not risk any chance of injury to underlying viscera.

Another comparison between the two techniques is the rate of false-positive or, even worse, false-negative results (which are fortunately very few because sensitivity is more than 98%). Although many authorities report that open DPL offers reliable guidance of the catheter into the pelvis under direct visualization, I believe that closed DPL can be done just as reliably. It is, however, important to have a low threshold to convert closed DPL to open technique if there is reason to suspect that the catheter is not well placed.

Subcutaneous rather than intra-abdominal placement of the DPL catheter is the most frequent pitfall of the technique. This occurs—particularly in obese patients—during insertion if the catheter is directed toward the suprapubic symphysis rather than the coccyx. There will be no flow of fluid through the catheter, which should be withdrawn completely and re-

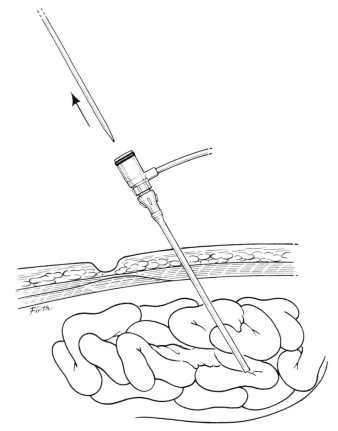

FIGURE 10–10. The dilator and the J-wire are removed, and the catheter is left in place.

placed. A DPL catheter can also be misplaced into a pelvic hematoma if a pelvic fracture is not suspected and the catheter is inserted below rather than above the umbilicus.

Both closed DPL techniques are valid, and choice of technique rests with the individual physician's preference. The Arrow kit offers a more controlled insertion by the Seldinger technique but has a softer catheter, which may be compressed or kinked easily, resulting in no fluid return. Familiarization with all techniques is essential for the physician who is treating acute or critically ill patients.

Suggested Readings

1. Advanced Trauma Life Support Manual: Abdominal Trauma. Chicago, American College of Surgeons, 1993, p 155.
2. Lazarus HM, Nelson JA: A technique for peritoneal lavage without risk or complication. Surg Gynecol Obstet 1979;149:889–892.
3. Lopez-Viego MA, Mickel TJ, Weigelt JA: Open versus closed diagnostic peritoneal lavage in the evaluation of abdominal trauma. Am J Surg 1990;160:594–597.
4. Root HD, Hauser CW, McKinley CR, et al: Diagnostic peritoneal lavage. Surgery 1965;5:633–636.
5. Velmahos GC, Demetriades D, Stewart M, et al: Open versus closed diagnostic peritoneal lavage: A comparison on safety, rapidity, efficacy. J R Coll Surg Edinb 1998;43:235–238.

11 Assisted Ventilation and Intubation

Michael J. Sullivan

A human is an obligate aerobe. Complete cessation of a continuous supply of oxygen will cause death in about 4 minutes. All other elements needed to maintain an organism's viability (e.g. water, glucose) can be obtained in a discontinuous manner. Management of an airway centers on ensuring that the supply of oxygen is constant. The most secure means we have of ensuring an oxygen supply by means other than extracorporeal oxygenation is placing a tube into the trachea. The mouth or the nose is the usual starting point, and localization or visualization of the glottic opening is the goal in endotracheal tube placement. Surgical securing of an airway is generally achieved by one of two methods: cricothyroidotomy or tracheostomy. This chapter reviews how to assess the airway and presents basic airway management maneuvers and various techniques for securing the airway. Time is always a factor to consider. Complete airway obstruction requires rapid airway management, whereas there is much more time to prepare for securing the airway in patients with spontaneous ventilation and oxygenation.

Anatomy of the Airway

The aerodigestive tract is divided into the nasopharynx, the oropharynx, and the laryngopharynx (hypopharynx). The arrangement of the structures allows the three competitive activities of deglutition, respiration, and phonation to occur, generally without overlapping the functional activities of any other process.

The Nose

The nose is the beginning of the respiratory pathway; its function is to warm, humidify, and filter inspired air. Orotracheal or nasotracheal intubation bypasses these functions and delivers cool, dry gases to the lungs. The nose begins as the triangular or pyramidal structure affixed to the face and continues posteriorly into the nasopharynx, ending at the choanae or the posterior nasal apertures at the posterior aspect of the septum. The nasal cavities are at a right angle to the face. When an artificial airway is placed through the nasal cavities, the airway should be advanced into the nasal cavity parallel to the hard palate, not cephalad to it. The nasal septum divides the nasal cavity into two compartments. A roof, a floor, and medial and lateral walls define each compartment. The roof begins with the mucosal surface of the external nose and continues as the cribriform plate of the ethmoid bone, located beneath the anterior cranial fossa; it finishes as part of the sphenoid bone. The medial wall is the nasal septum; deviations are common, so that one of the nares may accept an artificial airway more easily than the other. The lateral wall has three turbinates or conchae: superior, middle, and inferior. The floor of the nose begins just inside the external nares and is formed by the palatine process of the maxilla; the horizontal plate of the palatine bone forms the posterior segment.

The blood supply is derived from the internal and the external carotid arteries. The internal carotid artery feeds the ophthalmic artery, which gives rise to the anterior and the posterior ethmoidal arteries. These supply the anterosuperior aspect of the nasal septum and the lateral wall. The external carotid artery feeds the maxillary artery, which gives rise to the sphenopalatine artery. This supplies blood to the posteroinferior aspect of the nasal septum and the lateral wall. The nares or the nasal vestibule receives the terminal branches of the anterior ethmoid, the sphenopalatine arteries, and the superior labial artery, which is a branch of the facial artery. Kisselbach's plexus is the anastomotic site between the anterosuperior and posteroinferior blood supply.

The trigeminal nerve (cranial nerve V) supplies the sensory innervation of the nasal cavity via its ophthalmic division (V1) and its maxillary division (V2). The anterior ethmoidal nerve supplies the superoanterior aspect of the nasal septum. The nasopalatine nerve innervates the remainder, or the majority of the nasal septum. The floor of the nose is innervated anteriorly by the anterior superior dental branch of the infraorbital nerve and posteriorly by the greater palatine nerve. The anterior segment of the lateral wall is innervated by the same nerve as the anterior aspect of the nasal septum, the anterior ethmoidal nerve. The posterior aspect of the lateral wall is innervated by the sphenopalatine nerve, and the skin overlying the nose is innervated by branches of the anterior ethmoidal nerve. The infraorbital nerve supplies the nasal vestibule and the skin lateral to and below the vestibule.

The Mouth

The external part of the mouth comprises the lips and the cheeks. The internal part consists of the hard and the soft palates, the maxillary and the mandibular alveolar processes, the gums, the teeth, and the tongue. The anterior two thirds of the palate is a bony vault that arises from the palatine plates of the maxillas and the horizontal plates of the palatine bone. This also forms the structure of the maxillary alveolar bone. Teeth are anchored to this structure by means of various types of support tissue. The soft palate is the posterior third and is contiguous with the hard palate. It is composed of the palatine aponeurosis, which is a tough fibrous sheath. The free posterior edge forms the uvula in the midline, and laterally it becomes part of the anterior and the posterior pillars of the lateral pharyngeal walls. Several groups of muscles act on the palate to close off the nasopharynx from the oropharynx during swallowing and phonation. Paralysis of these muscles permits food to be regurgitated into the nasopharynx.

The mandible is a horizontal U-shaped structure with vertical rami at each end. The teeth are anchored to the alveolar bone of the mandible via supporting tissues. The angle of the jaw is formed by the intersection of the horizontal section and the vertical ramus. The head of the ramus forms the temporomandibular joint in the mandibular fossa of the temporal bone. Two types of motion occur at this joint (hinge and forward gliding), which allow the mouth to open. The normal opening distance is about three fingerbreadths (4 cm between upper and lower incisors). Dysfunction of this joint can lead to a limited range of motion and can affect the ability to secure an airway.

In the adult, full dentition includes 32 teeth: incisors, canines, premolars, and molars. Starting from the front and moving backward, each side of the mouth contains one frontal incisor, one lateral incisor, one canine, two premolars, and three permanent molars. Many factors can affect the number of teeth, and in managing the airway, teeth can be damaged.

The tongue is a muscular appendage. Its anterior two thirds occupy the floor of the mouth, and its posterior third forms the anterior aspect of the oropharynx. The intrinsic muscle groups alter the shape of the tongue, whereas the extrinsic muscle groups move the tongue as a whole. The bony attachments are the symphysis of the mandible, the hyoid bone, and the styloid process. The palatoglossus muscle attaches the tongue to the soft palate. All muscles of the tongue are innervated by the hypoglossal nerve (cranial nerve XII) except for the palatoglossal muscle, which is innervated by cranial nerve XI.

Sensation and taste are a function of the lingual branch of cranial nerve V for the anterior two thirds of the tongue. The glossopharyngeal nerve (cranial nerve IX) supplies common sensation and taste to the posterior third. Unfortunately, the pressure receptors in the posterior third are submucosal and cannot be anesthetized topically.

The Pharynx

The pharynx comprises the naso-, oro-, and laryngopharynx. It begins at the base of the skull, lies in apposition to the anterior aspect of the cervical vertebrae, and becomes continuous with the esophagus at the level of the sixth cervical vertebra. The nasopharynx traverses the posterior choanae to the uvula, occupying the space above the soft palate and behind the nasal cavities. The oropharynx is the space bordered by the soft palate above, the tip of the epiglottis below, the pharyngeal wall on one side, and the mouth cavity and the posterior third of the tongue on the other. The laryngopharynx extends from the epiglottis to the lower border of the cricoid cartilage, where it becomes continuous with the esophagus. The epiglottis, the aryepiglottic folds, the arytenoid cartilages, and the posterior commissure define the larynx. The larynx bulges backward into the laryngopharynx.

The muscular investments of the pharynx are three sets of constrictor muscles: superior, middle, and inferior. All the constrictor muscles are innervated by the vagus nerve (cranial nerve X). The uppermost attachment is to the base of the skull at the pharyngeal tubercle. The remainder of the attachments are to a midline raphe along the anterior aspect of the cervical vertebrae. From these attachments, the constrictors fan out bilaterally to insert on various bony and cartilaginous structures of the pharynx. The superior constrictor attaches to the medial pterygoid plate, the pterygomandibular raphe, and the mandible. The middle constrictor attaches to the hyoid bone. The inferior constrictor attaches to the thyroid cartilage, the cricoid cartilage, and the tendinous arch over the cricothyroid muscle. The cricothyroid muscle can be considered a detached portion of the inferior constrictor and is the only muscle of speech found outside the larynx.

Cranial nerves IX, X, and XI form the pharyngeal plexus. The muscles of the superior and the middle constrictors are innervated by motor fibers from cranial nerves X and XI. The inferior constrictor receives motor fibers from the recurrent laryngeal nerve. Sensory nerve fibers from cranial nerve IX supply the afferent nerve apparatus for the nasopharynx and the oropharynx. The internal branch of the superior laryngeal nerve supplies sensation to the laryngopharynx and to the larynx above the level of the false vocal cords. This nerve can be located where it pierces the thyrohyoid membrane inferior to the greater cornu of the hyoid bone. Externally on the neck, one should feel for the most superolateral aspect of the thyroid cartilage, then continue one fingerbreadth superolaterally until the inferior aspect of the hyoid bone is appreciated. It is here that a deposit of local anesthetic will anesthetize this nerve. The epiglottis is dually innervated. The superior aspect, which is visualized during direct laryngoscopy, is innervated by the glossopharyngeal nerve; the inferior aspect receives sensory fibers from the vagus.

The Larynx

The larynx provides the ability to have a common aerodigestive tract and prevents breathing food into the trachea as well as preventing intestinal distention as a result of ingestion of copious amounts of air. In humans, the tract of inspired air crosses that of ingested food. In other mammalian species, the larynx is high in the neck next to the nasopharynx. This anatomic arrangement allows for almost simultaneous feeding and olfactory sampling of the air by predators.

Table 11-1 shows the innervation of upper airway structures.

Assessment of the Airway

Assessment of the airway centers on searching for historical and anatomic factors associated with difficulty in visualizing the glottis. It is the responsibility of the health care professional to recognize a difficult intubation. The assessment is done before direct laryngoscopy to determine the ease or the difficulty of viewing the glottis during direct laryngoscopy.

Viewing the glottis is central to airway assessment. The Cormack-Lehane scoring system grades the view of the glottis during laryngoscopy. A grade 1 score represents full visualization of the glottis; grade 2 is a partial view; grade 3 is visualization of only the epiglottis; and grade 4 indicates that no laryngeal structures can be seen. Three bedside examinations can be performed to determine if a difficult airway is present. One is the determination of the relationship of tongue size to pharynx size. The size of the tongue correlates with the ease of glottic exposure during laryngoscopy.

TABLE 11–1. Sensory Innervation of Upper Airway Segments

Structure	Innervation
Nose	Trigeminal (V)
Tongue	Anterior lingual (V)
	Posterior glossopharyngeal (IX)
Pharynx	Glossopharyngeal (IX)
	Vagus (X)
Larynx	Superior laryngeal (X)
	Recurrent laryngeal (X)
Vocal cords	Recurrent laryngeal (X)
Trachea	Vagus (X)

The patient is instructed to open the mouth while in the sitting position. In a class I airway, visible structures are the soft palate, the fauces, the uvula, and the anterior and posterior tonsillar pillars. A class II airway shows the soft palate, the uvula, and the fauces. Only the soft palate and the base of the uvula are visible in a class III airway, whereas in a class IV airway, the soft palate is not visible.

The second examination is assessment of atlanto-occipital joint extension; this is how well the patient can assume the "sniff" position. A line drawn along the upper molars should intersect the floor at least at a 30-degree angle. The third examination is assessment of the mandibular space. Displacement of the soft tissues into the mandibular space is necessary for successful glottic visualization. A thyromental distance of less than 6 cm suggests that routine laryngoscopy may be difficult.

The Pediatric Airway

There are several differences in head and neck anatomy in children that make visualization of the glottis technically more difficult. A small child may have a prominent occiput, bringing the mouth to a position that is too far anterior to the larynx. A shoulder roll compensates for the increased occiput size. Readily available materials, such as a towel, a hospital gown, or an intravenous fluid bag, may be used. The infant has a relatively large tongue in relation to the size of the oropharynx. This increases the risk of obstruction caused by a lax tongue and thereby requires more technical expertise. In addition, the larynx is higher in the neck, creating a more acute angle between the oropharynx and the larynx. To compensate for this anatomic difference, one should use straight blades rather than curved blades. Gentle external pressure on the thyroid cartilage displaces the larynx posteriorly, aiding in visualization. The epiglottis is short, stubby, and soft, obstructing the view of the vocal cords. The narrowest part of the infant's larynx is below the level of the vocal cords. The endotracheal tube may pass through the vocal cords only to meet resistance. If this occurs, the tube size should be changed to one size smaller. Uncuffed endotracheal tubes are preferred for children younger than 10 years of age. A leak should be present around the tube at peak airway pressures greater than 20 mm Hg.

The ability to estimate an infant's weight quickly and accurately, base drug dosages on this weight, and determine endotracheal tube size and depth and depth of insertion is helpful in pediatric airway management. The following are guidelines. Weight can be estimated for a child 1 to 10 years of age by the following equation: [patient's age $\times$ 2] + 9 = weight in kilograms. The approximation can be adjusted depending on the overall body habitus of the child. Endotracheal tube size is calculated by the following formula: [age + 16]/4. A 4-year-old may require a size 5.0 endotracheal tube, but tubes that are one size larger (5.5) and one size smaller (4.5) should be immediately available as well. The distance of endotracheal tube insertion is roughly three times the tube size. Using the previous example, a size 5.0 endotracheal tube would be inserted to a distance of 15 mm from the lips.

The Adult Airway

When assessing the airway, one should look at both the mouth and the neck. Each has characteristics that can increase the difficulty of intubation. A short neck is associated with difficulty in visualizing the glottis. A receding mandible, defined as the inability to place three fingerbreadths between the mandibular symphysis and the hyoid bone, limits the space available to displace the tongue. Prominent upper incisors or a small mouth limits viewing when a laryngoscope and an endotracheal tube are placed in the oropharynx. Limited jaw opening can prevent placement of the laryngoscope in the mouth. Limited range of motion of the cervical vertebra prevents alignment of the neck to facilitate viewing the glottis.

If the patient is coherent, ask if there is a history of previous attempts to place a breathing tube that resulted in difficulty. Look for evidence of surgical scars on the neck; it is appropriate to palpate the neck gently. This will also aid in locating the cricothyroid membrane if needle cricothyroidotomy or emergent cricothyroidotomy is required.

Traumatic facial and laryngeal injury can add to the aforementioned problems. Any disease process that manifests as swelling or edema of the lips, the tongue, the pharyngeal tissues, and the epiglottis may create a difficult airway. Examples are angioneurotic edema, Ludwig's angina, peritonsillar abscesses, hot vapor inspiration, hematoma, surgery, and epiglottitis. Failed intubation attempts traumatize the oropharyngeal tissue, increasing secretions and producing swelling. Fractures of the mandible usually do not increase the difficulty of intubation. A closed injury with suspected partial or complete laryngotracheal separation requires an immediate secure surgical airway (i.e., awake tracheostomy). In difficult airways, one must remember never to take away what cannot be given back. A traumatized airway that still allows ventilation is better than an airway that is lost secondary to iatrogenic interventions.

Assisted Ventilation

The majority of traumatized patients require only endotracheal intubation. Initial interventions include ba-

sic airway maneuvers. A variety of objects can cause partial or complete airway obstruction mechanically, which must be quickly overcome. The tongue, vomitus, blood, dentures, swollen or distorted tissues, and foreign bodies are common causes of obstruction. Clearing these objects with suction reestablishes the airway. Positioning a patient on his or her side facilitates external drainage of secretions, vomitus, or blood, which would pool in the oropharynx in a supine patient. Reflex clenching of the jaw and cervical spine precautions may hinder the ability to place the patient on his or her side and to clear the airway.

Working suction is absolutely essential. Several types of suction catheters are available; the most common in the emergency department is the tonsil tip suction catheter. The tip is designed to prevent tissue and clots from obstructing the suction orifice in the presence of hemorrhage or secretions. The large-bore lumen is routinely used in the operating room to remove secretions that have accumulated in the posterior oropharynx. The rounded tip is less traumatic to the soft mucosa. The dental tip suction catheter is for large particulate debris such as food, clots, and teeth. Flexible, slender, small-bore suction catheters have no role in suctioning out the airway in a critical situation.

Lax pharyngeal musculature and tongue occlusion can be managed with one of three maneuvers. For all techniques, the patient must be in the supine position. The first is the neck lift–head tilt. Suspected cervical spine injury is a contraindication to the use of this technique. One hand is placed on the back of the neck, and the other is placed on the forehead. Upward movement of the hand on the neck performed simultaneously with downward motion of the hand on the forehead opens the mouth and relieves the airway obstruction. The chin lift maneuver can be used with possible cervical spine injury (Fig. 11–1). The thumb is placed just below the border of the lower lip, and several fingers of the same hand are placed on the volar surface beneath the patient's chin. As the mandible is gently lifted by the fingers, the mouth is opened by downward traction on the lower lip. In the jaw thrust maneuver, usually the index and the middle finger are placed on the section of the mandible that is superior to the angle of the mandible and inferior to the ear (Fig. 11–2). Forward displacement of the mandible is done, and opening of the mouth is achieved with downward displacement of the lower lip by the thumbs. The chin lift and jaw thrust methods rely on forward displacement of the mandible to relieve airway obstruction. The bony attachment of the tongue is to the mandible, and forward displacement "pulls" the lax anterior oropharyngeal tissue off the posterior aspect, increasing or creating a lumen for passage of oxygen.

Bag-mask assisted ventilation or complete bag-mask ventilation can be used in conjunction with the chin

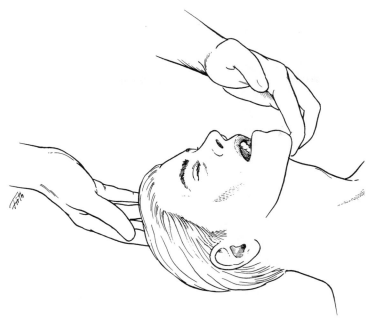

FIGURE 11–1. The chin lift maneuver.

lift or the jaw thrust maneuver. A common mistake in bag-mask ventilation is to apply extreme downward pressure to create a tight seal between the mask and the face (Fig. 11–3). The upward displacement of the mandible is lost, and high tidal volumes and pressures are required to offset the inadequate ventilation. This forces air into the stomach, reduces the ability to ventilate, and increases the risk of aspiration. To prevent this common mistake, the first priority is to relieve the oropharyngeal obstruction by forward displacement of the mandible (Fig. 11–4). A tight mask seal can then be accomplished with minimal pressure.

Two adjunctive artificial airways that improve assisted ventilation are the oropharyngeal and the nasopharyngeal devices (Fig. 11–5). The oropharyngeal airway is shaped like a question mark (**?**). The curved portion follows the contour of the tongue and lifts the lax tongue off the posterior wall of the pharynx,

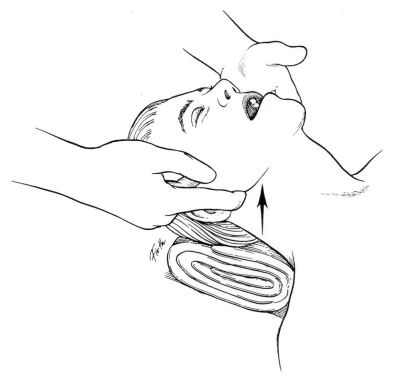

FIGURE 11–2. The jaw thrust maneuver.

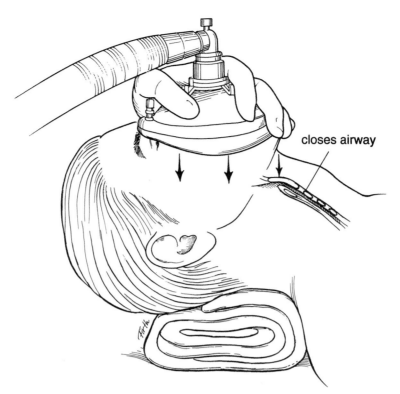

FIGURE 11–3. The wrong way to ventilate via mask.

relieving or preventing obstruction. The most common means of insertion is to position the curve of the oropharyngeal airway in the opposite direction of the tongue. After advancing the airway into the mouth for one third to one half of its length, rotate the device 180 degrees so that the curve of the tongue and the airway are approximated. Another method is to use a tongue blade to depress the tongue and to slide the airway over the tongue blade and into the final position that it will assume in the oropharynx. Once the airway is in place, look in the mouth to verify that the tongue appears to be in the normal anatomic position,

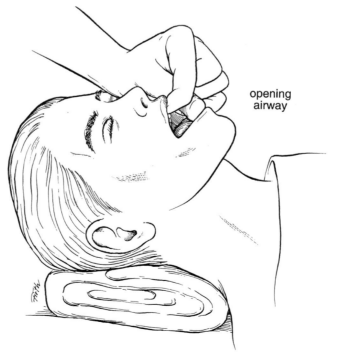

FIGURE 11–4. Opening the airway with the digits before intubation.

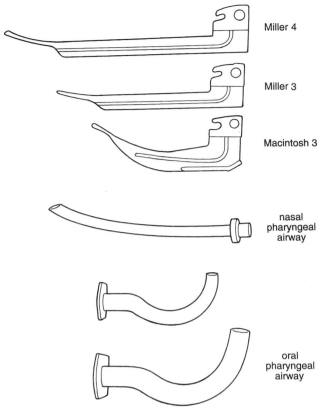

Miller 4

Miller 3

Macintosh 3

nasal pharyngeal airway

oral pharyngeal airway

FIGURE 11–5. Different blades and airways.

with the edge of the tongue filling the space defined by the inside border of the lower teeth (or gums if the patient is edentulous). If the tongue appears depressed, the device is probably worsening the obstruction by forcing the tongue against the posterior pharyngeal wall. Reposition the airway to relieve the obstruction.

The nasopharyngeal airway is a soft tube that is flared at one end. The nonflared end is inserted into the naris, and the entire length of the tube is advanced until the flared end rests at the nasal opening. Surgical gel lubrication facilitates this maneuver. The tube should always be inserted parallel to the hard and the soft palates. Occasionally, resistance is met when about one third of the tube has been inserted. Maintain constant forward pressure, but do not force the tube past the obstruction; after several seconds, the tube will advance into the proper position. Patience and gentle pressure will prevent epistaxis. Gagging is not common with this device, and its correct use will alleviate airway obstruction.

These basic airway manipulations can be used alone or in combination. In a semiobtunded patient, placement of a nasopharyngeal airway may be all that is required. Bag-mask assisted ventilation with or without the chin lift maneuver can also be applied. These devices do not substitute for tracheal intubation and do not protect against pulmonary aspiration.

Intubation

Four techniques of airway management are described in this chapter: (1) tracheal intubation by direct laryngoscopy, (2) intubation using a light wand, (3) fiberoptic-assisted intubation, and (4) placement of a laryngeal mask airway (LMA). Studies of the use of various techniques in the management of difficult airways by anesthesiologists showed that the majority used either direct laryngoscopy or flexible fiberoptic-assisted endotracheal tube placement.

Direct Laryngoscopy

The handle of the laryngoscope is about 6 inches long; a short handle is available if the chest or the breasts make it technically difficult to position the laryngoscope. Two basic blades are used: the curved MacIntosh blade or the straight Miller blade (see Fig. 11–5). Choice of blade is primarily dictated by the user's experience. Attachment of a blade to the handle makes the handle a left-handed instrument; it is held in the left hand with the blade on the ulnar side of the hand facing inward toward the operator. MacIntosh and Miller blades come in sizes 1 to 4 (the larger the number, the larger the blade). Usually, size 3 or 4 blades are used for adult patients. An old adage is that too big a blade and too small a tube is better than too small a blade and too big a tube. Endotracheal tube size is also given a numerical description, ranging from 3 to 8 in increments of ½. The number is the internal diameter of the tube in millimeters. The larger the number, the larger the size. Average-sized adult women need a 7.0- to 7.5-mm tube, and average-sized adult males need a 7.5- to 8.0-mm tube.

Success in tracheal intubation using direct laryngoscopy starts with correct preparation of equipment and positioning of the patient. Essential items include a bag-mask device, a secure working intravenous line, a suction catheter, a working laryngoscope with multiple blade types and sizes, and an appropriately sized endotracheal tube with larger and smaller tubes immediately available. Pharmacologic adjuncts such as an induction agent and a muscle-paralyzing agent are drawn into labeled syringes at the correct doses.

The bed should be at a good height, and the patient should be placed in the sniff position—neck flexion with head extension (Fig. 11–6). With the patient in the supine position, create as much vertical distance as possible between the chest and the point of the chin. Placement of towels underneath the occiput of the head facilitates proper positioning. If a patient's body mass index is increased, place a shoulder roll that is 6 to 8 inches in height underneath the shoulder blades, and place towels underneath the head so that the chin is higher than the chest. An induction agent

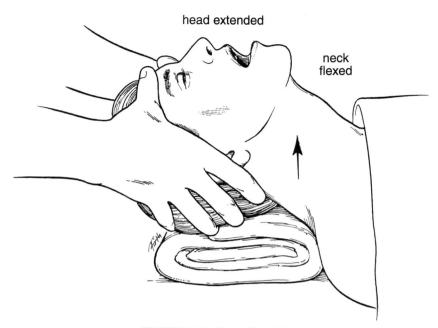

"sniff position"

head extended

neck flexed

FIGURE 11–6. The sniff position.

is given after the patient is in proper position and the laryngoscopist is standing at the head of the bed. The patient enters the anesthetized state and becomes apneic; use of a bag-mask device and the chin lift maneuver now easily supports ventilation. The muscle relaxant is given, and after the appropriate interval, the patient's muscles become lax.

The following procedure is for the MacIntosh blade. Step one is to open the mouth as widely as possible by pushing on the premolars with the finger and the thumb of the right hand. The mouth is opened without changing the position of the head. A common mistake is to flex the head on the neck when pushing the mandible open. Use the upper premolars to stabilize the head while opening the jaw.

Next, the tip of the laryngoscope blade is positioned at the tip of the tongue. The laryngoscope handle should be parallel to the floor and should point to the patient's right nipple. Keeping the handle parallel to the floor and pointing at the right nipple, insert the blade in the right side of the mouth, sliding the blade over the right side of the tongue (Fig. 11–7). As the blade pushes the tongue to the left and out of the field of vision, rotate the handle so that it points to the umbilicus instead of the nipple. Continue to insert the blade until the handle gently touches the lower lip. The blade will come to rest in the proper position in the vallecula anterior to the epiglottis (Fig. 11–8). The handle should now be parallel to the floor, pointing to the patient's umbilicus, and should be inserted into the mouth for the length of the blade. The right hand can be removed from the teeth. Keeping the handle parallel to the floor and the midline, "dislocate" the jaw by pushing the handle away from oneself and by shortening the distance between the end of the handle and the umbilicus (horizontal vector). The next motion is to lift the handle up while keeping it parallel to the floor (vertical vector). Connecting the point that is the beginning of the horizontal vector with the point that is the end of the vertical vector describes a third vector that is the sum of the first two. Its force and direction are about a 45-degree angle to the floor and toward the patient's feet.

If visualization of the vocal cords is still not optimal, continue to lift the laryngoscope in the vertical direction. The head may be lifted up off the towels if necessary; it will not slip and fall off the blade. The vocal cords will then come into view. Use of these motions will prevent the common tendency to "crank back on the laryngoscope handle" to try to visualize the vocal cords better. Teeth are not damaged, and all the tissues blocking the laryngoscopist's view are displaced out of the field of vision. The endotracheal tube can now be placed in the trachea (Fig. 11–9).

Lighted Stylet

The lighted stylet is a semirigid "wire" that can be shaped into the desired form and placed inside the endotracheal tube. The distal end of the stylet has a light source; the proximal end has a power source. The lighted stylet is best suited for an anesthetized patient who can be easily ventilated via the bag-mask

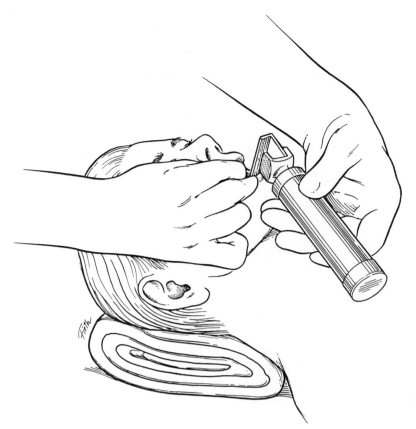

FIGURE 11–7. Inserting the laryngoscope.

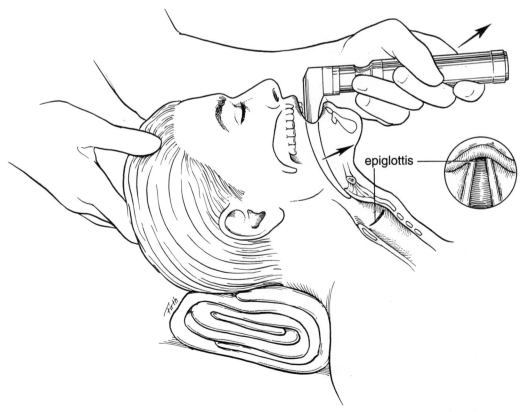

FIGURE 11–8. The epiglottis should be displaced upward by the blade to visualize the vocal cords *(inset)*.

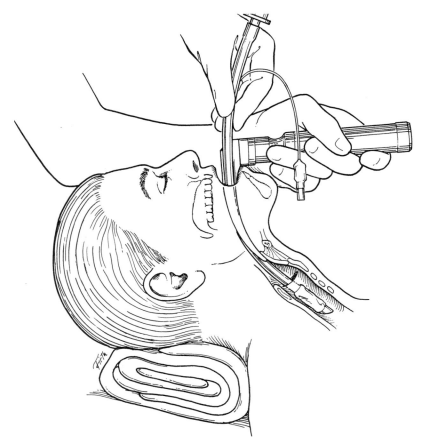

FIGURE 11–9. Inserting the endotracheal tube.

method and who has normal pharyngeal anatomy but whose vocal cords were not able to be visualized with direct laryngoscopy. The first step is to place the stylet inside the endotracheal tube with the distal lighted end advanced beyond the end of the endotracheal tube about 1 cm. The stylet with the endotracheal tube is then shaped to form an L or a hockey stick, with the bend at the level of the endotracheal tube cuff. The L shape, along with the plastic surfaces of the stylet and the endotracheal tube, creates frictional forces. Hold the endotracheal tube and remove the stylet; if frictional forces seem excessive, a coating of mineral oil or surgical lubricant applied to the shaft of the stylet will facilitate removal.

Unlike laryngoscopy, intubation with the lighted stylet can be performed with either the right or the left hand. The hand used must hold both the proximal end of the endotracheal tube and the shaft of the stylet where it enters the proximal end of the endotracheal tube. The shaft of the stylet and the proximal end of the endotracheal tube have to be held simultaneously by the same hand to function as a unit. Holding one and not the other while attempting intubation will change the relationship between the light source and the distal end of the endotracheal tube. The highest probability for success occurs if the light source remains extended about 1 cm beyond the distal end

of the endotracheal tube. Check and make sure that the light source is bright.

The patient's head and neck should be in a neutral position, with the person performing the intubation standing at the head of the bed. Insertion of the light wand begins with one of two starting positions. If the right hand is used, the proximal end of the tube and the shaft of the stylet are held in the right hand, and the distal end of the tube and the stylet distal to the bend are placed in the mouth in the midline of the tongue, with the light pointing to the floor (otherwise termed "illuminating the back of the throat"). The main shaft of the stylet can be directly over the sternum, or it can be at a 90-degree angle to the patient's body, exiting the side of the mouth. In either position, the main body of the shaft is parallel to the floor. From the sternal starting position, the stylet, which is kept in the midline of the tongue, is rotated so that it is no longer parallel to the floor but points upward at the ceiling while the distal end is advanced into the mouth. This advances the lighted end into the laryngopharynx and places the bend in the stylet at the natural curve of the oropharynx into the laryngopharynx.

From a starting position at the side of the mouth, the lighted end is advanced into the mouth while the main body of the stylet is rotated to point to the roof. Room lights in the area should be turned off or dimmed to enhance visualization of the stylet through the anterior neck tissues. The light should be visible as a well-circumscribed dot at the level of the hyoid bone on the external surface of the neck. A common mistake is to begin with the stylet inserted too deeply into the throat. The vocal cords are behind the thyroid shield; positioning the light at the level of the hyoid bone ensures that the stylet is not already below the level of the cords. Once it has been noted that the light source is in the proper position, the instrument is advanced forward deeper into the throat.

The light source may deviate off the midline to either side; if this occurs, pull back to the initial starting point, the midline at the hyoid bone. If the light stays in the midline but diffuses outward and loses its well-circumscribed borders as it travels toward the sternal notch, the esophagus has been entered. Pull back and try again. If the light stays in the midline and is well circumscribed to the level of the sternal notch, advance the endotracheal tube forward off the stylet several centimeters. The tube should slide forward without resistance. Now withdraw the stylet from the endotracheal tube, being careful not to pull the tube out with the stylet. Inflate the endotracheal tube cuff, and verify tube placement. Lighted stylet intubation can be performed more rapidly than any other intubation technique. It is limited to patients in whom bag-mask assisted ventilation can easily be used and whose laryngopharyngeal reflexes are blunted. Endotracheal tube sizes of 7.0 or 7.5 are easiest to use.

Laryngeal Mask Airway

The LMA is an airway management device intended as an alternative to use of a face mask. It is inserted without instrumentation of the oropharynx, and visualization of the vocal cords is not required. It can provide a clear airway and can be inserted with minimal stimulation if the pharyngeal reflexes are sufficiently depressed. The LMA has a section that is a large silicone rubber mask. This section is oval, with the distal segment forming a tip and the proximal end having a rounded contour. An airway tube attaches to one side of the mask with an aperture that opens to the other side, allowing ventilation of the airway at the level of the vocal cords when the mask is inserted in the proper position. The distal tip lies in the hypopharynx immediately proximal to the esophagus. The aperture apposes the vocal cords. The sides of the mask are in contact with the piriform fossa, whereas the proximal segment rests against the base of the tongue (Fig. 11–10). The breathing tube follows the posterior pharyngeal wall into the oropharynx and out of the mouth. The proximal end of the breathing tube has a standard adapter for attachment to a breathing circuit. An inflation line is present that is about the same

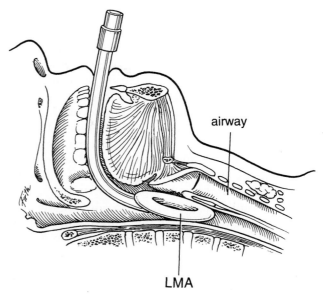

FIGURE 11–10. The laryngeal mask airway (LMA) sits against the tracheal opening but at the same time obstructs the esophageal opening.

length as the breathing tube. The distal end attaches to the laryngeal mask, and the proximal end, which is outside the mouth, acts as a port and a valve for inflation and deflation of the mask.

The LMA does not protect the airway against the risk of regurgitation or aspiration. It can be used for an unexpected difficult airway. In a profoundly depressed patient or a catastrophic airway event (e.g., inability to ventilate or intubate), the risk of aspiration is less than the risks associated with the immediate hypoxic insult, and ventilation with an LMA may be lifesaving. The incidence of aspiration with use of the LMA in outpatient general anesthesia is low and is comparable to that associated with use of an endotracheal tube or a face mask. The LMA comes in several sizes: Size 3 is for children weighing more than 30 kg and for small adults; size 4 is for normal and large adults; and size 5 is for large adults.

There are several methods of insertion of the LMA. The use of fiberoptic observation to provide better final placement is described. The person performing LMA insertion is positioned at the patient's head, which is positioned with the neck flexed and the head extended. Anesthetic induction is performed to blunt protective airway reflexes. The LMA can be inserted with either the right or the left hand. The thumb and the index finger are used to grasp the distal segment of the airway tube just proximal to its insertion into the mask. The index finger should be snug between the cuff and the tube. The greater curve of the tube should rest close to the web between the thumb and the index finger. A black line runs the length of the airway tube along the greater curve for orientation. If the tube were to be cut along this line, it would divide into mirror-image halves. This black line is oriented anteriorly toward the upper lip.

Place the tip of the mask against the hard palate. The wrist will need to be flexed to achieve this starting position. Advance the LMA along the hard palate toward the soft palate, directing the force of the index finger into the hard palate and the movement of the hand into the mouth. This will slide the LMA from the oropharynx into the laryngopharynx, following the contour of the mouth. It follows the same trajectory as a bolus of food, which enters the mouth at the lips and travels upward and backward to exit via the posterior oropharynx. Continue to advance the LMA until resistance is felt. Using the other hand, grasp the proximal end of the breathing tube section to stabilize the LMA, and remove the "insertion hand" from the patient's mouth. This will prevent displacement of the LMA. Inflate the cuff with just enough pressure to obtain a seal. The LMA may appear to back out of the patient's mouth with cuff inflation; this is caused by the tube settling into position in the hypopharynx. It can now be connected to a breathing circuit to ventilate the patient with gentle positive pressure, not to exceed 20 cm H$_2$O. Difficulty in insertion may be encountered when advancing the LMA around the turn from the posterior exit of the oropharynx into the laryngopharynx. If this occurs, withdraw the LMA back to the starting position at the front of the hard palate, and try again.

Fiberoptic Assisted Intubation

The fiberoptic scope (FOS) has three continuous sections: the body, which consists of the tip deflector control lever, the eyepiece, the focusing ring, and a working channel sleeve for suction or insufflation; a light transmission cord, which extends from the light source to the body; and the insertion cord, which contains the fiberoptic bundles that transmit light and receive images as well as a working channel. The insertion cord diameter ranges from 1.8 to 4.9 mm, and the length varies from 550 to 600 mm. The FOS can be used for nasotracheal or orotracheal intubation in an awake or an asleep patient. Two adjuncts assist with orotracheal intubation: the Ovassapian fiberoptic oral airway and the LMA. The Ovassapian airway serves as a bite block and as a conduit to protect the fiberoptic bundle, allowing placement of the distal end of the FOS just above the vocal cords. The airway can be removed without dislodging the tracheal tube and will accommodate up to an 8.5-mm endotracheal tube. The airway tube of the LMA can accommodate an FOS with an endotracheal tube threaded over it. Once the FOS has passed through the vocal cords into the trachea, the endotracheal tube is advanced into the LMA over the FOS into the trachea. The FOS is removed,

but both the endotracheal tube and the LMA are left in place.

An adjunct to nasotracheal fiberoptic intubation is use of the nasopharyngeal tube. This is a soft rubber tube that comes in various sizes. After the tube has been split down its length, it is lubricated and is placed into the nasopharynx. The FOS is then passed into the lumen of the nasopharyngeal airway and exits the distal end in the proximity of the vocal cords. After successful passage through the cords, the nasopharyngeal airway can be removed from the nose and off the scope without dislodging the FOS. The preloaded endotracheal tube can be advanced along the FOS into the nose and through the vocal cords.

Awake fiberoptic intubation is generally easier to perform for two reasons: (1) The soft tissue tone is maintained, and (2) the patient can be placed in the sitting position, allowing gravity to keep the insertion cord in the midline in the oropharynx. The nasal route is technically easier. If the patient is sitting up, the endoscopist is facing the patient; if the patient is supine, the endoscopist is at the head of the bed (Fig. 11–11).

Intubation in the supine anesthetized patient is more challenging in that the pharyngeal tissue is lax and may narrow or occlude the posterior pharyngeal space. The sniff position causes the epiglottis to touch the posterior pharyngeal wall, making passage of the FOS difficult. The head should be in a neutral position or extended if possible.

Administering sedatives builds on the "verbal anesthesia." Several benzodiazepines provide excellent sedation and antegrade amnesia. Sedation is adequate if the patient is still responsive to verbal commands. Butyrophenones provide sedation and antiemetic properties. Narcotics provide sedation and analgesia. Antisialogogues are given to dry the airway. Copious secretions can hinder the endoscopist's view and can prevent topical anesthetics from working. Commonly used agents are glycopyrrolate and atropine. If there is a history of gastric reflux or a full stomach, aspiration prophylaxis is beneficial. Metoclopramide given 15 to 30 minutes before the procedure improves forward gastric motility and helps empty the stomach. Nonparticulate antacids (sodium citrate [Bicitra]) increase the pH of the gastric contents, and H$_2$ antagonists reduce gastric acid production.

Topical anesthesia can be used for the nasal and the oropharyngeal mucosa. Good results can be obtained with the use of cotton-tip applicators (Q-tips), which are soaked in an anesthetic solution and a vasoconstrictor, placed into the nares, and gently advanced deeper into the nares over 5 to 10 minutes. A nasal trumpet coated in 2% lidocaine gel is then placed to facilitate nasal intubation. The oropharynx is anesthetized topically using sprays, atomizers, or nebulizers that can

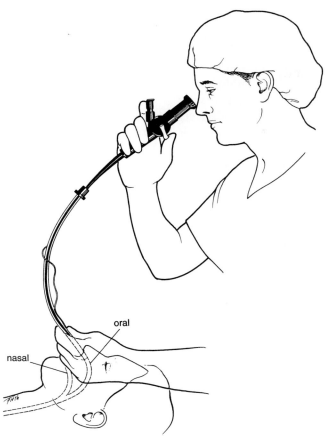

FIGURE 11–11. Bronchoscopic nasotracheal intubation.

reach the trachea. Any residual is suctioned to prevent toxicity.

Complications and Pitfalls

The main complication is inability to reinstate ventilation and oxygenation after removing the patient's innate respiratory ability. With complete cessation of ventilatory function, the time course is short before significant morbidity and mortality occur. The incidence of completely failed mask ventilation and endotracheal intubation in the general surgical population is estimated to be 0.01 to 2.0 in 10,000 patients.

Direct Laryngoscopy

Proper positioning and preparation reduce the risk of failure. If one is unable to view the glottic opening during direct laryngoscopy, the following maneuvers should be performed:

1. Check that the patient is in the sniff position (flexion of the neck and extension of the head). Placing towels underneath the head to accentuate the sniff position improves the sight axis from the mouth to the vocal cords.

2. Manually move the larynx by external pressure on the thyroid cartilage. An assistant, under direction of the laryngoscopist, manually moves the thyroid cartilage and, thus, the vocal cords into a position for better visualization. The thyroid is pushed straight down to the floor (with the patient supine), then to the patient's right side, and finally up toward the patient's head. This moves the vocal cords into a better position for visualization.

3. Increase the size of the laryngoscope blade. If a MacIntosh No. 3 (curved) blade is used initially, try a MacIntosh No. 4 blade.

4. Change the style of blade from a MacIntosh to a Miller (straight) blade.

Another complication not involving interruption of gas exchange is damage to any structure that is in the field during direct laryngoscopy. Teeth can be loosened from their sockets, chipped, or broken. Poor dental hygiene increases the risk of damage. The lips may be lacerated. The soft tissue of the mouth or the pharynx can be traumatized, leading to swelling, hematoma, or even laceration. The vocal cords are a mobile structure that can be disarticulated, causing dysfunction. Edema or pressure necrosis can occur anywhere the endotracheal tube is in prolonged contact with the airway tissue. In addition, the mandible can be dislocated from its position in the temporomandibular joint. Fracture-subluxations of the cervical spine can occur. Another devastating complication is manipulation of an unstable cervical spine during intubation, increasing the cervical spinal cord injury.

Medications chosen for induction and paralysis have both side effects and idiosyncratic effects. The most common and problematic are cardiovascular effects, such as hypotension and arrhythmias in an unstable patient.

The incidence of minor complications increases as the difficulty of placing an endotracheal tube increases. Normal airways undergoing direct laryngoscopy and intubation under direct vision are associated with about a 5% incidence of minor trauma. In patients with anticipated difficult airways, the incidence of minor trauma increased to 17%. In patients actually found to be difficult to intubate, the incidence increased to 63%. As experience is gained through repetition, the incidence of minor trauma will decrease.

Lighted Stylet

The lighted stylet should be avoided in patients with known distortion of the upper airway due to tumors, abscesses, polyps, infection, or facial trauma. Foreign bodies in the airway are a contraindication. Obese patients may have excess neck tissue, which diminishes the ability to transilluminate. Novice users should not attempt this technique in an emergent situation, such as a rapid-sequence induction for traumatic injury, or in an uncooperative awake patient. As experience is gained, these contraindications are less relevant, and the light wand can be used as a rescue technique.

Laryngeal Mask Airway

Difficulty arises during placement of an LMA in a supine patient when the advancing tip moves from the vertically oriented oral cavity to the horizontally oriented posterior pharynx. The tip may not follow the contour of the pharynx into the larynx but may fold back on itself and jam against the posterior pharyngeal wall. Partially inflating the laryngeal mask or using an alternative insertion technique alleviates this problem. Rotating the LMA 180 degrees from the standard position to face the patient's head and then rotating it back to the regular position once the tip has entered the hypopharynx is an alternative. The conventional technique results in the highest rate of correct placement in adults.

An LMA with a folded tip that is advanced into the hypopharynx can push the epiglottis into a position that obstructs the airway. Minimal to no ventilation will ensue. Removal of the LMA and reinsertion are required.

There is about a 1% to 5% incidence of failed intubation with the LMA. Selection of the correct size, adherence to insertion technique, ensuring adequate depth of anesthesia, and experience with placement are important factors in maximizing success.

Fiberoptic Intubation

Oropharyngeal secretions, inadequate patient preparation, and unfamiliarity with the FOS are causes of failure. Giving an agent that will dry the mouth, such as glycopyrrolate, 15 to 30 minutes before attempting intubation decreases secretion of saliva. Care must also be taken when inserting the FOS through the nasal passages. Laceration of nasal mucous membranes causes bleeding that pools in the posterior pharynx, obstructing the viewing lens. Using a suction catheter separate from the FOS or using the working channel as a suction port or an insufflation port are methods of removing secretions from the immediate area of the viewing lens. Ruptured abscesses and regurgitated gastric contents are also sources of secretions.

Repeated use of the FOS on mannequins and in the surgical suite decreases the feeling that the FOS is an unwieldy instrument and increases its versatility. Choosing the appropriate application of this technique in managing the airway increases the likelihood of success.

Suggested Readings

1. Benumof JL: Management of the difficult airway. With special emphasis on awake tracheal intubation. Anesthesiology 1991;75:1087–1110.
2. Benumof JL, Scheller MS: The importance of transtracheal jet ventilation in the management of the difficult airway. Anesthesiology 1989;71:769–778.
3. Bogdonoff DL, Stone DJ: Emergency management of the airway outside the operating room. Can J Anaesth 1992;39:1069–1089.
4. Brimacombe J, Berry A: Insertion of the laryngeal mask airway—a prospective study of four techniques. Anaesth Intensive Care 1993;21:89–92.
5. Eichhorn JH: Documenting improved anesthesia outcome. J Clin Anesth 1991;3:351–353.
6. Hirsch IA, Reagan JO, Sullivan N: Complications of direct laryngoscopy: a prospective analysis. Anesthesiology Review 1990; 17:34–40.
7. McGovern FH, Fitz-Hugh GS, Edzeman LJ: The hazards of endotracheal intubation. Ann Otol Rhinol Laryngol 1971;80:556–564.
8. McIntyre JWR: Laryngoscope design and the difficult adult tracheal intubation. Can J Anaesth 1989;36:94–98.
9. Salem MR, Mathrubhutham M, Bennett EJ: Difficult intubation. N Engl J Med 1976;295:879–881.
10. Silverman SM, Culling RD, Middaugh RE: Rapid-sequence orotracheal intubation: A comparison of three techniques. Anesthesiology 1990;73:244–248.

12 Flexible Bronchoscopy

Gail T. Tominaga

Indications

In the critically ill patient, the most common indications for fiberoptic bronchoscopy are airway management, intubation, aspiration of mucus plugs, re-expansion of atelectatic lung, removal of aspirated foreign bodies, and diagnosis of bronchopleural fistula. A list of all indications is presented in Table 12–1.

Flexible bronchoscopy is a useful adjunct in establishing an airway in difficult situations (e.g., cervical spine injury, cervical fusion, or hemoptysis) or in patients with unfavorable laryngeal anatomy. Placement of double-lumen endotracheal tubes can be aided by bronchoscopy. The flexible bronchoscope can also be used to inspect the vocal cords before intubation of patients in whom there is a high suspicion of cord edema or to evaluate the vocal cords before extubation.

Flexible bronchoscopy is an important adjunct in assessing and managing inhalational lung injury. Endotracheal tube placement in this setting can be aided by bronchoscopy. Additionally, bronchoscopic removal of sloughing mucus membranes or heavily viscous airway secretions 4 to 7 days after the injury can minimize complications in inhalational injuries.

In respiratory insufficiency, flexible bronchoscopy can help differentiate between atelectasis secondary to secretions and that caused by obstructing foreign bodies. Flexible bronchoscopy has a central role in the diagnosis of major bronchial injuries after chest wall trauma. The flexible bronchoscope is also used as an adjunct in performing safe percutaneous tracheostomy.

Hemoptysis usually requires rigid bronchoscopy and is not covered in this chapter. Aspiration of particulate matter or foodstuffs may require immediate fiberoptic bronchoscopy with lavage to aspirate or remove foreign matter directly.

In the intensive care unit, a common problem in the intubated sedated patient is the inability to clear retained secretions. In selected cases, fiberoptic bronchoscopy can be beneficial in clearing thick secretions and mucus plugs. Inhaled bronchodilators and chest physiotherapy should be the initial treatment for acute lobar collapse or segmental atelectasis. Bronchoscopy may be needed if these measures are not effective. Fiberoptic bronchoscopy can be used to diagnose ventilator-associated pneumonia. Direct examination of the bronchial tree can aid in the diagnosis of nosocomial pneumonia in the ventilated patient.

Bronchoalveolar lavage (BAL) and protected specimen brushing can be directed to areas of maximum radiographic infiltrate to obtain specimens for analysis of potential pathogens. BAL is particularly useful in diagnosing opportunistic infections in the immunocompromised patient and obtaining samples from specific alveoli. Biopsies and brushings should be avoided before BAL.

Airway secretions should be aspirated gently. The bronchoscope channel should be rinsed, and the suction trap should be changed. The distal tip of the bronchoscope is then wedged into the desired segmental or subsegmental bronchus. This can be confirmed by means of fluoroscopy. Aliquots of 20 mL of normal saline solution are infused, and suction is applied. A total of 100 to 300 mL is usually instilled, and the return volume is usually 40% to 60% of the total instilled. The fluid collected is separated into aliquots and is submitted for microbiologic and cytologic analysis.

Technique

Preparation for Bronchoscopy

Preparation of both the patient and the equipment is key to successful performance of flexible bronchos-

TABLE 12–1. Indications for Fiberoptic Bronchoscopy

Airway management
  Airway establishment
  Atelectasis
  Mucus plugs
  Acute lobar collapse
  Acute inhalational injury
Diagnostic/therapeutic uses
  Biopsy
  Brushings/washings
  Bronchoalveolar lavage
  Foreign body removal
  Hemoptysis
  Trauma
Interventional uses
  Brachytherapy catheter placement
  Transbronchial needle aspiration biopsy
  Cryotherapy
  Argon plasma coagulation

copy. Most patients, whether intubated or not, will require premedication for anxiolysis, antegrade amnesia, and analgesia. Midazolam (usually at a dose of 0.07 mg/kg) is ideal because of its rapid onset, short duration, and amnesic properties. Opiates are also useful for their analgesic and antitussive properties. When these agents are being used, flumazenil, a benzodiazepine antagonist, and naloxone, an opioid antagonist, should be readily available. Blood pressure, heart rate, respiratory rate, and respiratory excursion should be monitored closely. In selected cases, antisialagogues such as atropine or glycopyrrolate can be used to reduce secretions, prevent bradycardia, and inhibit vagal responses.

Topical airway anesthesia is often needed to inhibit the gag reflex and coughing, particularly in the nonintubated patient. Hurricaine (20% benzocaine) spray is often used to anesthetize the oropharynx before endoscopy. Benzocaine has a rapid onset of action (30 seconds), a short duration of action (5 to 15 minutes), and minimal systemic absorption. The recommended dose is one 1-second or 2-second spray. The tracheobronchial tree can be topically anesthetized with 5-mL aliquots of 1% lidocaine through the irrigation channel of the bronchoscope. The duration of action is 20 to 30 minutes. Toxicity presents as seizures or respiratory arrest and occurs when the maximum total dose exceeds 400 mg. Patients receiving high doses of lidocaine should be monitored for a minimum of 90 minutes following drug administration because the peak plasma concentration occurs between 5 and 90 minutes. Drugs and equipment necessary for the treatment

of arrhythmias, seizures, and hypotension and for intubation should be readily available when these agents are used for premedication.

After the patient has been premedicated, the bronchoscopist should don a mask covering the nose and the mouth, eye protection, and gloves. The head of the bed should be raised 30 degrees, and the fraction of inspired oxygen (FIO_2) should be 100%. Blood pressure, heart rate, pulse oximetry, end-tidal CO_2 (if available), tidal volumes, and airway pressures should be closely monitored throughout the procedure. A majority of patients requiring bronchoscopy in the intensive care unit are endotracheally intubated. A fiberoptic bronchoscope swivel adapter (SIMS Portex, Keene, NH) is placed at the end of the endotracheal tube and is connected to the ventilator tubing. This allows an airtight system so that mechanical ventilation can continue during bronchoscopy.

The equipment required for flexible bronchoscopy includes a bronchoscope (Fig. 12–1), a light source, and suction apparatus. Biopsy tools and a camera may also be needed. Before each use, the bronchoscope should be inspected thoroughly. The external surface should be checked for any irregularities. The angulation control lever should be tested to ensure that the bending section bends smoothly and correctly. The optical system should also be checked. The single-use suction valve should be inspected to identify any cracks and to verify that the rubber valve is correctly attached to the main body. After completing the abovementioned procedures, the suction line should be connected to the scope, and the light-guide connector

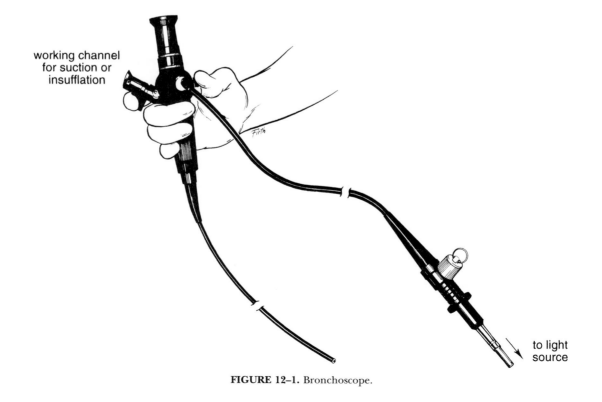

working channel for suction or insufflation

to light source

FIGURE 12–1. Bronchoscope.

should be plugged into the light source. The suction mechanism should be checked by dipping the distal end of the scope into clean water. The biopsy valve should be removed, and a syringe should be filled with clean water attached to the biopsy port. Water should come out of the channel outlet when the plunger is pressed. If water leaks into the suction line, replace the suction valve with a new one.

Performing Bronchoscopy

Care must be taken when handling the scope. Any bending or twisting of the bending portion of the scope could result in damage to the optical glass fibers. The operator's left hand should be used to hold the control section of the scope. The index finger is used to activate the suction valve, and the thumb is used to control the angulation lever (see Fig. 12–1). The operator's other hand is used to manipulate the insertion tube while an assistant holds the endotracheal tube in place (Fig. 12–2). The scope can be placed transnasally, transorally, or through the endotracheal tube. A bite guard must be used to prevent the scope from being bitten (Fig. 12–3). The scope should not be advanced if the lumen cannot be visualized.

On introduction of the scope through the endotracheal tube, the trachea and the carina are visualized. The trachea bifurcates both to the right and, more acutely, to the left mainstem bronchi at the carina (Fig. 12–4). Approximately 2 cm from the carina, the right upper lobe bifurcates from the right wall of the main bronchus (Fig. 12–5). The length of the left main bronchus is approximately 4 cm. The bifurcation to the left upper and lower lobe bronchi can be sharp or blunt.

The anatomy of the bronchial segments is reviewed in detail before bronchoscopy. The trachea, the carina, and the bronchial segments should be systematically inspected for secretions, mucosal abnormalities, or endobronchial lesions. If excessive coughing occurs, additional aliquots of topical lidocaine can be given though the biopsy port of the scope. Aspiration of pulmonary secretions is performed by pressing down on the suction valve. The aspiration pressure should be less than 50 mm Hg. Irrigation with sterile saline solution or N-acetylcysteine may be required to loosen thick mucus secretions before aspiration. Diagnostic procedures such as BAL, bronchial brushings or washings, or biopsies may be performed during flexible bronchoscopy.

When a sputum specimen is needed for culturing, a 40-mL specimen trap (Sherwood Medical, St. Louis,

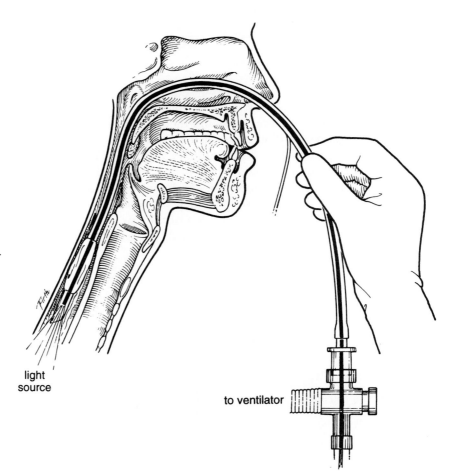

FIGURE 12–2. Advancement of bronchoscope.

light source

to ventilator

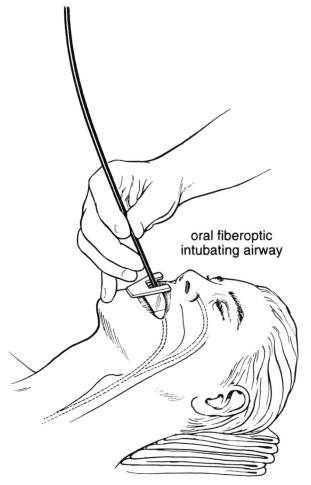

FIGURE 12–3. A mouthpiece can be used in intubated or nonintubated patients.

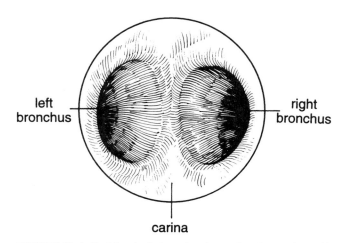

FIGURE 12–4. Endoluminal view of carina and mainstem bronchi.

Mo) is connected to the suction valve and the suction tubing. Normal saline solution is instilled via the biopsy port, and the suction valve is depressed to aspirate mucus into the collection chamber.

When the scope is being withdrawn, the lumen is viewed through the scope to avoid damage to the tracheobronchial tree. The correct location of the distal end of the endotracheal tube is confirmed, or the end is repositioned above the carina before withdrawing the bronchoscope. After removing the scope, the distal end should be placed in a container of clean water, and 50 to 100 mL should be aspirated through the suction channel to clear out any remaining pulmonary secretions within the scope. Each facility should have a standardized procedure for cleaning and disinfecting the bronchoscope.

Pitfalls

Early studies reported a major complication rate of 0.8% to 5%, with half of these related to premedication. A retrospective review of 4273 flexible bronchoscopy procedures reported in 1995 had a major complication rate of 0.5% and a minor complication rate of 0.8%. Anesthetic complications include respiratory failure, hypoxia, hypotension, syncope, seizure, methemoglobinemia, and arrhythmias. Complications of bronchoscopy include respiratory arrest, pneumothorax, bronchospasm, fever, pneumonia, hemoptysis, syncope, and arrhythmias. Pneumothorax is rare in routine bronchoscopy but has been reported in 7% to 14% of transbronchial biopsies.

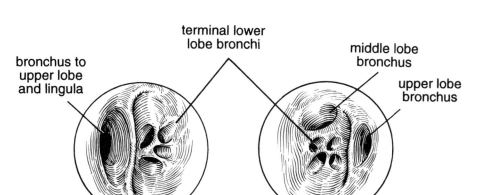

FIGURE 12–5. Endoluminal view of bronchial branching.

Hypoxemia is seen frequently following flexible bronchoscopy. A fall in the arterial oxygen tension of 10 to 20 mm Hg during the procedure is common. In patients with extremely poor pulmonary function, the bronchoscope should not be inserted for more than 15 to 20 seconds at a time, with a rest period of 30 to 60 seconds between insertions. Hypoxemia during or immediately following bronchoscopy correlates significantly with the development of arrhythmias.

Laryngospasm can occur as the bronchoscope is passed between the vocal cords and is usually due to inadequate topical anesthesia. This can be reduced with atropine premedication.

Reflex sympathetic discharge caused by mechanical intubation of the larynx and the bronchi can cause hemodynamic changes (increased heart rate, increased mean arterial pressure, increased mean pulmonary arteriolar occlusion pressure, and increased cardiac index). Cerebral hemodynamics are also altered during bronchoscopy and should be monitored closely throughout the procedure. Intracranial pressure rises during bronchoscopy in the patient with severe head injuries, but cerebral perfusion is usually maintained owing to an increase in the mean arterial pressure. When the intracranial pressure becomes dangerously high, the bronchoscope should be pulled out of the endotracheal tube until cerebral hemodynamics improve.

Improper technique in the use of the fiberoptic bronchoscope can lead to mechanical complications. Perforation or hemorrhage can result from forceful insertion of the scope without a clear view of the lumen or from blind withdrawal of the scope. Prolonged suctioning with the distal tip in contact with mucosal surfaces will result in bleeding and suction artifact. Thermal injury to the mucosa can be caused by prolonged close-up observation of the mucosal surface with excess illumination. Finally, an improperly cleaned instrument can result in cross-contamination and infection.

Suggested Readings

1. Fulkerson WJ: Fiberoptic bronchoscopy. N Engl J Med 1984;311:511–515.
2. Helmers RA, Pisani RJ: Bronchoalveolar lavage. In Prakash UBS (ed): Bronchoscopy. New York, Raven Press, 1994, p 154.
3. Heyland DK, Cook DJ, Marshall J, et al: The clinical utility of invasive diagnostic techniques in the setting of ventilator-associated pneumonia. Chest 1999;115:1076–1084.
4. Kvale PA: Bronchoscopic biopsies and bronchoalveolar lavage. Chest Surg Clin North Am 1995;6:205–221.
5. Oho K, Amemiya R: Instrumentation and technique. In Oho K, Amemiya R: Practical Fiberoptic Bronchoscopy, 2nd ed. Tokyo, Igaku-Shoin Ltd, 1984, pp 27–67.
6. Pereira W, Kovnat DM, Snider GL: A prospective cooperative study of complications following flexible fiberoptic bronchoscopy. Chest 1978;73:813–816.
7. Prakash UB, Offord KP, Stubbs SE: Bronchoscopy in North America: The ACCP survey. Chest 1991;100:1668–1675.
8. Shennib H, Baslaim G: Bronchoscopy in the intensive care unit. Chest Surg Clin North Am 1996;6:349–361.
9. Silver MR, Balk RA: Bronchoscopic procedures in the intensive care unit. Crit Care Clin 1995;11:97–109.
10. Timsit JF, Misset B, Azoulay E, et al: Usefulness of airway visualization in the diagnosis of nosocomial pneumonia in ventilated patients. Chest 1996;110:172–179.

13 Intra-abdominal Pressure Monitoring

Juan A. Asensio, José Ceballos, Walter Forno, and Jack Sava

Compartment syndrome is a well-described condition in which increased pressure in a defined anatomic space adversely affects regional circulation, causing a state of poor tissue perfusion and ischemia and threatening tissue viability. The importance of the abdominal compartment syndrome has been increasingly recognized as more and more trauma patients sustain massive injuries, protracted episodes of shock, or massive fluid replacement and survive long enough to develop reperfusion injury, which causes massive abdominal visceral swelling and leads to the development of this syndrome.

The abdominal cavity can be considered a single compartment; thus, any change involving the viscera can significantly elevate intra-abdominal pressure. Normal intra-abdominal pressures range from 2 to 10 cm H_2O. There is a normal pattern of fluctuation in intraperitoneal pressure during quiet respiration. Pressures between 10 and 20 cm H_2O are abnormal but are usually acceptable in postoperative patients. Pressures of more than 20 cm H_2O are clearly abnormal and usually require treatment.

Clinically significant increases in intra-abdominal pressure have been observed in a variety of clinical conditions in which acute increases in volume have developed within the abdominal cavity. Abdominal compartment syndrome can occur after any abdominal operation complicated by postoperative hemorrhage or bowel edema.

Pathophysiology

Elevated intra-abdominal pressure affects multiple organ systems in a graded fashion. An associated decrease in cardiac output is seen consistently with intra-abdominal pressures greater than 20 mm Hg. This decrease is directly related to diminished venous return secondary to compression of the inferior vena cava and the portal vein. Venous return has been shown to be impaired with intra-abdominal pressures as low as 15 mm Hg. Similarly, it is well known that hypovolemia in the presence of elevated intra-abdominal pressure contributes to significant decreases in cardiac output. This can be reversed by the administration of intravenous fluids.

An increase in intrathoracic pressure secondary to diaphragmatic elevation is responsible for reductions in ventricular compliance. If combined with an increase in systemic vascular resistance, which produces increased afterload, it results in decreased cardiac contractility at intra-abdominal pressures greater than 30 mm Hg. Diaphragmatic elevation markedly elevates intrapleural pressures. This increase is transmitted in a retrograde fashion to the heart and the central venous system, which may lead to spurious elevations of central venous pressure, pulmonary artery pressure, and pulmonary artery wedge pressures.

The respiratory system is also affected by increases in intra-abdominal pressure. The peak inspiratory pressure increases as a result of elevation of the diaphragm, resulting in reduced pulmonary compliance. Consequently, the functional residual capacity decreases and the partial oxygen tension worsens.

The renal system is directly impaired by elevations of intra-abdominal pressure. Oliguria progressing to anuria accompanied by prerenal azotemia that does not respond to volume expansion characterizes the renal dysfunction associated with the abdominal compartment syndrome. Oliguria can usually be demonstrated at pressures of more than 20 mm Hg, whereas pressures consistently higher than 30 mm Hg lead to anuria. Two mechanisms have been postulated to account for this phenomenon. First, decreases in cardiac output lead to decreases in renal perfusion pressure and renal arterial blood flow and increases in renovascular resistance, resulting in changes in intrarenal regional blood flow. Similarly, increases in intra-abdominal pressure may cause direct compression of the kidney, producing an obstruction of renal venous outflow. Because blood is shunted away from the cortical glomeruli, this results in a reduction in renal plasma flow and glomerular filtration rates.

Increases in intra-abdominal pressure also cause other abdominal visceral abnormalities. Mesenteric and hepatic arterial, intestinal mucosal, and hepatic microcirculatory blood flows have all been shown to decrease with abdominal hypertension. Concomitantly, there is also a definite and significant decrease in portal and mesenteric venous outflow.

Abdominal compartment syndrome can occur after

any abdominal operation that is complicated by postoperative hemorrhage. It is well known to occur in post-traumatic patients who have undergone extensive abdominal surgical procedures, particularly those who have suffered prolonged episodes of shock. It is also known to occur in patients requiring thoracic or abdominal aortic cross-clamping secondary to profound shock. Patients who have experienced the syndrome of hypothermia, acidosis, and coagulopathy are particularly susceptible to the development of this syndrome. Intra-abdominal or retroperitoneal packing as temporizing means to control abdominal hemorrhage may cause a pseudosyndrome because of direct compression of the inferior vena cava and obstruction of the venous outflow.

Chronic causes of abdominal compartment syndrome and elevated intra-abdominal pressures include chronic hepatic disease or cirrhosis producing tense ascites, large abdominal or retroperitoneal tumors, and severe pancreatitis. The abdominal compartment syndrome can also develop in patients with a history of extensive resuscitation for cardiac arrest, septic shock, or burns and profound hypothermia, even in the absence of abdominal injuries or operations.

Diagnosis

The diagnosis of abdominal hypertension is based on clinical signs and objective measurements of intra-abdominal pressure. Clinically, any patient with a tense and distended abdomen following a major abdominal operation and massive blood volume replacement is at risk. Elevated peak airway pressures, decreasing urine output, and hemodynamic instability in the presence of a tense distended abdomen establish the diagnosis.

Because abdominal compartment syndrome can develop intraoperatively, the surgeon should never close the abdominal wall under undue tension. Severe bowel swelling, extensive packing, or profound hemodynamic instability are risk factors for acute development of the syndrome. The intraoperative method of diagnosis consists of pulling the fascia together with Kocher clamps and observing for significant elevations of the peak airway pressure or deterioration of hemodynamic values. Such patients require temporary abdominal wall closure with prosthetic materials. Even if the patient undergoes fascial closure, the risk of development of the syndrome continues with ongoing postoperative resuscitation.

Objective measurements of intra-abdominal pressure are important in the definitive diagnosis of this syndrome. Intra-abdominal pressures can be measured directly or indirectly, although direct measurement is usually not feasible. Therefore, indirect measurement is the method of choice. The latter can be obtained from rectal, gastric, and urinary bladder pressures, which are measured across the wall of these organs via a manometer. All except the rectal method have been shown to correlate well with directly measured intra-abdominal pressures in animal models. Measurement of intra-abdominal pressures is indicated in the following patients:

1. Postoperative patients with a distended and tense abdomen and with other signs of organ dysfunction consistent with the abdominal compartment syndrome.
2. Patients with intra-abdominal or retroperitoneal packing.
3. Patients temporarily closed via a prosthetic abdominal wall, who are still undergoing massive postoperative fluid resuscitation.
4. Patients who have not undergone laparotomy but who have received large volumes of fluid resuscitation.

Measurements

The only direct way to measure intra-abdominal pressure is to place a catheter directly into the femoral vein and to advance it to the inferior vena cava. The catheter is then connected to a transducer. This direct method is not used because of its invasiveness and potential risks.

There are two methods of indirect intra-abdominal pressure measurement: gastric pressure measurement and urinary bladder pressure measurement. Of the two, the latter is almost always used.

Measurement of Gastric Pressure

This method of measurement is predicated on the concept that the stomach when partially filled is both a distensible and a compressible bag lying within the abdominal cavity. Therefore, it follows that intra-abdominal pressure can be transmitted to the stomach. With a patient lying supine, a nasogastric or a gastrostomy tube can be used. Fifty to 100 mL of saline solution is then instilled into the stomach. A water manometer or a pressure transducer is attached to the tube, and the midaxillary line is considered zero. The cavity pressures are noted in centimeters of water at the end of expiration. Alternatively, a ruler can be used to measure the height of the column of the fluid in the nasogastric tube (Fig. 13–1). This method is used only rarely.

Measurement of Urinary Bladder Pressure

This measurement can be done by two techniques.
Standard Technique. In the standard technique, with

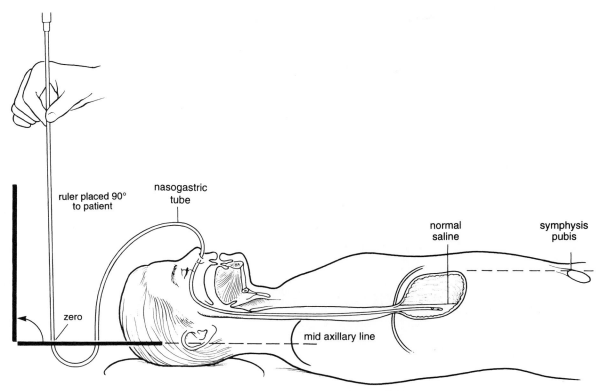

FIGURE 13–1. Measurement of gastric pressure.

the patient lying supine, the bladder is emptied of all urine via a Foley catheter. The drainage tube connected to the Foley catheter is double clamped. A pressure measurement apparatus is then rigged, which consists of an 18-gauge needle attached to a three-way stopcock; a 50-mL syringe is attached to one of the ports, and a manometer is attached to a third port. After the bladder has been drained of all fluid, 50 to 100 mL of normal saline solution is instilled into the Foley catheter via the aspiration port. The three-way stopcock is then opened to the manometer, which has previously been set to zero at the level of the symphysis pubis, and the bladder pressure is measured in centimeters of water (Fig. 13–2).

U-tube Technique. The U-tube technique is a simplified approach that measures bladder pressure without requiring an additional apparatus and that prevents violation of the continuity of the Foley catheter. It requires raising the Foley catheter above the patient, allowing a U-shaped loop to develop, and measuring the height of the column of fluid (urine) in the catheter from its meniscus to the symphysis pubis. Catheter continuity remains intact, thus reducing the risk of infection (Fig. 13–3).

Measurement of intra-abdominal pressure can have several pitfalls, which may lead to abnormal values. Intra-abdominal pressure in patients who are agitated, thrashing, or fighting the ventilator or who are not perfectly supine may be falsely elevated. The patient must be calm and sedated. The most accurate measure-

ments of intra-abdominal pressure are obtained in patients who are chemically paralyzed and sedated.

Treatment of Abdominal Compartment Syndrome

A grading system has been established for measuring intra-abdominal pressures and selecting therapeutic interventions (Table 13–1).

If the intra-abdominal pressure is between 10 and 15 cm H_2O (grade I), abdominal decompression is not indicated. If the intra-abdominal pressure is between 15 and 25 cm H_2O (grade II), treatment should be based on the patient's clinical condition. Obviously, in the absence of oliguria, abnormally elevated peak airway pressures, hypoxemia, or hemodynamic derangements, abdominal decompression is not justified. These patients require close monitoring, however. In patients whose bladder pressures are 25 to 35 cm H_2O (grade III), abdominal decompression is indicated in the majority of cases even in the absence of overt

TABLE 13–1. Grading of Intra-abdominal Pressure

Grade	Bladder Pressure, *cm H_2O*
I	10–15
II	15–25
III	25–35
IV	>35

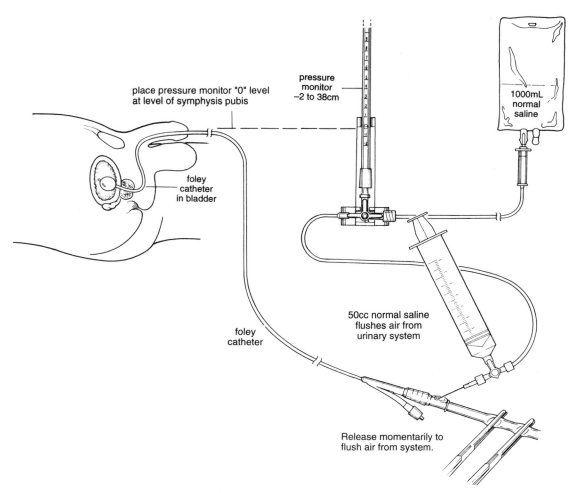

place pressure monitor "0" level
at level of symphysis pubis

pressure
monitor
−2 to 38cm

1000mL
normal
saline

foley
catheter
in bladder

50cc normal saline
flushes air from
urinary system

foley
catheter

Release momentarily to
flush air from system.

FIGURE 13–2. Measurement of bladder pressure.

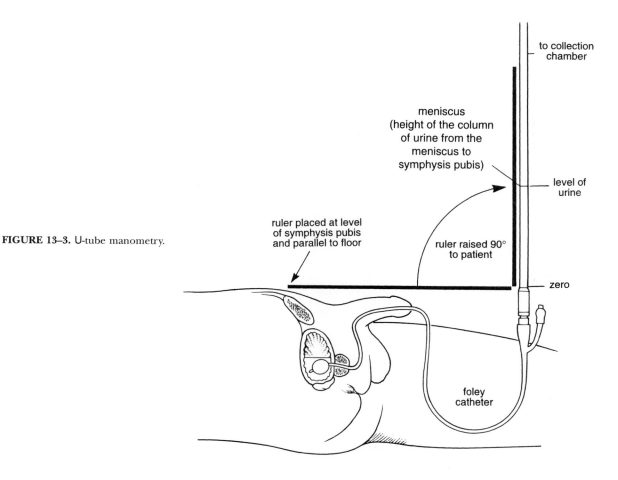

FIGURE 13–3. U-tube manometry.

signs, because the signs and symptoms of abdominal compartment syndrome may develop insidiously. In patients with pressures measured at greater than 35 cm H_2O, immediate abdominal decompression is indicated because these patients are at risk of developing cardiovascular collapse.

Rapid abdominal decompression is the only known treatment for the abdominal compartment syndrome and demands immediate surgical intervention. Often, these patients are critically ill (in the intensive care unit) and cannot be moved to an operating suite without considerable risk. Abdominal decompression can be performed in the intensive care unit if proper planning is instituted. Closure of the abdominal wound is achieved by using a prosthetic device, usually an intravenous fluid bag or some type of prosthetic mesh.

Suggested Readings

1. Burch JM, Moore EE, Moore FA, et al: The abdominal compartment syndrome. Surg Clin North Am 1996;76:833–842.

2. Diebel LN, Wilson RF, Dulchavsky SA, et al: Effect of increased intra-abdominal pressure on hepatic, arterial, portal, venous and hepatic microcirculatory blood flow. J Trauma 1992;33:279–283.

3. Gross R: A new method for surgical treatment of large omphaloceles. Surgery 1948;24:277–292.

4. Iberti TS, Kelly KM, Gentilli DR, et al: A simple technique to accurately determine intra-abdominal pressure. Crit Care Med 1987;15:1140–1142.

5. Ivatury RR, Simon RJ, Islam S, et al: Intra-abdominal hypertension, gastric mucosal pH and the abdominal compartment syndrome [abstract]. J Trauma 1997;43:194.

6. Kron IL, Harman PK, Nolan SP: The measurement of intra-abdominal pressure as a criterion for abdominal re-exploration. Ann Surg 1984;199:28–30.

7. Lee SH, Anderson JT, Kraut EJ, et al: U-tube manometry accurately measures intra-abdominal pressure [abstract]. Proceedings of the 71st Annual Meeting of the Pacific Coast Surgical Association, February 19–22, 2000, San Francisco, California.

8. Richard WO, Scovill W, Shin B, Reed W: Acute renal failure associated with increased intra-abdominal pressure. Ann Surg 1983;197:183–187.

9. Saggi BH, Sugerman, HJ, Ivatury R, et al: Abdominal compartment syndrome. J Trauma 1998;45:597–609.

10. Sugrue M, Buist MD, Lee A, et al: Intra-abdominal pressure measurement using a modified nasogastric tube: A description and validation of a new technique. Intensive Care Med 1994;20:588–590.

14 Intracranial Pressure Monitoring

Ali Salim and Larry Khoo

Measurement of intracranial pressure (ICP) was first performed in the early 1900s indirectly by measuring lumbar cerebrospinal fluid (CSF) pressure. It was not until 1951 that the direct measurement of ICP by means of ventricular cannulation was introduced, and it subsequently came into routine use in 1960. ICP monitoring provides information on the likelihood of cerebral herniation and allows calculation of the cerebral perfusion pressure (CPP). CPP is an important clinical indicator of cerebral blood flow. An elevated CPP implies diminished cerebral blood flow, which may lead to further brain injury. Because CPP equals mean blood pressure minus ICP, and because significant intracranial hypotension has been associated with as much as a 50% increase in mortality rate, ICP monitoring is essential to ensure adequate cerebral perfusion and to optimize outcome. When the device is capable of external ventricular drainage, ICP monitoring can also be used to assay the CSF, to treat elevated ICP directly, and to maximize CPP. There are substantial data supporting the finding that the absolute level of ICP affects outcome and the ability to reduce ICP improves it.

Currently, ICP monitoring is a standard intervention in the management of severe head injury. Normal ICP ranges from 5 to 20 mm Hg. Transient elevations of the ICP up to 40 mm Hg can occur with normal actions such as coughing, sneezing, or the Valsalva maneuver. Persistent elevation above 20 to 25 mm Hg should be actively treated in a timely fashion.

Indications

The indications for placement of an ICP monitor are based on the guidelines for the management of severe head injury published in 1996 by the Joint Section on Neurotrauma and Critical Care of the American Association of Neurological Surgeons. Though there was little scientific evidence from randomized prospective clinical trials, guidelines were produced based on available data. According to these guidelines, ICP monitoring is appropriate in patients with severe head injury with abnormal findings on an admission computed tomography (CT) scan. Severe head injury is associated with a Glasgow Coma Scale score of 3 to 8 after cardiopulmonary resuscitation. Abnormal find-

ings on a CT of the head include hematomas, contusions, edema, or compressed basal cisterna.

Additionally, ICP monitoring is appropriate in patients with severe head injury and a normal CT scan when two or more of the following features are noted on admission: age of more than 40 years, unilateral or bilateral motor posturing, or systolic blood pressure of less than 90 mm Hg. ICP monitoring is not indicated in the majority of patients with mild or moderate head injury. A physician may choose to monitor ICP in such patients with traumatic mass lesions based on individual risk factors. If alcohol, drug use, or toxic or metabolic factors cloud the clinical examination, ICP monitoring should be used judiciously for only a limited period of time.

To date, there are no randomized prospective trials of the impact of ICP monitoring on outcome. Until more class I data are available, the abovementioned guidelines remain the standard of care.

Contraindications

Absolute contraindications include severe coagulopathy or other conditions associated with an unacceptably high risk of intracranial hemorrhage due to passage of the catheter (e.g., platelet or coagulation disorders such as hemophilia A or B or von Willebrand disease). Relative contraindications include severe infection, severe hemodynamic instability, open wounds of the scalp and the skull around the planned site of insertion, immunosuppression, and small or effaced ventricles (in regard to ventriculostomy) as visualized on CT or magnetic resonance imaging.

Intracranial Location and Catheter Device

Intracranial pressure devices can be placed in epidural, subdural, subarachnoid, parenchymal, or ventricular locations. Ventricular ICP has been the gold standard and is used as the reference for comparing the accuracy of ICP monitoring in other intracranial locations. It has the therapeutic advantage of allowing CSF drainage in intracranial hypertension and CSF assay for evidence of infection, tumor, or inflammation. Direct parenchymal or subdural monitoring can also be done and is quicker and technically easier. Subdural and parenchymal transduction has been reported to be similar to ventricular ICP monitoring but precludes CSF examination and drainage.

To measure ICP, pressure transducers are required. There are three types: external strain gauge, catheter-tip strain gauge, or catheter-tip fiberoptic technology. External strain-gauge transducers are coupled to the patient's intracranial space via fluid-filled lines, whereas catheter-tip transducers are placed intracranially. External strain-gauge transducers are generally accurate and can be recalibrated, but obstruction of the fluid-filled lines can cause inaccuracy. Such fluid-coupled systems have a minimum of drift during extended monitoring. The external transducer must be consistently maintained at a fixed point relative to the patient's head to avoid measurement error (Fig. 14–1).

Catheter-tip strain gauge or fiberoptic devices are calibrated before intracranial insertion and cannot be recalibrated once inserted (without an associated ventricular catheter). This may lead to inaccurate measurements if the device drifts and is not recalibrated. Overall, these non–fluid-filled systems with fiberoptic or catheter-tip strain-gauge technology are easier to use because ICP measurement is independent of head elevation. Without recalibration, however, these devices have the potential for measurement drift. Several studies have demonstrated significant temperature and measurement drift of these devices over time.

Preoperative Evaluation

Either CT or magnetic resonance imaging of the brain should be performed to assess the location of the ventricular system. Ventricular shift, obstruction, anatomic variation, contusion, or hemorrhage should be noted. A reasonable attempt should be made to determine the patient's complete blood count and bleeding indices (prothrombin time, partial thromboplastin time, bleeding time) as well as his or her infectious and immune status before the procedure. Informed consent from either the patient or an appropriate legal designee should be obtained when possible. Preprocedural consultation with a neurologic surgeon or other qualified physicians experienced in ICP monitoring is advised as well.

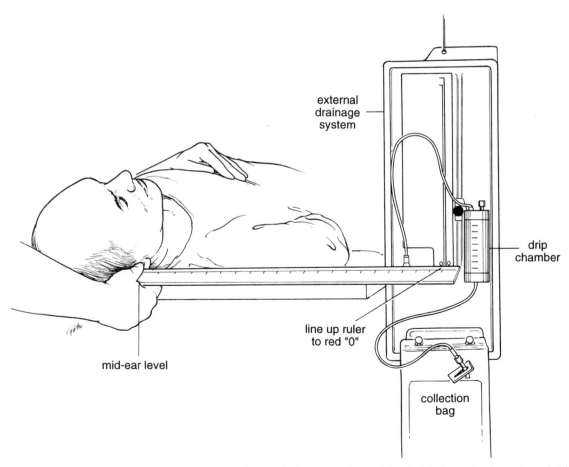

FIGURE 14–1. The external drainage system connected to the ventriculostomy catheter is level with the patient's ear to maintain accurate and consistent measurements.

Procedure

Surgical Planning. The patient's cranium is examined, and the entry site is identified. In general, the ventricular catheter should enter the cranium and should pass through the frontal lobes, thereby avoiding injury to the motor cortex and the somatosensory cortex, which are immediately adjacent and posterior. Because the left frontal lobe is dominant in all right-handed individuals and in up to 70% of left-handed individuals, right-sided placement of the catheter is preferred. Parenchymal and subdural monitoring devices should also be placed in the frontal region if possible.

Kocher's point is the most commonly used superficial landmark for entry of the catheter into the brain.

It lies at the junction of the plane 1 cm anterior to the coronal suture at the midpupillary line (Fig. 14-2A). Other sites include the occipitoparietal region (i.e., Frazier's point; Fig. 14–2B), Dandy's point (2 cm lateral to the midline, 3 cm above the inion; Fig. 14–3A), and Keen's point (2.5 to 3 cm posterior and 2.5 to 3 cm superior to the pinna; see Fig. 14–2C). From Kocher's point, the catheter is then aimed perpendicular to the surface of the skull, toward the ipsilateral medial canthus and the contralateral external auditory canal (Figs. 14–4 and 14–5). The insertion depth is typically 5 to 7 cm but will vary from case to case.

The use of prophylactic antibiotics in patients without infection is left to the discretion of the individual surgeon. For patients with infection, appropriate intravenous antibiotic therapy should be implemented be-

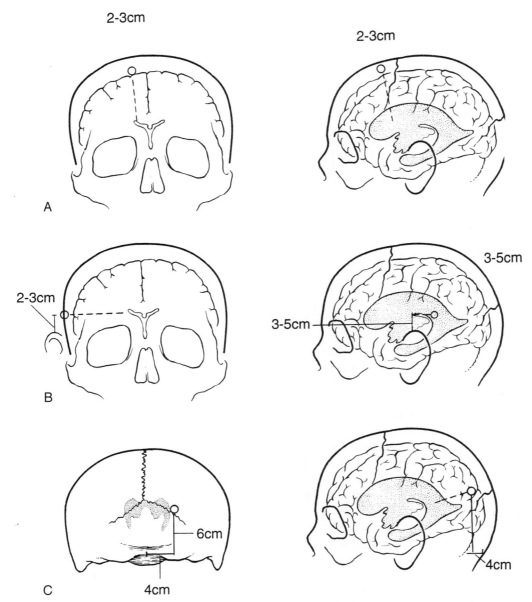

FIGURE 14–2. *A,* Kocher's point (1 cm to the coronal suture and 2 to 3 cm lateral to the midline). *B,* Frazier's point (occipitoparietal region). *C,* Keen's point.

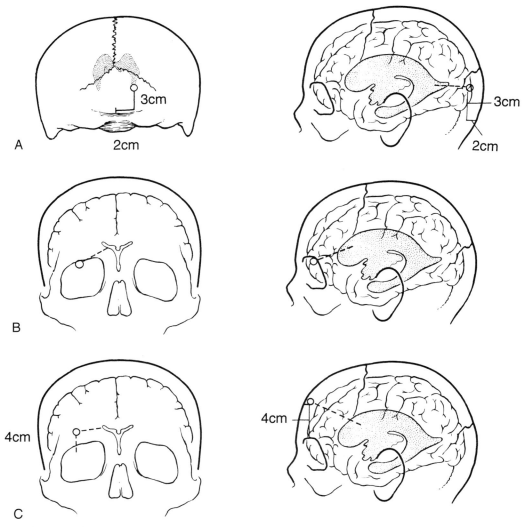

FIGURE 14–3. *A*, Dandy's point. *B* and *C*, Different sites for anterior placement of ventricular catheter.

fore the procedure. For patients with coagulopathy, preprocedural transfusions with appropriate blood products are warranted.

Surgical Preparation. The ipsilateral hemicranium should be fully shaved and wiped clean with water and diluted alcohol. The head can also be loosely held in place with tape or by an assistant. The hemicranium is painted with iodine, and a sterile drape is applied.

Anesthesia. Appropriate sedation can typically be achieved with the use of intravenous analgesics (2 to 6 mg of morphine sulfate) and sedatives (1 to 2 mg of lorazepam). The sedatives should be tailored to the neurologic status of the patient. Appropriate equipment for emergent resuscitation should be nearby. Local anesthesia and hemostasis are facilitated with the use of 1% to 2% lidocaine with epinephrine at the operative site.

Equipment. Necessary equipment includes a sterile ventricular catheter (varying lengths from 15 to 30 cm are commonly available; Fig. 14–6), ventricular drainage apparatus (allows for drainage and monitoring of

ICP; see Fig. 14–1), a surgical tray (including twist drill with various drill bits; Fig. 14–7), sterile towels, sutures (typically 2–0 or 3–0 nylon), and dressing material.

Technique. After injection of local anesthetic with epinephrine, either a horizontal or a vertical incision is made with a No. 10 blade at the entrance site down to the level of bone. The blade is then used to sweep the periosteum off the skull. Because the scalp is highly vascular, hemostasis should be obtained with either a ligature or cautery before proceeding further. A twist drill or a mechanical perforator is then used to penetrate the skull, aiming orthogonal to the skull and toward the ipsilateral medial canthus. Frequent assessment and confirmation of the depth of the drill hole with a probe or a needle are warranted. After penetration of the skull, a sharp durotomy is made with a Tuohy needle, a No. 11 blade, or the tip of the catheter-passing trocar. Caution is necessary to avoid dissecting the dura off the overlying bone, thereby causing an iatrogenic epidural hematoma. The wound is irrigated with sterile normal saline solution or Ringer's

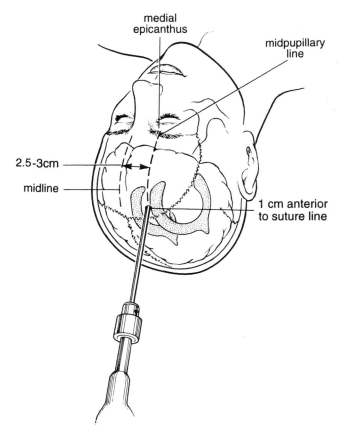

FIGURE 14–4. The catheter is inserted into Kocher's point 1 cm anterior to the coronal suture at the midpupillary line and 3 cm lateral to the midline toward the ipsilateral medial catheters.

lactate solution to remove accumulated blood or bony debris. The ventricular catheter is inserted gently with the metal stylus to the appropriate depth, typically 5 to 7 cm (Fig. 14–8).

In many cases, the ventricular lining or ependyma is firmer and can provide a tactile response or a "pop" on entry. After entrance into the ventricle, the stylus is removed, and the return of CSF is confirmed. In patients with normal or decreased ICP, this may require gentle aspiration with a saline-filled syringe. Care should be taken to avoid excessive loss of CSF. The trocar is then passed beneath the galea to a point 2 to 4 cm distal to the incision (Fig. 14–9). Tunneling helps decrease the incidence of infection during extended monitoring. Next, the catheter is secured to the skin. The original incision is closed with a simple running 2–0 or 3–0 nylon stitch, and a sterile dressing is applied. The catheter is connected to the transducer and the drainage apparatus (Fig. 14–10). The opening pressure, the quality of the waveform, and the CSF characteristics (color, quality, and amount of blood) are recorded. Several commonly used ventricular catheter monitoring systems and parenchymal/subdural monitoring systems use a bolt-type device, which is screwed directly into the twist drill hole and is not tunneled. Although such devices are much quicker to install, they are often more susceptible to breakage, accidental disconnection, and infection.

Complications

Complications of ICP device use include infection (local wound infection, ventriculitis, meningitis, cerebritis), hemorrhage, malfunction, obstruction, malposition, seizures, and injury to the brain parenchyma or the cerebral vasculature. These complications rarely cause long-term morbidity but may require device replacement or may lead to inaccurate ICP readings.

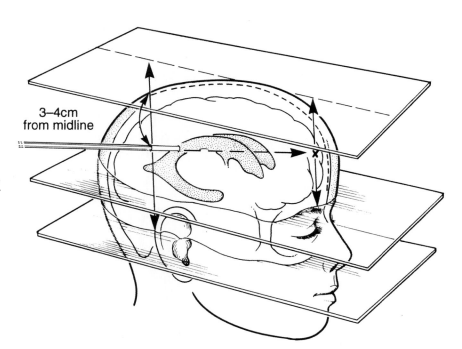

FIGURE 14–5. Lateral view of Kocher's point, with insertion aiming toward ipsilateral medial catheters.

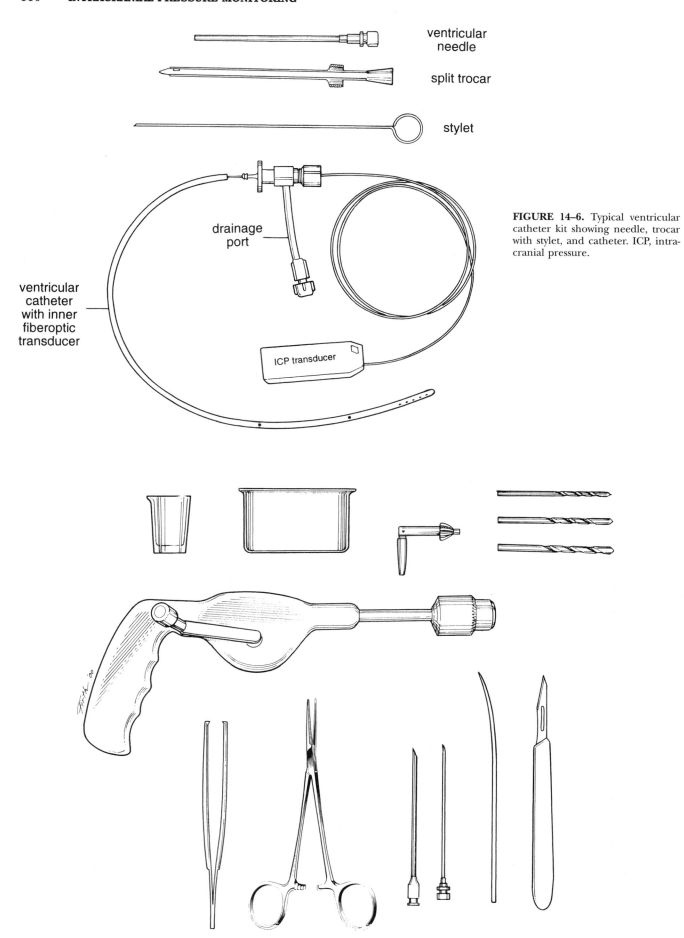

ventricular
needle

split trocar

stylet

drainage
port

ICP transducer

ventricular
catheter
with inner
fiberoptic
transducer

FIGURE 14–6. Typical ventricular catheter kit showing needle, trocar with stylet, and catheter. ICP, intracranial pressure.

FIGURE 14–7. Surgical tray shows basic requirements for ventricular catheter insertion.

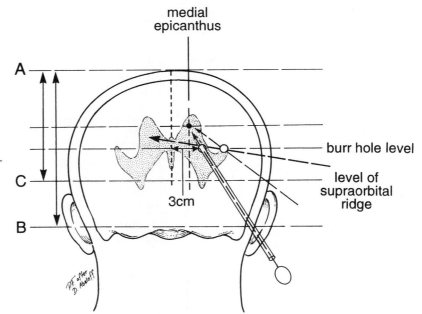

FIGURE 14–8. Catheter with stylet entering the ventricle at Kocher's point.

Infection. Infection is defined as a positive CSF culture of a specimen from the ventricular or the subarachnoid monitors or a positive culture of a specimen from the explanted intracranial device. Some argue that a better term would be colonization rather than infection because there are no reports of clinically significant intracranial infections associated with ICP monitoring device use in large prospective studies. Nevertheless, the incidence of infection of ICP devices increases significantly after 5 days of implantation. Treatment is removal of the device. Appropriate antibiotics should be implemented as well. Colonization rates, according to intracranial location, are as follows:

intraventricular, 5% (range, 0% to 9.5%); subarachnoid, 5% (range, 0% to 10%); subdural, 4% (range, 1% to 10%); intraparenchymal, 12% with catheter-tip strain gauge and 17% with fiberoptic device.

Prolonged ICP monitoring beyond 7 to 10 days is typically not advised. For patients requiring persistent ventricular drainage to control ICP, permanent diversion in the form of a ventriculoperitoneal or a ventriculopleural shunt should be used.

Hemorrhage. Hemorrhage associated with ICP monitor placement is reported in terms of hematoma, with an incidence of 1.4% to 5% in study patients who underwent postprocedural CT. Significant hematomas

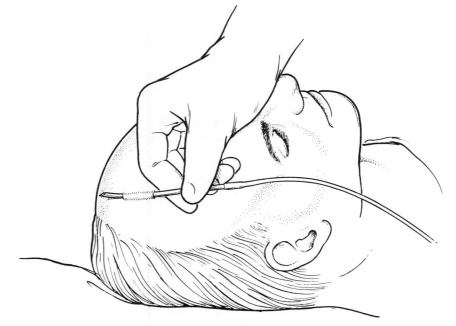

FIGURE 14–9. The catheter is tunneled approximtely 2 to 4 cm distal to the incision.

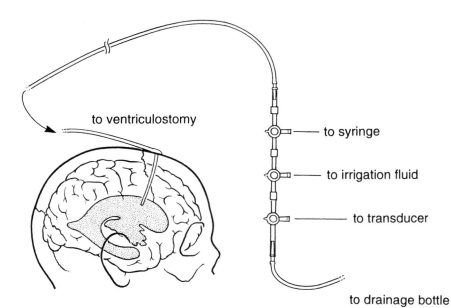

to ventriculostomy

to syringe

to irrigation fluid

to transducer

to drainage bottle

FIGURE 14–10. Ventricular catheter connected to drainage apparatus and transducer.

requiring surgical evacuation occur in 0.5%. The incidence of delayed hematomas after 24 hours is extremely rare (<0.1%) and typically occurs in the face of systemic hypertension and underlying coagulopathy.

Malfunction, Obstruction, and Malposition. Rates of malfunction, obstruction, and malposition vary according to the location: ventricular catheters, 6%; subarachnoid bolts, 16%; subdural catheters, 10%. With ICP measurements of more than 50 mm Hg, higher rates of obstruction may be noted. A CT scan may be helpful in assessing the location of the catheter tip. Treatment involves redirection and may require insertion of a new catheter. Approximately 3% of patients will need operative revision. Severe brain injury with high ICP can cause complete effacement or collapse of the ventricular lining around the ICP catheter. When this occurs, pressure readings of strain-gauge or fluid-coupled systems are no longer accurate. Furthermore, drainage of the CSF is also no longer possible. Fiberoptic systems are advantageous in that they are not susceptible to this phenomenon. Each type of pressure transduction system and location of the monitor has its own set of potential complications. Careful insertion, monitoring for infection, and checking for obstruction are necessary and will ensure optimal ICP monitoring.

Follow-up

Serial assessment of the surgical site and sampling of the CSF should be performed for infection surveillance. As previously noted, prolonged use (>5 days) is associated with increased rates of infection. Prophylactic ventriculostomy at a new site may be warranted when prolonged use is needed. Interval CT scans should be obtained if there are any concerns regarding hemorrhage, catheter obstruction, catheter misplacement, or new neurologic deficits.

Suggested Readings

1. Fortune JB, Feustel PJ, Graca L, et al: Effect of hyperventilation, mannitol, and ventriculostomy drainage on cerebral blood flow after head injury. J Trauma 1995;39:1091–1099.
2. Ghajar J: Intracranial pressure monitoring techniques. New Horiz 1995;3:395–399.
3. Guidelines for the management of severe head injury. Brain Trauma Foundation, American Association of Neurological Surgeons, Joint Section on Neurotrauma and Critical Care. J Neurotrauma 1996;13:641–734.
4. Lang EW, Chesnut RM: Intracranial pressure and cerebral perfusion pressure in severe head injury. New Horiz 1995;3:400–409.
5. Marion WD, Spiegel PT: Changes in the management of severe traumatic brain injury: 1991–1997. Crit Care Med 2000;28:16–18.
6. White JR, Likavec JM: The diagnosis and initial management of head injury. N Engl J Med 1992;327:1507–1511.
7. Wilberger JE Jr: Outcomes analysis: Intracranial pressure monitoring. Clin Neurosurg 1997;44:439–448.

15 Jugular Bulb Oximetry

Julio Cruz

In the history of cerebral hemometabolic monitoring, arteriovenous differences in oxygen content ($AVDO_2$), in glucose concentration, and in lactate concentration were first reported in normal volunteers in 1942. A few years later, quantification of cerebral blood flow (CBF) and of cerebral metabolic rate of oxygen ($CMRO_2$) was introduced. Continuous monitoring of intracranial pressure (ICP) in humans started in 1951; in 1965, cerebral perfusion pressure (CPP, the difference between mean arterial pressure and mean ICP) was reported.

Background

Basic Cerebral Hemometabolic Interrelationships

Conventionally, the basic interrelationships between cerebral hemodynamics and metabolism have assumed that CBF is a direct function of CPP. Cerebrovascular resistance (CVR), however, is inversely related to CBF and acts as the opponent force to CPP, as follows:

$$CBF = CPP/CVR$$

Accordingly, no matter how high CPP is, CVR will modulate cerebral perfusion (either globally or regionally). This circumstance is well understood in patients with acute ischemic stroke, who are frequently hypertensive on hospital admission and have no intracranial disease to account for increased ICP. Nevertheless, despite high CPP, clinical and radiologic signs of profound cerebral ischemia may be found (because CVR is pathologically increased). The same applies to patients with cerebral vasospasm following aneurysmal subarachnoid hemorrhage.

Thus, normal CPP does not guarantee adequate cerebral metabolism. Conversely, relative decreases in CVR may yield a condition of relative cerebral hyperemia (in which CBF is normal) or absolute cerebral hyperemia (in which CBF is increased). The normal CBF is 50 mL per 100 grams per minute.

By using accurate CBF measurement, it has been shown that acutely comatose patients with cerebral hyperperfusion (either relative or absolute hyperemia) have a worse long-term clinical outcome than patients with low CBF (normally coupled with low oxygen consumption).

The $CMRO_2$ is the product of CBF and $AVDO_2$, as follows:

$$CMRO_2 = (CBF \times AVDO_2)/100$$

We have found that under circumstances of either moderate or profound acute anemia in the face of a severely injured brain, the arteriojugular oxyhemoglobin saturation difference (CEO_2) is far more reliable than $AVDO_2$.

Accordingly, we have also proposed that CCO_2 (cerebral consumption of oxygen) is a more reliable parameter than the conventional $CMRO_2$. In calculation of the CCO_2, CEO_2 replaces $AVDO_2$, thus yielding stable and reliable values for cerebral oxygen consumption in both anemic and nonanemic conditions (unlike the conventional $CMRO_2$). The CCO_2 calculation is as follows:

$$CCO_2 = (CBF \times CEO_2)/100$$

For practical bedside management, this equation must be rearranged, as follows:

$$CEO_2 = (CCO_2/CBF) \times 100$$

Accordingly, without the need to measure CBF and CCO_2, just maintaining normal or therapeutically normalized CEO_2 values will imply adequate coupling between flow and consumption.

Both CEO_2 and CCO_2 are practical and reliable in comparison with the conventional parameters ($AVDO_2$ and $CMRO_2$) in most circumstances. CEO_2, in turn, is calculated as follows (where SaO_2 is the oxygen saturation in arterial blood and SjO_2 is the oxygen saturation in jugular blood):

$$CEO_2 = SaO_2 - SjO_2$$

The normal CEO_2 ranges from 24% to 42% in adults and is estimated to be 7% lower in children. These ranges are used for therapeutic normalization, especially with optimized hyperventilation and optimized mannitol dosing (see later). The goal is the maintenance of approximately normal mean values (33% in adults and 26% in children).

113

Coupling and Uncoupling between Cerebral Blood Flow and Cerebral Consumption of Oxygen

It has been shown that a better long-term clinical outcome can be achieved in severely brain-injured patients with reduced CBF throughout the acute comatose period (i.e., when normal [spontaneous] coupling exists between reduced CBF and pathologically decreased cerebral oxygen consumption).

Accordingly, we have long adopted CEO_2 monitoring and management as the means of therapeutically restoring the normal coupling between CBF and CCO_2. By doing so, we have routinely attempted to reproduce the natural history of physiologic homeostasis during the acute comatose period, aiming at favorable long-term clinical outcome. Obviously, to calculate CEO_2, we monitor SjO_2 by means of jugular bulb catheterization and SaO_2 by means of pulse oximetry.

Technique of Jugular Bulb Catheterization

For either continuous fiberoptic or frequent intermittent SjO_2 and CEO_2 monitoring, catheter insertion is performed at bedside, *without* turning or lowering the patient's head. Under sterile conditions, the common carotid pulse is felt at the level of the cricoid cartilage. Just lateral to the carotid pulse, a thin needle and local anesthesia should be used, with the needle pointing approximately 30 degrees cephalad (Fig. 15–1). The internal jugular vein should be located easily no deeper than approximately 2 to 3 cm from the skin surface. Once the vein has been located, the thin needle should be left temporarily in place to guide the placement of a larger (intracatheter) needle.

After the internal jugular vein has been punctured with a large-bore needle, blood should be aspirated easily and should be reinjected once or twice as a means of ensuring that the tip of the insertion device is not abutting the vessel wall. A guidewire is inserted through the needle (Fig. 15–2), and after the needle has been removed, a special peel-away introducer is advanced over the guidewire (Fig. 15–3). Then the guidewire is removed, and the jugular bulb catheter can be *gently* introduced cephalad until resistance is felt, which corresponds to the superior wall of the jugular bulb (Fig. 15–4). Next, the introducer is peeled away (Fig. 15–5). The catheter should be pulled out-

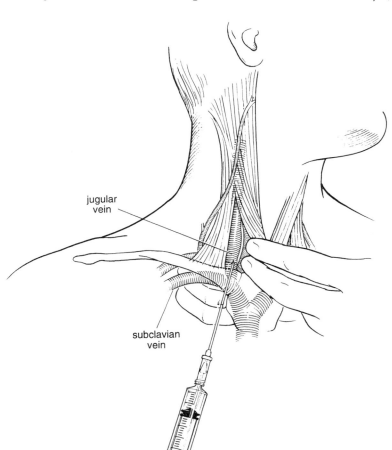

jugular vein

subclavian vein

FIGURE 15–1. Location and puncture of jugular vein.

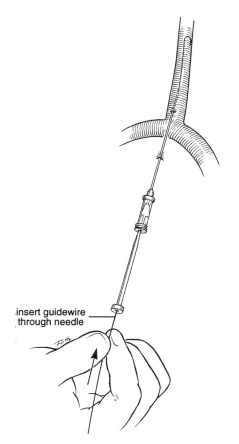

FIGURE 15–2. Insertion of guidewire through needle.

ward approximately 0.5 cm to prevent endothelial damage (and eventually thrombosis) as well as artifactual recordings (when a fiberoptic catheter is used).

The right internal jugular vein is usually broader than the left and is therefore chosen for monitoring under most circumstances (irrespective of lesion side on computed tomography of the head). This approach is used because both right and left internal jugular veins drain bilateral intracranial blood. Although the right-sided vein drains predominantly bilateral supratentorial cortical and subcortical blood, the left-sided vein drains bilateral blood from deeper (centrencephalic) structures as well as from posterior fossa elements.

For continuous fiberoptic monitoring, proper anatomic positioning of the head and the neck is paramount to prevent motion artifacts. Therefore, patients *must* be selected who can be kept sedated and immobile for prolonged periods.

The use of a cervical collar may also be considered (especially in patients with brain trauma). With proper patient selection and immobilization, we have found excellent agreement between the results of conventional jugular bulb oximetry and the results of fiberoptic jugular bulb oximetry.

Once the jugular bulb catheter has been properly positioned, adequate gentle but firm stitching must be carried out to prevent unintentional outward mobiliza-

tion (especially during nursing procedures), which will eventually result in extracranial "contamination" of jugular blood and falsely low CEO_2 (false-high SjO_2) values.

Management Protocols

Our cumulative treatment protocol is based not only on normalizing ICP (<20 mm Hg in adults, <15 mm Hg in children) and perfusion pressure but also on therapeutically inducing normal coupling between CBF and CCO_2. The protocol consists of the following treatment modalities, employed with the patient's head elevated approximately 30 degrees:

1. Nonbarbiturate sedation.
2. Neuromuscular junction blockade (which has been used less frequently and has been replaced by more profound sedation if necessary).
3. Optimized hyperventilation (for elevated ICP and decreased CEO_2 or for relative cerebral hyperperfusion).
4. Optimized fast intravenous boluses of hypertonic mannitol (for elevated ICP and increased CEO_2 or for relative cerebral hypoperfusion), up to a serum osmolality of approximately 315 mOsm/L.

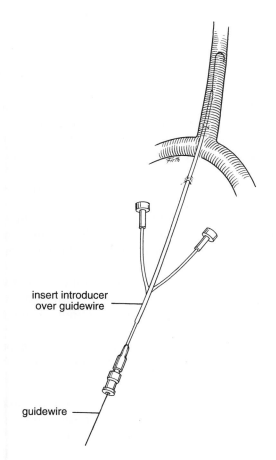

FIGURE 15–3. Insertion of dilator and introducer over guidewire.

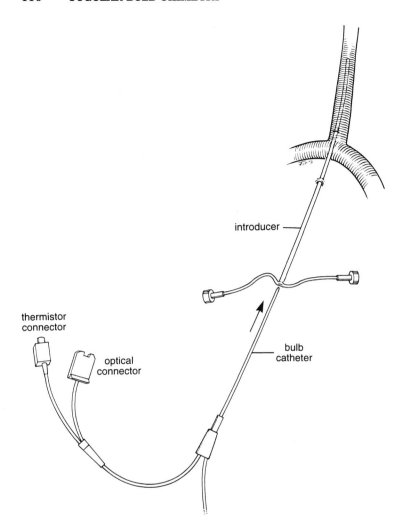

thermistor
connector

optical
connector

introducer

bulb
catheter

FIGURE 15-4. Insertion of jugular bulb catheter through introducer.

5. Cerebrospinal fluid drainage (essentially abandoned over the years as we have learned to select patients with small lateral ventricles and have adopted ICP monitoring from the brain surface instead).

6. Barbiturate therapy (which frequently requires the concomitant use of vasopressors).

7. Hypothermia (essentially abandoned over the years because of our frequent experience with unmanageable pneumonia related to hypothermia-induced immunosuppression).

8. "Extreme" mannitol administration (irrespective of high serum osmolality) if patients display pupillary widening despite the abovementioned ongoing measures.

9. Decompressive craniotomy (before bilateral pupillary widening is found to be irreversible by nonsurgical means).

Our tendency has been *not* to wait for pupillary widening before adopting decompressive surgery. In most patients with severe acute brain injuries, the described protocol has been implemented in the presence of induced normovolemia. We reserve induced hypervolemia (and eventually vasopressors) for patients without brain trauma in whom clinically relevant cerebral vasospasm is suspected or confirmed, such as in those with aneurysmal subarachnoid hemorrhage.

Thus, our comprehensive approach to the management of severely brain-injured patients can be adopted for a variety of acute intracranial insults besides brain trauma (Table 15-1). This is because phasic cerebral hemometabolic changes may be expected in many circumstances associated with acute coma. Accordingly, either low or high SjO$_2$ values may require proper management, in light of concomitant ICP abnormalities.

Optimal dosing of mannitol and optimized hyperventilation represent the basic and most practical means of managing intracranial hypertension and restoring the physiologic coupling between CBF and CCO$_2$. Under more challenging conditions—when barbiturate therapy is required for control of refractory ICP problems—we have found that intravenous pentobarbital boluses have undesired effects, because the blood pressure may fall markedly (even transiently) and trigger an abnormal decrease in SjO$_2$ in some of these patients. We believe that these patients present with grossly defective cerebral pressure autoregulation, so that they cannot

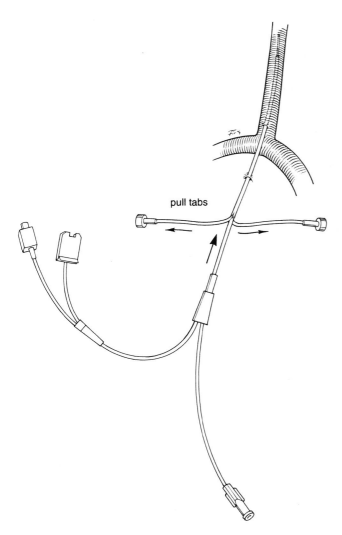

FIGURE 15–5. Introducer is peeled away, and jugular bulb catheter is pulled slightly back.

pull tabs

TABLE 15–1. Indications for Arteriojugular Monitoring

Severe acute brain trauma with suspected or confirmed intracranial hypertension and brain swelling
Some forms of spontaneous intracranial hemorrhage with suspected or confirmed intracranial hypertension and brain swelling (either pre- or postoperatively)
Some forms of meningitis or meningoencephalitis with suspected or confirmed intracranial hypertension and brain swelling
Some forms of hypoxic-ischemic encephalopathy with suspected or confirmed intracranial hypertension and brain swelling
Hepatic encephalopathy and coma
Uremic encephalopathy and coma
Other metabolic encephalopathies
Near-drowning and coma
Severe septic encephalopathy
Eclamptic encephalopathy
Selected general anesthetic procedures

Figure 15–6 illustrates the general SjO_2 profile throughout the acute phase in optimally hyperventilated patients. As seen, despite marked PCO_2 variations (to normalize ICP and CEO_2 simultaneously), the SjO_2 remains predominantly within the normal range (i.e., both profoundly and moderately optimized hyperventilation effectively offset the pathologic condition of relative cerebral hyperperfusion, which would have been associated with abnormally high SjO_2 values had the patients been kept normocapnic).

Potential Pitfalls of Jugular Monitoring

True limitations of either continuous or intermittent arteriojugular monitoring are rare. In patients with regional lesions detected on computed tomography of

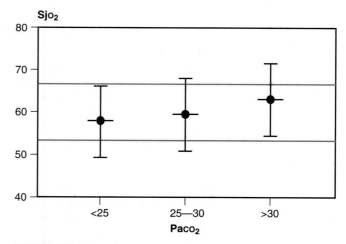

FIGURE 15–6. Jugular bulb oxyhemoglobin saturation (SjO_2, in percent) plotted against arterial PCO_2 ($PaCO_2$, in torr) in a large series of patients who underwent optimized hyperventilation therapy for combined normalization of intracranial pressure and cerebral extraction of oxygen. *Vertical bars* represent one standard deviation from the mean. *Horizontal lines* indicate the upper and the lower normal limits for SjO_2. Despite marked intentional PCO_2 variations, the SjO_2 remained essentially within its normal range. (See text for further details.)

maintain stable CBF (and therefore SjO_2 and CEO_2) as the blood pressure drops within the normal range. Therefore, unlike mannitol administration and hyperventilation, pentobarbital administration (especially bolus injections) has not yet been optimized by use of the jugular monitoring technique. Future studies are required, perhaps involving administration of vasopressors even before barbiturate boluses.

In contrast to indiscriminate hyperventilation, our approach has involved optimized hyperventilation, a dynamic process of ventilatory manipulations (frequently combined with mannitol administration). In this approach, we initially adopt moderate hypocapnia (partial pressure of carbon dioxide [PCO_2] levels close to 26 to 30 torr) on the first day, followed by profound hypocapnia ($PCO_2 < 26$ torr), usually on days two through four. By days five through seven, we *slowly* reverse the profound hypocapnic process toward near-normocapnic PCO_2 levels, so that ICP monitoring can be safely discontinued by the end of 1 week in most patients.

the head, jugular monitoring is also useful. This is particularly true when regional lesions (e.g., hemorrhagic contusions) are not manageable nonsurgically, as is frequently the case. The overall philosophy underlying jugular monitoring is that it provides information about cerebral hemometabolism from 90% to 98% (or more) of the brain in most selected patients. Therefore, global brain monitoring and management have resulted in ultrahigh rates of globally well-recovered brains.

Conversely, when a primarily regional vascular insult is suspected or confirmed (e.g., regional cerebral vasospasm in aneurysmal subarachnoid hemorrhage), the global monitor is not expected to help. As listed in Table 15–1, however, a broad spectrum of acute intracranial insults is associated with *predominantly* (not necessarily exclusively) global abnormalities, insofar as cerebral hemometabolic patterns are concerned.

Furthermore, ICP and CPP are also global measurements, and over the years a large variety of therapeutic approaches have become available for global ICP and CPP management. Normal-to-increased CPP, however, totally lacks information regarding cerebral metabolic activity, as we have unequivocally demonstrated. Arteriojugular monitoring and management are therefore necessary to supplement ICP and CPP assessment properly.

Alternative Monitoring Modalities

For bedside monitoring, some alternative modalities to arteriojugular monitoring have been proposed. First, noninvasive near-infrared spectroscopy has been contemplated. This monitoring modality, however, is being abandoned because of several limitations, as follows:

1. Any layer of blood between the probe and the brain tissue will generate artifactual values.
2. The monitor assumes a normal arteriolovenular compartmental oxygen distribution in pathologic brain tissue, which is not a true reflection of the state of the brain in several circumstances.
3. Skin burns may frequently develop.
4. Marked variations in SjO_2 may not be detected by the near-infrared monitor.

Highly invasive, transcranially placed monitors are also available for measurement of the partial pressure of oxygen (PO_2) in brain tissue or for the assessment of a variety of cerebral metabolic elements with microdialysis. In this respect, acute placement of brain tissue probes produces focal microvascular compression and distortion, with resulting *false* low tissue oxygen values relative to the global brain. This limitation may have catastrophic implications for patient care because attempts to increase CBF or cerebral blood

volume (e.g., by increasing the PCO_2 or the blood pressure) may induce intracranial herniation and death if patients present with compromised basilar cisterns. Moreover, not even normal values are known for brain tissue PO_2 in humans (because healthy humans will not volunteer to have a monitor placed transcranially).

In the case of microdialysis, in addition to focal microvascular compression, disruption of the blood-brain barrier may also occur. Therefore, it is not surprising to find artificially low tissue PO_2 and high tissue lactate values with these probes. The same applies to other elements, such as glutamate. Again, just as for brain tissue PO_2, normal values in humans are not known for elements evaluated by microdialysis.

An additional positive feature of arteriojugular monitoring is that virtually any element measurable in blood (besides oxygen) can be evaluated from arteriojugular samples. Therefore, for bedside monitoring, the arteriojugular technique is the most solid. For regional (or focal) monitoring, however, bedside techniques are much too limited and are even dangerous, as described earlier. It therefore remains for positron emission tomography or functional magnetic resonance imaging to provide information on regional abnormalities. These two techniques, however, *do not* apply to unstable patients, whose best environment is the intensive care unit during the acute phase of illness.

Suggested Readings

1. Bouma GJ, Muizelaar JP, Choi SC, et al: Cerebral circulation and metabolism after severe traumatic brain injury: The elusive role of ischemia. J Neurosurg 1991;75:685–693.
2. Cruz J: On-line monitoring of global cerebral hypoxia in acute brain injury. Relationship to intracranial hypertension. J Neurosurg 1993;79:228–233.
3. Cruz J: Adverse effects of pentobarbital on cerebral venous oxygenation of comatose patients with acute traumatic brain swelling: Relationship to outcome. J Neurosurg 1996;85:758–761.
4. Cruz J: The first decade of continuous monitoring of jugular bulb oxyhemoglobin saturation: Management strategies and clinical outcome. Crit Care Med 1998;26:344–351.
5. Cruz J, Gennarelli TA, Alves WM: Continuous monitoring of cerebral hemodynamic reserve in acute brain injury: Relationship to changes in brain swelling. J Trauma 1992;32:629–635.
6. Cruz J, Jaggi JL, Hoffstad OJ: Cerebral blood flow, vascular resistance, and oxygen metabolism in acute brain trauma: Redefining the role of cerebral perfusion pressure? Crit Care Med 1995;23:1412–1417.
7. Cruz J, Minoja G, Mattioli C, et al: Severe acute brain trauma. In Cruz J (ed): Neurologic and Neurosurgical Emergencies. Philadelphia, WB Saunders, 1998, pp 405–436.
8. Cruz J, Miner ME, Allen SJ, et al: Continuous monitoring of cerebral oxygenation in acute brain injury: Injection of mannitol during hyperventilation. J Neurosurg 1990;73:725–730.
9. Jaggi JL, Obrist WD, Gennarelli TA, et al: Relationship of early cerebral blood flow and metabolism to outcome in acute head injury. J Neurosurg 1990;72:176–182.
10. Kiening KL, Unterberg AW, Bardt TF, et al: Monitoring of cerebral oxygenation in patients with severe head injuries: Brain

tissue Po$_2$ versus jugular vein oxygen saturation. J Neurosurg 1996;85:751–757.

11. Lewis SB, Myburgh JA, Thornton EL, et al: Cerebral oxygenation monitoring by near-infrared spectroscopy is not clinically useful in patients with severe closed-head injury: A comparison with jugular venous bulb oximetry. Crit Care Med 1996;24:1334–1338.

12. Marion DW, Darby J, Yonas H: Acute regional cerebral blood flow changes caused by severe head injuries. J Neurosurg 1991;74:407–414.

13. Muizelaar JP, Marmarou AM, Ward JD, et al: Adverse effects of prolonged hyperventilation in patients with severe head injury: A randomized clinical trial. J Neurosurg 1991;75:731–739.

14. Obrist WD, Langfitt TW, Jaggi JL, et al: Cerebral blood flow and metabolism in comatose patients with acute head injury. Relationship to intracranial hypertension. J Neurosurg 1984; 61:241–253.

15. Rosner MJ, Rosner SD, Johnson AH: Cerebral perfusion pressure: Management protocol and clinical results. J Neurosurg 1995;83:949–962.

16 Cardiac Pacemaker Placement

Ismael N. Nuño

Major advances have occurred in recent years in every aspect of care provided in intensive care units. It is important for any intensivist or physician caring for the critically ill to know how to insert and manage a pacemaker, either temporary or permanent.

Types of Pacing

Temporary pacing is done for a short period of time (hours, days, or weeks) with the expectancy that at some point it will no longer be required. Temporary pacing devices include externally applied gum patches and internally inserted pacing transvenous catheters, which may be secured to the right ventricular endocardium. Access for these catheters can be via the right or the left internal jugular vein, the right or the left subclavian vein, the right or the left cephalic or basilic vein, or the right or the left femoral vein. If the chest is open for other reasons (median sternotomy or lateral thoracotomy), temporary epicardial pacing wires may also be placed. Current endovascular cardiopulmonary bypass techniques have used temporary esophageal atrial pacing with good success. Permanent pacing systems should be inserted once the need for long-term therapy (more than 2 weeks) has been definitively established. The usual accepted access site for permanent pacemaker systems is through either the left or the right subclavian vein.

Current batteries employ lithium. Their sizes and thicknesses may vary, but they are usually approximately 3 cm in diameter and ¼ to ½ cm in thickness. The battery needs to lie in a flat nonmobile tissue such as the anterior chest wall in order not to dislodge the lead-battery connections, fray the lead, and thereby reduce the life expectancy of the implanted system. Historically, permanent pacemakers were inserted via the cephalic veins through a cutdown at the deltopectoral groove (Fig. 16–1). The approach was safe with minimal risk of complications (e.g., pneumothorax).

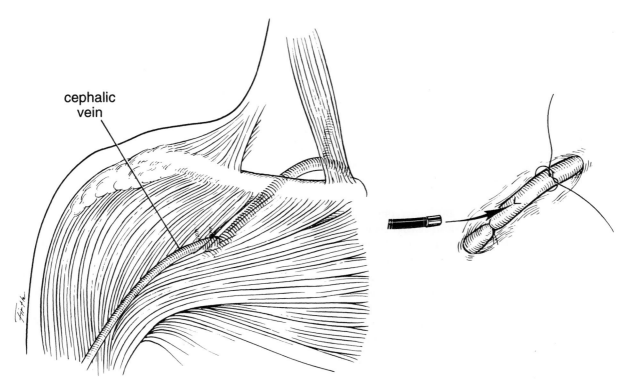

cephalic vein

FIGURE 16–1. Use of the cephalic vein via dissection of the right deltopectoral groove. *Inset,* Distal ligation of vein and insertion of catheter centrally.

With modern disposable insertion kits, the subclavian veins can be safely and readily used.

In a temporary situation, the right ventricle is usually paced to ensure ventricular contraction and maintenance of cardiac output. Atrial pacing in these situations is also feasible but is not as safe as right ventricular pacing because the atrioventricular (AV) node may fail and result in no ventricular contraction at all.

Permanent pacemakers may employ right ventricular, right atrial, or right AV two-chamber pacing. The North American Society of Pacing and Electrophysiology and the British Pacing and Electrophysiology Group have developed an internationally accepted nomenclature classifying pacemakers by mode of function: AOO (atrial pacing), VVI (ventricular demand pacing), DVI (AV sequential pacing), and DDD (AV sequential demand pacing). For most patients in intensive care units, permanent pacing is usually limited to atrial, ventricular, or AV sequential modes.

Technique

Temporary or permanent pacemakers can be inserted either at the bedside or in the radiology or cardiology suite. Sterile technique is important and should include full skin preparation and use of sterile sheets, gowns, gloves, hats, and facemasks. Perioperative antibiotics should also be given. Fluoroscopy may or may not be used for insertion of a temporary pacer but should always be used for insertion of a permanent system. Protection of the patient and the physician from unnecessary radiation is essential.

Temporary pacing leads (e.g., Cordis) are used at our institution. Placement of the lead is carried out with either electrocardiographic monitoring or fluoroscopy, depending on the urgency of the clinical situation and the availability of equipment. The pacing lead is introduced into the right ventricle and is manipulated to lie at or near the apex of the right ventricle (Fig. 16–2). Once the lead has been properly placed in the right ventricular endocardium, it is hooked up to a pacing box. We use the Medtronic (Redmond, Wash) pacing system. The usual settings for the pacemaker are heart rate of 60 to 90 beats per minute (bpm), output of 0.1 to 20 mA, and asynchronous, or 20 to 1 mV, sensitivity. If the patient is bradycardic or asystolic, the best attempt should be to pace the patient at 80 bpm. If the patient has a rhythm but has occasional episodes of bradycardia or asystole, it is better to leave the existent rhythm but to place the pacer as a backup at around 60 bpm. The pacing threshold should be tested. Gradually lower the mA until there is no capture. If the mA necessary to generate electrical activity alarms exceeds 10 mA, consider relocating the endocardial leads or the epicardial pacing wires.

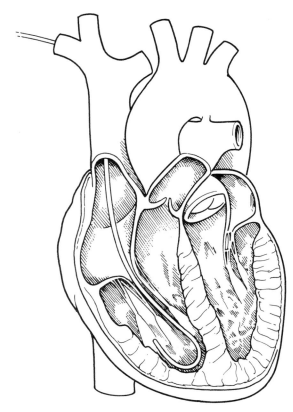

FIGURE 16–2. Passage of an endocardial lead (temporary or permanent) into the right ventricular chamber.

The insertion of a permanent pacer will employ the abovementioned basic techniques. Venous access should be via the right or the left subclavian vein. The battery will need to rest on the anterior surface of the chest wall in a subcutaneous or submuscular position. Access into the subclavian vein is obtained with percutaneous puncture. We use the "Peel-away" Introducer Set (Cook Critical Care, Bloomington, Ind). It has a split-sheet sheath system by which the lead can be introduced intravenously. The sheath is split and is removed, leaving the lead in its proper place. The patient may require one lead (ventricular) or two leads (atrial and ventricular) (Fig. 16–3). Once the leads are in proper position and tested, they are secured to the muscle with silicone holding sheaths, are sutured to the muscle fascia with interrupted 2–0 silk stitches, and are securely tied down (Fig. 16–4). The leads are inserted into the battery pack, and the battery is buried in the chest wall (Fig. 16–5). The wound is then closed in various layers after antibiotic irrigation, and hemostasis is secured. Scarpa's fascia is closed with running or interrupted 3–0 Vicryl sutures, and the skin is approximated with running 4–0 Vicryl sutures. Sterile dressings are applied.

Incisions for the insertion of a permanent pacemaker should be kept meticulously clean. Nursing care should include application of topical antibiotics to the

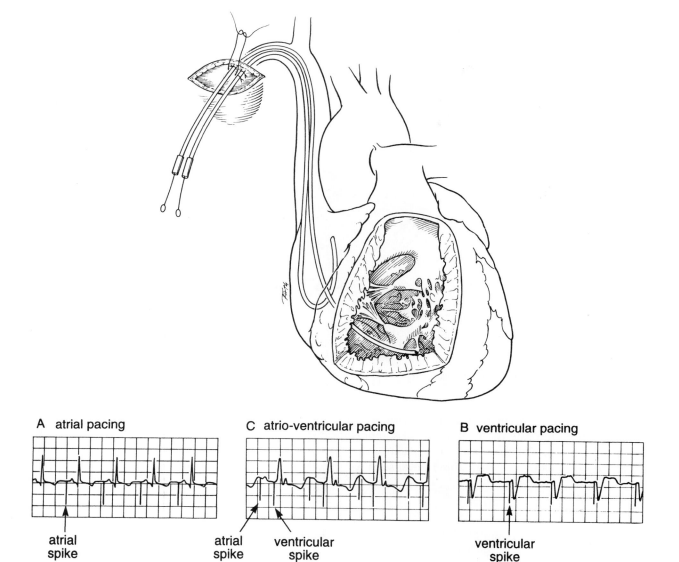

A atrial pacing

atrial
spike

C atrio-ventricular pacing

atrial
spike

ventricular
spike

B ventricular pacing

ventricular
spike

FIGURE 16–3. Proper positioning of atrial and ventricular endocardial leads for dual-chamber systems.

wound and coverage with a clear transparent dressing for 2 days. Thereafter, the wound should be painted daily with Betadine (povidone-iodine) solution and allowed to air dry. The implanted leads and the generator must be registered with the manufacturer.

For various reasons, on occasion the critically ill patient may have undergone open median sternotomy or thoracotomy. Episodes of bradycardia or asystole can be controlled by the immediate placement of epicardial pacing wires connected to an external pacing box via intermediary cables (Fig. 16–6). Two intramuscular wires can be placed quickly by piercing the epicardium. This technique will pace the ventricles but not the atria. If the lack of atrial contraction results in a low cardiac output syndrome with hypotension, two atrial wires may also be placed, and AV pacing may be carried out. In this way, atrial contraction supplements cardiac output by nearly 20%.

Indications

Atrial Pacing

Atrial pacing requires a normal sinus rhythm or sinus bradycardia. The AV node must be functioning satisfactorily. The indications for atrial pacing include the following:

1. Sinus bradycardia (fewer than 60 bpm).
2. Premature ventricular complexes (bigeminy, trigeminy, or quadrigeminy or more than 10 premature ventricular contractions per minute).
3. Premature atrial complexes (atrial fibrillation, atrial flutter, or more than 10 premature atrial contractions per minute). In these cases, one can manage the patients by overdrive pacing (i.e., selecting a rate on the pacer 10 beats faster than the patient's

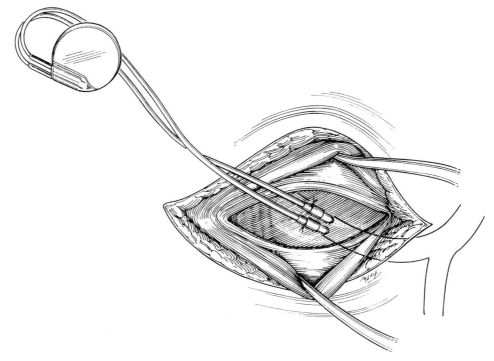

FIGURE 16–4. Atrial and ventricular leads attached to a battery generator and well secured to the pectoral muscle fascia.

own rhythm with the arrhythmias). For example, if the atrial fibrillation rate is 135 bpm, select a generator box rate of 145 bpm. Once it is pacing, decrease the rate to a more reasonable figure, such as

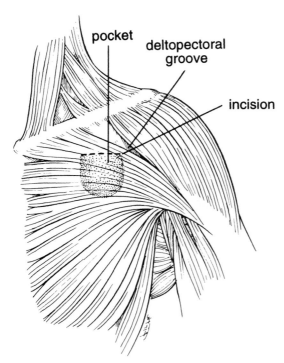

FIGURE 16–5. Positioning of generator pack either anterior to pectoral fascia or buried behind the pectoral muscle. To avoid pocket seromas and hematomas, hemostasis should be meticulous, and the size of the pocket should be no larger than the size of the battery.

60 to 80 bpm. Another option is to turn the generator off suddenly and allow the patient's own rhythm to be regained, hopefully without the arrhythmia.
4. Slow junctional rhythm (fewer than 45 bpm).
5. Postoperative use after cardiac surgery (temporary epicardial wires).

Ventricular Pacing (VVI Mode)

Ventricular output should be on demand mode. Otherwise, it may discharge on the T wave and trigger ventricular fibrillation. Indications include the following:

1. Atrial fibrillation or flutter with ventricular response of fewer than 60 or greater than 130 bpm.
2. Failure of atrial pacing to transmit through the AV node, resulting in lack of ventricular contraction.
3. Overdrive pacing of ventricular tachycardia, as in atrial pacing.
4. Postoperative use after cardiac surgery (temporary epicardial wires).
5. Bradycardia of fewer than 60 bpm in cardiac injuries (temporary epicardial wires).

Dual-Chamber Pacing (Sequential Atrioventricular Pacing)

Indications for dual-chamber pacing include the following:

1. Complete heart block.
2. Second-degree heart block to achieve 1:1 conduction.

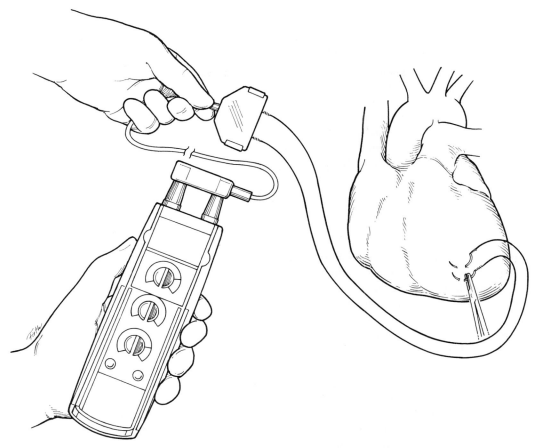

FIGURE 16–6. Two epicardial wires are placed on the anterior surface of the right ventricle. Both wires are attached to a connecting cable and to the external battery box.

3. First-degree heart block if 1:1 conduction cannot be achieved at a faster rate because of a long PR interval.
4. Postoperative use after cardiac surgery (temporary).
5. Bradycardia of fewer than 60 bpm in cardiac injuries (temporary pacing).
6. DDD pacing for fast atrial rates of greater than 120 bpm with second- or third-degree heart block.

Atrioventricular pacing is preferable to ventricular pacing because of the atrial contribution to ventricular filling. If sudden hemodynamic deterioration occurs during AV pacing, atrial fibrillation may have occurred.

Contraindications to Implantation of Permanent Pacemakers

The implantation of temporary pacing leads or wires in a critically ill patient will most likely occur in an emergency situation rather than as prophylaxis. In these cases, even in the presence of sepsis, there is an emergent need to treat asystole or severe and symptomatic bradycardia or heart block. Insertion of a permanent pacemaker in patients in the intensive care unit should be delayed until good control of sepsis has been obtained. Also, if an accurate diagnosis of bradycardia or arrhythmia cannot be made with certainty, electrophysiologic studies may be carried out by specially trained cardiologists to ascertain the true need for a pacemaker.

Pitfalls

Poor contact or lack of contact at connection sites is a common problem encountered in pacemaker implantation. There may be poor contact involving the lead in the endocardium or the wire at the epicardium. The contact between the wire or the lead and the connecting cables may be faulty. The insertion of the cables into the pulse generator may be loose, or the pulse generator battery may be low in voltage. The development of new atrial fibrillation may cause failure of atrial capture. Electrodes located in areas of poor electrical contact and high threshold will lead to poor function. Competition between the patient's own intrinsic rhythm and the pulse generator signal may become a problem and may lead to arrhythmias or frequent ectopic atrial or ventricular beats.

Solution. Check all connections. You may even need to change the connecting cable. Also, to increase or obtain capture, increase the output of the pulse generator to a maximum current of 20 mA. Use a different wire electrode as the negative (conducting) electrode. Unipolarize the pacemaker by attaching the positive lead to a surface electrocardiography electrode or a skin pacing wire. Convert to ventricular pacing if the atrial lead fails to capture. If there is competition between the patient's intrinsic rhythm and the pacemaker signal, either turn off the pacemaker generator or reduce the generator rate to less than the patient's rhythm.

Tips and Precautions

1. Serum potassium levels greater than 5.5 to 6 mEq/ L may lead to poor capture and conduction of paced signals. Certainly, levels greater than 6.5 to 7 mEq/L will lead to a near-catastrophic lack of conduction of electrical signals.
   Solution: Institute immediate treatment of hyperkalemia with medical therapy.
2. Poorly placed or secured leads (temporary or permanent) will lead to dislodgement and will result in either no pacing or irregular pacing. This may result in death if the patient is 100% dependent on pacing for any cardiac function. Irregular or intermittent pacing may result in a ventricular arrhythmia, such as ventricular fibrillation.
   Solution: Under fluoroscopic guidance, place or reposition endocardial leads, which should be securely sutured to surrounding tissues. Replace epicardial wires to muscular areas of the heart.
3. Sudden loss of pacemaker artifact on electrocardiography is usually caused by connection problems. Oversensing by the generator may be at fault, or disconnection may have occurred anywhere along the electrical circuit from endocardium or epicardium to generator box.
   Solution: Check all cable and wire connections, including batteries. For oversensing, turn the sensitivity knob all the way to the left to asynchronous pacing.
4. Connected and functioning temporary or permanent pacemaker generators may be deprogrammed by interference with static signals from other equipment, such as electrocautery.
   Solution: In these cases, thermal cautery is preferable. If a permanent generator is deprogrammed,

immediate reprogramming should be done. If there are no recognizable signals from the pulse generator, external pacing may be started until reprogramming can be accomplished.

5. A sudden change in normal pulse and rhythm in a patient with either a temporary or a permanent pacemaker should alert the clinician that either the patient has developed a supraventricular arrhythmia (atrial fibrillation or flutter) or frequent premature atrial or ventricular contractions are occurring. The pacemaker may become ineffective. Multiple ectopic beats may signal competition between the patient's own rhythm and the paced impulse.
   Solution: Correct arrhythmias medically with antiarrhythmogenic drugs. Sometimes just stopping the pacing reverts the patient back to a regular rhythm. If the pacer is competing with the patient's own underlying rhythm, stop the pacing completely or decrease the pacer rate to below that of the patient's own heart rate. The backup pacer rate is usually set at 50 to 60 bpm.
6. Occasionally, a patient being paced may sustain an episode of ventricular fibrillation. The ABCs of cardiopulmonary resuscitation (airway, breathing, circulation) should be initiated. If the pacer is still on, the electrical stimulus may prolong the episode of fibrillation.
   Solution: Turn the pace generator off immediately. Cardiovert the patient electrically. If the patient becomes asystolic or bradycardic after cardioversion, restart pacing.

Suggested Readings

1. Atlee JL, Pattison CZ, Mathews EL, Hedman AG: Transesophageal atrial pacing for intraoperative sinus bradycardia or AV junctional rhythm. J Cardiothorac Vasc Anesth 1993;7:436–441.
2. Bojar R, Warner K: Manual of Perioperative Care in Cardiac Surgery, 3rd ed. Boston, Blackwell Science, 1999, pp 274–284.
3. Broka SM, Ducart AR, Caolard EL, et al: Hemodynamic benefit of optimizing atrioventricular delay after cardiopulmonary bypass. J Cardiothorac Vasc Anesth 1997;11:723–728.
4. Dreifus LS, Fisch C, Griffin JC: Guidelines for implantation of cardiac pacemakers and antiarrhythmic devices. A report of the American College of Cardiology/American Heart Association Task Force on Assessment of Diagnostic and Therapeutic Cardiovascular Procedures (Committee on Pacemaker Implantation). J Am Coll Cardiol 1991;18:1–13.
5. Heger J, Niemann J, Roth F, Criley M: Cardiology, 4th ed. Philadelphia, Lippincott Williams & Wilkins, 1998, pp 373–380.
6. Kusumoto FM, Goldschlager N: Cardiac pacing. N Engl J Med 1996;334:89–97.

17 Inferior Vena Caval Filter Placement

Vincent L. Rowe and Douglas B. Hood

Pulmonary embolism (PE) continues to contribute to morbidity and mortality in hospitalized patients. Plentiful evidence linking PE with deep venous thrombosis (DVT) led to the development of multiple methods of DVT prophylaxis. The main methods that have reduced the incidence of DVT include anticoagulation (either low-molecular-weight or unfractionated heparin), the use of sequential compression devices, and early mobilization after surgery. Despite these, there remains a subgroup of patients at high risk of developing DVT and PE, namely, neurosurgical, orthopedic, and multitrauma patients. In these high-risk patients, reluctance to prescribe anticoagulation because of the fear of bleeding complications and poor use of sequential compression devices secondary to long bone fractures treated with fixation devices can limit prophylaxis. As such, this subdivision of patients requires a more aggressive approach to treatment and prophylaxis of thrombotic and embolic events. Additionally, patients with recurrent episodes of venous thromboembolism despite anticoagulant treatment, congenital coagulation tendency, or unstable myocardial function who are at risk of thromboembolism may need aggressive measures to reduce the likelihood of death following an acute episode.

Vena caval interruption has been an effective method of PE prophylaxis for more than 30 years. Advances in technology have allowed insertion of inferior vena caval (IVC) filters percutaneously, simplifying their placement. Until recently, percutaneous IVC filter placement was routinely performed in the interventional radiology suite or the operating room under fluoroscopic guidance. In most circumstances, transportation to these treatment areas is easily accomplished. For patients in the intensive care unit, however, transportation may be difficult and in some cases dangerous owing to ventilator dependency; the presence of intravenous lines and medications, drains and tubes, and invasive monitors; and immobilization of spinal or orthopedic injuries. Bedside placement of IVC filters alleviates transportation risks and has been shown to be a safe and more cost-effective treatment. Placement using duplex ultrasonography and fluoroscopic guidance is described here.

Indications

Indications for bedside IVC filter placement are identical to those for placement in any other location.

Absolute Indications

1. Presence of a contraindication to anticoagulation in patients with a known PE or DVT. Major contraindications include active hemorrhage; recent hemorrhagic stroke; recent ocular, spinal, or neurosurgical procedures; recent major trauma; and intracranial tumor.
2. Recurrent PE despite adequate anticoagulation.
3. Inability to anticoagulate or the presence of complications resulting from anticoagulation.
4. Previous pulmonary embolectomy.

Relative Indications

1. Chronic PE in patients with pulmonary hypertension.
2. Large free-floating iliofemoral thrombus.
3. Significant cardiopulmonary disease and poor reserve in a patient who cannot tolerate a PE of any magnitude.
4. Septic embolus.

Prophylactic Indications

1. Multisystem high-risk trauma requiring prolonged immobilization. Risk factors include extensive long bone fractures treated with fixation devices, spinal cord injuries, older age, and need for multiple blood transfusions. Patients in this category must be selected on an individual basis.

Filter Types

Since the introduction of caval interruption, manufacturers have produced IVC filters with variations in design but one common purpose: clot capture. In most cases, filter type selection should be based on operator and hospital preference and cost (Fig. 17–1).

Stainless Steel Greenfield Filter. Greenfield has been one of the leaders in pioneering vena caval interruption devices. The stainless steel Greenfield filter (Medi-Tech/Boston Scientific, Watertown, Mass) was first introduced in 1972 and has the longest reported follow-

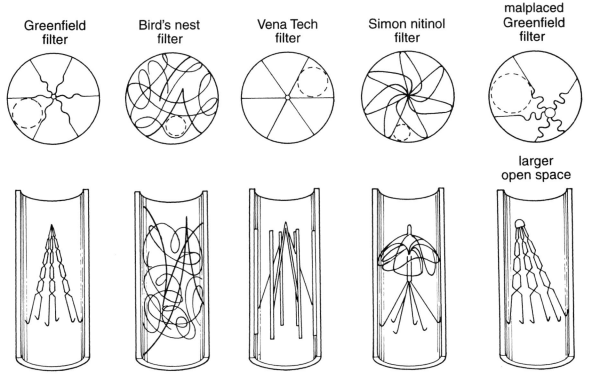

FIGURE 17-1. Various types of inferior vena caval filters. Note the orientation of the struts on the malpositioned Greenfield filter, which potentially allows clots to flow through.

up in the literature. The filter is 4.6 cm in length from the apex to the base. Fixation occurs via six angled struts with small curled hooks at the end. Caval patency and recurrent PE rates with long-term follow-up are 98% and 4%, respectively. The frequency of initial problems (e.g., a high rate of insertion site thrombosis) has decreased with the use of lower-profile carrier systems.

Titanium Greenfield Filter. The titanium Greenfield filter (Medi-Tech/Boston Scientific, Watertown, Mass) is the most recent version of the original stainless steel model. It has a similar conical shape but has the following modifications:

1. Titanium metal construct. Titanium is felt to help increase strut strength and diminish strut fatigue.
2. Slightly larger size: 0.5 cm taller and 0.8 cm wider.
3. Increased curvature of the hooks to reduce IVC wall penetration and filter migration.

Follow-up studies show recurrent PE and IVC patency rates similar to those associated with the stainless steel model but with reduced migration rates.

Vena Tech Filter. The Vena Tech filter (B. Braun Medical Division, Evanston, Ill) was introduced in 1986 and is made from a metal alloy similar to that used for cardiac pacing wires. The filter construct consists of six angled prongs connected to six vertically oriented siderails for vessel wall adherence. The total filter length is 3.8 cm. This design is felt to improve centralization of the filter in the IVC. Recurrent PE and IVC

patency rates are comparable to those associated with Greenfield filters in small studies.

Simon Nitinol Filter. The Simon nitinol filter (Nitinol Medical Technologies, Woburn, Mass; Bard Inc., Billerica, Mass) was approved for use by the United States Food and Drug Administration in 1990. The filter has six fixation struts with hooks that support a 28-mm dome of seven overlapping circular loops. The filter is made from a combination of nickel and titanium and has the unique feature of thermal memory. At cool temperatures (4°C to 10°C), the filter wires are aligned in a straight, tight configuration. Once warmed to body temperature, the filter resumes its predetermined shape. Because of this property, it is recommended that the filter be flushed with cold saline solution before deployment. When compared with the previously discussed filters, equivalent recurrent PE rates but lower caval patency rates have been reported. (Note: Comparison was not done in a randomized prospective study.)

Bird's Nest Filter. The name of the bird's nest filter (Cook Critical Care, Bloomington, Ind) comes from the resemblance of the mesh configuration within the IVC to the nest of a bird. The filter was introduced clinically in 1982 and consists of an array of four 25-cm wires, each attached to a securing strut with fixation hooks. The potential advantages of this device are the following:

1. The complex array of wires will capture smaller emboli.

2. Veins up to 4 cm in diameter can be accommodated.
3. No intraluminal centering is required.
4. A longer segment of IVC is protected (7 cm); therefore, potential emboli from collateral veins will be eliminated.

With recent revisions in the construct, the frequency of earlier problems (e.g., filter migration) has been considerably reduced. Recurrent PE rates are reported to be less than 3%.

Technique

Fluoroscopically Guided Placement

With the availability of high-quality imaging via portable fluoroscopy, bedside fluoroscopically guided placement of IVC filters can be performed safely without significant difficulty. The advantages of fluoroscopic placement over duplex-directed placement are (1) precise and more easily interpreted visualization of the IVC and the iliac veins is possible, and (2) bony landmarks can be used for filter positioning if needed. The disadvantages include exposure to ionizing radiation and the need for intravenous contrast material. Although the use of carbon dioxide as the contrast agent can eliminate the deleterious effects of intravenous administration, this technique is very difficult at the bedside and is currently better performed in a dedicated angiography suite.

Screening

A screening duplex ultrasound to check for thrombosis of the IVC and the iliofemoral venous system should be performed to help determine a proper access site.

Insertion

Preparations similar to those described for duplex-directed placement are made. Fluoroscopy is used to define the L2-L4 vertebral body region. Seldinger technique is used to cannulate the desired common femoral vein. A 4- to 5-Fr pigtail angiographic catheter is advanced over a guidewire in the IVC to the L2 region under direct fluoroscopic visualization. Contrast venography is performed to measure the IVC diameter and to document the location of the renal veins. For increased delineation of anatomy, selective cannulation of individual renal veins can be performed. The location of the renal veins may be correlated with a bony landmark to prevent improper filter placement with patient movement. If the renal veins cannot be accurately defined, the L2-L3 vertebral interspace may be used as a marker for safe filter deployment. The renal veins usually correspond to the L1-L2 vertebral bodies.

After venography has been completed, the pigtail catheter is exchanged over a wire for the dilator-sheath complex. The dilator is removed immediately after the sheath has been positioned just inferior to the renal veins. The filter carrier system is then put into position and is secured to the sheath (Fig. 17–2). Again, if any resistance is encountered during passage of the filter unit through the iliac veins, the filter unit and the sheath should be advanced simultaneously until the IVC is reached. The benefit is that this maneuver can be done with improved visualization. Before deployment, flushing with heparinized saline solution is performed to prevent thrombus accumulation. The IVC filter is then deployed in the standard fashion and with minimal delay to minimize clot adherence to the filter.

Completion venography is performed to confirm the technical adequacy of the procedure. The completion venogram should document the following: deployment at the desired level, no extravasation of contrast material through the wall of the IVC, complete opening of the filter, and minimal tilting.

Pitfalls

1. Poor visualization of the renal veins can be overcome by selective catheterization of each renal vein during preinsertion venography or by using the bony landmarks (L2-L3 vertebral bodies) to guide placement.
2. In IVCs larger than 2.8 cm, Greenfield filters cannot be used because it is difficult to secure the struts in the wall of the cava properly. An inferior vena cava of this size is usually seen in patients with right heart failure. If vena caval interruption is required, a bird's nest filter should be placed under fluoroscopic guidance. Deployment of this type of filter is best performed in a formal angiography suite. One other alternative for filter placement in a large IVC is use of the bilateral common iliac veins.

Duplex-Directed Placement

Duplex-directed bedside placement of IVC filters has received substantial attention recently. Advantages of using duplex guidance include avoidance of the need for intravenous contrast material and ionizing radiation, thus negating any side effects of these agents. This technique requires a skilled vascular technologist, however, because visualization of the vascular landmarks can be difficult or impossible in certain cases.

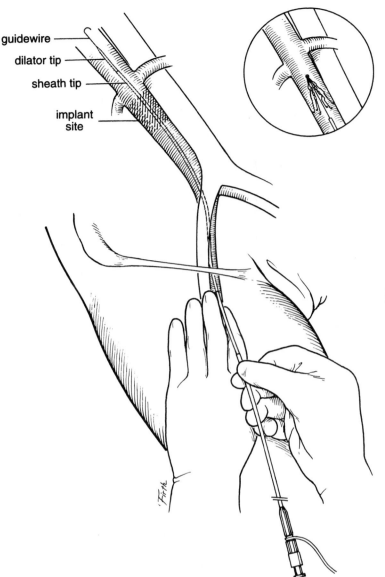

guidewire —
dilator tip —
sheath tip —
implant site —

FIGURE 17–2. Insertion of a filter via the femoral route. The filter is deployed below the level of the renal veins.

Screening

Once appropriate candidates for bedside IVC filter placement have been selected, screening duplex ultrasonography of the IVC and the iliofemoral veins is mandatory to assess proper visualization of the vascular landmarks used in the procedure. The duplex machine should be set on the "low-medium flow" selection. A low-frequency transducer is used to visualize the perirenal IVC for accurate measurements. Begin scanning transversely with color flow, and identify the celiac artery and the superior mesenteric artery. Just distal to the superior mesenteric artery, the left renal vein and the renal arteries can be visualized. This portion of the IVC should be the most carefully evaluated area. Measurements of the IVC are obtained in the longitudinal and the transverse planes. The IVC should not measure more than 2.8 cm in transverse diameter for placement of most currently available filters.

In the longitudinal view, the perirenal IVC with the right renal artery (RRA) passing posteriorly is imaged. The RRA serves as an important landmark for guiding filter positioning in the IVC inferior to the renal veins. If the landmarks are not seen or if any anomalies are present in the IVC (e.g., duplicate IVC) or the renal arteries, duplex-directed placement should be abandoned. The screening duplex ultrasound should ensure patency and the lack of thrombus formation in the IVC and at least one of the iliofemoral veins. If bilateral iliofemoral DVTs are present or passage through the iliac veins would be treacherous owing to the patient's condition, placement via the internal jugular vein is preferred (Fig. 17–3). In this case, screening duplex ultrasonography should ensure patency of the veins in the cervical region.

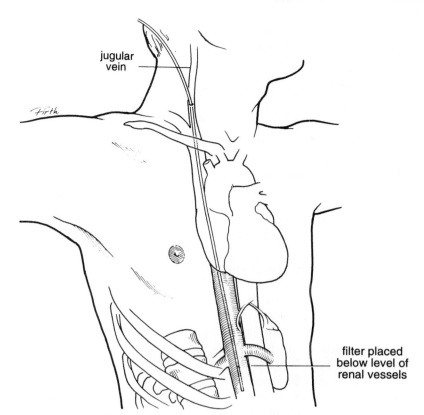

jugular
vein

Firth

filter placed
below level of
renal vessels

FIGURE 17–3. Insertion of a filter via the jugular route.

Insertion

If visualization is adequate, the patient is prepared for the procedure. Preoperative antibiotics are not routinely indicated. Also, continuous heparin infusions should be discontinued 1 to 2 hours before the procedure. Although an approach through either groin area may be used, the right groin is preferred for ease of cannulation. After administration of a local anesthetic agent, the common femoral vein is cannulated, and a 0.035-inch guidewire is passed into the upper regions of the vena cava using the Seldinger technique. Imaging of the IVC in the longitudinal position is maintained throughout the procedure. Gray-scale imaging of the IVC at this point may help with identification of the filter system hardware. By using the RRA as a landmark, the dilator-sheath complex is inserted over the wire, and the dilator is then removed. The tip of the delivery sheath should be positioned 1 to 2 cm inferior to the RRA. The filter carrier system is then placed in position and is secured to the sheath.

Occasionally, resistance is encountered during passage of the filter unit through the iliac veins. In this case, advance the filter unit and the sheath simultaneously until the IVC is reached. Before deployment, the unit is flushed with 5 to 10 mL of heparinized saline solution (10 units of heparin per 1 mL of normal saline mixture) to avoid thrombus accumulation. The IVC filter is then deployed in the standard fashion and with minimal delay to minimize clot adherence to the filter. After deployment, the sheath is removed, and digital pressure is placed at the puncture site until no bleeding is seen. The patient is maintained on bed rest for at least 2 hours. Completion duplex ultrasonography with color flow and plain radiography are performed to ensure proper filter positioning.

Pitfalls

1. Suboptimal visualization of the IVC (in approximately 10% of patients). Limitations to obtaining adequate visualization of the IVC include extensive bowel gas (postoperative ileus or bowel obstruction), obesity, retroperitoneal hematomas, and open abdominal wounds. Use of bowel cathartics and ensuring that the patient takes nothing by mouth for at least 8 hours before screening duplex ultrasonography may improve visualization. Also, avoid long delays between the screening duplex scan and filter placement to decrease the interval accumulation of unwanted bowel gas.
2. IVC larger than 2.8 cm.

Complications

Filter Tilting. There is approximately a 5% incidence of filter tilting, either at the time of placement or over a period of follow-up. The change in position can be due to migration of the filter or a fracture of one of the struts. Tilting is potentially dangerous because the change in position can create distortion of the natural filter shape. Enlarged gaps between the struts may decrease the clot-trapping ability of the filter. In vitro studies have shown that as few as 15 degrees of tilting off the vertical axis diminishes the clot-capturing capability of the filter, increasing the risk of PE. If the position is such that function of the filter is questioned, one option for correction is intraluminal manipulation under fluoroscopic guidance. This method carries the potential risk of further filter migration, endothelial damage, or IVC perforation. The other option would be to place a second IVC filter above the malpositioned one at the level of T12 via the internal jugular vein (see "Suprarenal Inferior Vena Caval Filter Placement").

Filter Malposition. In general, IVC filters should be placed in the IVC just caudal to the renal veins. This area, which is close to the confluence of the renal veins, is one of the highest-flow portions of the IVC. Placement of the filter in this high-flow region will decrease the incidence of complications due to venous stasis and will trigger the intrinsic thrombolytic cascade to dissolve captured thrombus. In situations in which a malpositioned filter will affect proper functioning of the device, a second filter should be placed.

Inferior Vena Caval Wall Penetration. Penetration of the IVC can occur during any step of insertion. The guidewire, the sheath-dilator complex, the filter carrier system, and the filters themselves have all been involved. The incidence ranges from 0.1% to 9% and is dependent on the type of filter system. If perforation is detected or suspected, conservative care is usually all that is required.

Caval Thrombosis. Caval thrombosis is reported in 3% to 9% of IVC filter placements. It usually occurs months to years after insertion and may present with lower extremity symptoms of venous stasis. Patients still at risk of PE should have a second filter inserted at the level of T12 via an internal jugular vein approach.

Pulmonary Embolism. The incidence of PE with an IVC filter in position can range from 0.1% to 10%. To date, the incidence of PE when an IVC filter is used prophylactically in high-risk trauma patients has been low.

Bleeding. Although the profile of IVC filters has been streamlined, percutaneous placement still creates a formidable hole in the insertion vein, leading to postprocedural bleeding. Therefore, patients should have adequate digital pressure applied after filter housing removal. For patients who have been previously anticoagulated, a longer duration of compression may be required.

Insertion Site Thrombosis. Common femoral vein thrombosis occurs during or after insertion of IVC filters approximately 3% of the time. This frequency has diminished with the use of more low-profile equipment, however.

Special Cases

Suprarenal Inferior Vena Caval Filter Placement

Patients with IVC occlusion or a malpositioned infrarenal IVC filter may require a second filter in the suprarenal IVC. This procedure should be performed under fluoroscopic guidance to ensure the clearest delineation of the anatomy. The approach for filter placement is through the internal jugular vein with proper positioning at the T13 vertebral body. Reports have documented no statistical difference in the incidence of suprarenal caval occlusion, renal dysfunction, and recurrent PE when compared with infrarenal filters.

Intravascular Ultrasound–Assisted Inferior Vena Caval Filter Placement

In intravascular ultrasonography, one of the most recent advances in vascular imaging, intraluminal visualization is captured through a small-diameter (7-Fr) ultrasound probe. Application of intravascular ultrasonography has expanded to IVC filter placement. The technique has the advantage of requiring no contrast agents. The machinery is quite cumbersome, however, and requires special training for accurate interpretation of anatomy.

References

1. Benjamin M, Sandager G, Cohn E, et al: Duplex ultrasound insertion of inferior vena cava filters in multitrauma patients. Am J Surg 1999;178:92–97.
2. Grassi CJ: Inferior vena cava filters: Analysis of five currently available devices. Am J Roentgenol 1991;156:813–821.
3. Greenfield LJ, Proctor MC: Twenty-year clinical experience with the Greenfield filter. Cardiovasc Surg 1995;3:199–205.
4. Greenfield LJ, Whitehill TA: Vena caval interruption and filters. In Raju S, Villavicencio L (eds): Surgical Management of Venous Disease. Baltimore, Williams & Wilkins, 1997, pp 497–511.
5. Katsamouris A, Waltman A, Delichatsios M, Athanasoulis C: Inferior vena cava filters: In vitro comparison of clot trapping and flow dynamics. Cardiovasc Radiol 1988;166:361–366.
6. Linsenmaier U, Rieger J, Schenk F, et al: Indications, management, and complications of temporary inferior vena cava filters. Cardiovasc Intervent Radiol 1988;21:464–469.
7. Nunn C, Neuzil D, Naslund T, et al: Cost-effective method for bedside insertion of vena caval filters in trauma patients. J Trauma 1997;43:752–758.
8. Sato D, Robinson K, Gregory R, et al: Duplex directed caval filter insertion in multi-trauma and critically ill patients. Ann Vasc Surg 1999;13:365–371.
9. Van Natta T, Morris J Jr, Eddy V, et al: Elective bedside surgery in critically injured patients is safe and cost-effective. Ann Surg 1998;227:618–626.
10. Tola J, Holtzman R, Lottenberg L: Bedside placement of inferior vena cava filters in the intensive care unit. Am Surg 1999;65:833–838.

18 Epidural Analgesia

Linda Rever

The discovery of opiate receptors in the dorsal horn of the spinal cord in the late 1970s has had a monumental impact on pain control in a large and varied patient population. The use of epidural and intraspinal opiates has continued to increase since the approval of preservative-free morphine by the United States Food and Drug Administration in 1984. Today, the use of epidural infusions to provide analgesia for labor, trauma, and postoperative patients is safe and cost effective. The benefits of superior analgesia include not only patient comfort but also earlier mobilization and improved pulmonary function, which decrease the frequency of complications, especially in the most critically ill patients. The focus of this chapter is on the use of epidural analgesia in critically ill and trauma patients.

Patient Selection

Continuous epidural analgesia is a highly effective method of pain control in patients with multiple trauma or rib fractures or in patients who have undergone thoracotomy or celiotomy in the critical care setting. The anesthesia-pain service should evaluate the patient after a discussion with all the specialists involved. A checklist should be completed to ensure that the patient is an appropriate candidate for the procedure (Table 18–1). Hemodynamic stability, normal coagulation status, absence of sepsis or bacteremia, absence of injury or infection at the proposed site of catheter placement, and absence of spinal or major head injury are prerequisites to epidural catheter placement. To proceed with epidural catheter placement, the prothrombin time and the activated partial thromboplastin time need to be within the normal range, the International Normalized Ratio should be less than 1.5, and the platelet count should be stable at 100,000/mm³ or greater. The last dose of subcutaneous heparin should be administered a minimum of 6 hours, and preferably 12 hours, before catheter placement. In the case of low-molecular-weight heparin, the last dose should be administered not less than 24 hours before epidural catheter placement. If any questions remain regarding the anticoagulant, the dose, or the administration time, coagulation studies and a platelet count should be obtained and

should be found to be in the normal range. If the patient is receiving thromboprophylactic therapy or full anticoagulation, epidural catheter placement must be delayed until all anticoagulant effects are reversed and coagulation studies are normal (as outlined previously).

The risks and the benefits of anticoagulation or thromboprophylactic therapy must be weighed against the risks and the benefits of epidural analgesia. Therefore, a patient who is to remain fully anticoagulated with intravenous heparin, oral warfarin, or low-molecular-weight heparin or who is to remain on low-dose, low-molecular-weight heparin for thromboprophylaxis is not a candidate for epidural catheter placement. This is based on a Pubic Health Advisory issued by the United States Food and Drug Administration on December 15, 1997, which noted an increased incidence of epidural hematomas in patients undergoing epidural or spinal anesthesia while receiving low-molecular-weight heparin for thromboprophylaxis. In particular, permanent neurologic injury occurred in some patients in spite of surgical decompression.

Blunt chest trauma, multiple fractured ribs, and flail chest are devastating injuries because they cause alterations in pulmonary function, which are compounded by the patient's inability to cough, clear secretions, and inspire deeply in the presence of excruciating pain. The morbidity and the mortality of severe chest wall trauma have been dramatically reduced by the routine use of epidural analgesia, which has shortened ventilator times, shortened intensive care unit stays, and decreased the number of pulmonary complications. Therefore, at our institution, thoracic epidural analgesia is a routine part of the management of all patients

TABLE 18–1. Patient Selection Checklist

Hemodynamic stability
Absence of bacteremia
Absence of infection or injury at site of catheter placement
Absence of head injury
Cervical spine clearance
Platelet count of 100,000/mm³
Normal PT and aPTT, INR <1.5
Last dose of subcutaneous heparin >12 hr
Last dose of low-molecular-weight heparin >24 hr
No anticoagulation planned during course of epidural therapy

aPTT, activated partial thromboplastin time; INR, International Normalized Ratio; PT, prothrombin time.

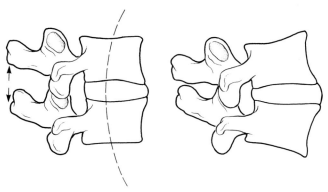

FIGURE 18–1. Anteria bending opens up the intervertebral spaces.

with flail chest and multiple fractured ribs, provided that no contraindications to catheter placement are present and the patient either is ready to be weaned from the ventilator or has not required intubation. In fact, our anesthesia-pain service is consulted urgently for initiation of epidural analgesia in some of these patients in the hope of preventing the need for mechanical ventilation. A caveat is that the patient's pain and overall status must be continually evaluated not only by the anesthesia-pain service but also by the trauma, surgical, or critical care team primarily responsible for the patient to diagnose promptly any underlying injury not previously evident.

Technique

The site for epidural catheter placement is selected according to the dermatomal location of the patient's injuries and the site of pain. The catheter tip should ideally be situated at the midpoint of the dermatomal distribution responsible for the pain. The major landmarks are the nipple at T4, the xiphoid at T6, the umbilicus at T10, the symphysis pubis at T12, and the knee at L3-L4. The approach to the epidural space may be either midline or paramedian below the T10 level. Above this level, however, only the paramedian approach is used owing to the occlusion of the interspace in the midline by the vertebral spinous processes.

Although the patient may be placed in the sitting position if not intubated, the lateral recumbent position is almost exclusively used for patients in the intensive care unit. Anteria bending (knee-to-chest position) opens up the intervertebral spaces (Fig. 18–1). The spine is palpated, and the chosen interspaces are marked if a midline approach is to be used. If a paramedian approach is necessary for midthoracic epidural analgesia, the spinous processes above and below the chosen level are marked. Sterile preparation with Betadine (povidone-iodine) and draping over this area are done. Local anesthesia with 1% lidocaine is infiltrated using a 1.5-inch 25-gauge needle through the skin 0.5 to 1.0 cm lateral and cephalad to the lower spinous process. This needle is advanced, and the local anesthesia is infiltrated until contact is made with the lamina. The 18-gauge Tuohy needle is advanced through this area of local anesthesia until the lamina is again contacted. The Tuohy needle is then walked off the lamina in a slightly cephalad direction (Fig. 18–2). As the cephalad edge of the lamina is sensed,

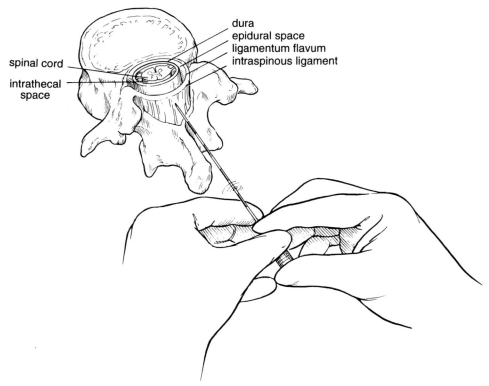

spinal cord
intrathecal space
dura
epidural space
ligamentum flavum
intraspinous ligament

FIGURE 18–2. The Tuohy needle is "walked off" of the lamina in a slightly cephalad direction.

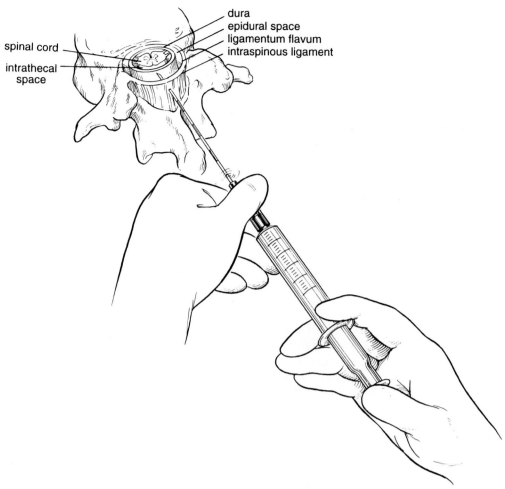

spinal cord

intrathecal space

dura
epidural space
ligamentum flavum
intraspinous ligament

FIGURE 18–3. Loss of resistance is sensed, and the saline solution is injected easily.

the stylet is withdrawn, and the saline-filled syringe is attached to the Tuohy needle. With constant pressure on the syringe, the Tuohy needle is advanced until a loss of resistance is sensed, and the saline solution is injected easily (Fig. 18–3). This is the epidural space, usually located approximately 4 to 7 cm deep to the skin. The syringe is disconnected from the needle, and the catheter is then threaded 4 to 8 cm into the epidural space (Fig. 18–4). If the patient experiences pain or any dysesthesia, the catheter should not be advanced farther. If the catheter does not thread easily at least 4 to 5 cm into the space, the needle and the catheter should be withdrawn entirely, and the procedure should be repeated.

The catheter should be aspirated for the presence of blood or cerebrospinal fluid. If none is aspirated, a test dose of 3 mL of 1.5% lidocaine is injected. The test dose is negative if the heart rate on electrocardiography or pulse oximetry does not increase more than 10 to 15 beats per minute and the patient does not begin to develop any numbness in the legs. The test dose should not be given if frank blood or cerebrospinal fluid is aspirated; in this instance, the catheter should be withdrawn. The entire procedure should be

repeated one level above or below the previous attempt. A sterile dressing is applied once the catheter is in place. The filter is attached to the Tuohy adapter, which is screwed onto the catheter. Labels are attached to the catheter and to all tubing between the patient

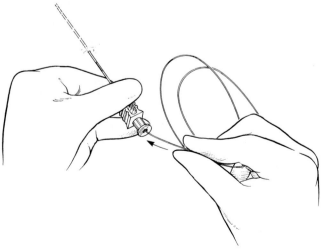

FIGURE 18–4. The catheter is threaded 4 to 8 cm into the epidural space.

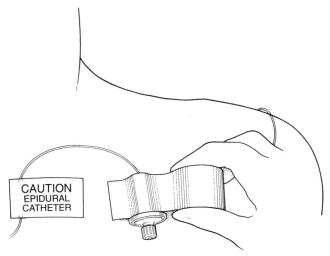

FIGURE 18–5. The epidural catheter and the pump must be clearly differentiated from all other intravenous lines and pumps.

and the infusion pump. The tubing must not contain any injection ports, and either a dedicated epidural patient-controlled anesthesia pump or a single-line infusion pump should be used. The epidural catheter and the pump must be clearly differentiated from all intravenous lines and pumps (Fig. 18–5).

Medications and Dosage Regimens

Initially, only opioids such as morphine and fentanyl were used for epidural analgesia because only lumbar epidural injections and catheters were in routine use. The remote possibility of spinal cord trauma at the thoracic level was considered too great a risk for there to be any possible benefit from thoracic epidural anesthesia or analgesia. As knowledge and expertise increased, however, thoracic epidural catheter placement for analgesia became safe and effective. The most common type of medication regimen is a combination of an opioid and a local anesthetic (Table 18–2). This combination exhibits a synergy owing to the different sites of action of the two drugs. The opioids bind to

opioid receptors in the dorsal horn of the spinal cord to inhibit pain transmission from peripheral nociceptors, whereas the local anesthetics block nerve fiber transmission by blocking the sodium channels. The synergy allows a lower concentration of each medication to be used with fewer unwanted side effects while providing more intense analgesia. With the addition of the local anesthetic bupivacaine, patients with thoracic trauma had greater improvement in vital capacity and forced expiratory volume than those receiving an opioid alone.

The opioids used most frequently are morphine, fentanyl, and hydromorphone (Table 18–3). The most hydrophilic opioid is morphine, followed by hydromorphone and fentanyl, which is highly lipophilic. The more hydrophilic the drug, the more it will spread in the cerebrospinal fluid and the longer it will take to diffuse into and out of it. This accounts for the increased incidence of nausea, vomiting, pruritus, urinary retention, and delayed respiratory depression as well as the increased onset and duration of action of morphine compared with hydromorphone or fentanyl.

The local anesthetics may cause hypotension as a result of sympathetic blockade. The sympathetic and C fibers are easily blocked by even dilute concentrations of local anesthetics because they are small and unmyelinated. The larger myelinated motor fibers are not easily blocked with dilute local anesthetics. Some numbness and weakness are possible, however, if higher concentrations of local anesthetics are used. In general, the sensory block may extend one or two dermatomal levels higher than the motor block, and the sympathetic block may extend one or two dermatomal levels above the sensory block.

Epidural infusions are dosed in milliliters per hour. Lumbar catheters require higher rates than thoracic catheters. For analgesia of each thoracic dermatomal level, a 1 mL/hour rate is required, whereas for analgesia of each lumbar dermatomal level, a 1.5 mL/hour rate is required. A patient with fractured ribs from T5 to T10 with an epidural catheter placed at the T8 level will require an infusion to run at 5 mL/hour. A patient with long bone fractures of the lower extremity with an epidural catheter placed at the L3 level will require an infusion to run at 7.5 mL/hour.

TABLE 18–2. Epidural Medication Side Effects

Opioids
  Sedation
  Respiratory depression, possibly delayed
  Pruritus
  Nausea
  Vomiting
  Urinary retention
Local anesthetics
  Hypotension
  Numbness
  Extremity weakness
  Toxicity—confusion, tinnitus, circumoral numbness, seizure, cardiovascular collapse

TABLE 18–3. Common Doses of Epidural Medications

Medication	Concentration
Narcotics	
Morphine	0.1 mg/mL
Fentanyl	5 μg/mL, 10 mg/mL
Hydromorphone	0.01–0.02 mg/mL
Local anesthetics	
Bupivacaine	0.1%–0.15%
Ropivacaine	0.1%–0.20%

TABLE 18–4. Continuous Epidural Infusion and/or Patient-Controlled Epidural Analgesia Orders

1. Implement continuous epidural infusion and patient-controlled epidural analgesia × _____ hr.
2. Discontinue all previously ordered narcotics and sedatives.
3. Medication/concentration: _____

   Continuous rate _____ mL/hr. PCEA bolus dose _____ mL. Lockout interval _____ min. Four-hour dose limit _____ mL. _____ Off. Loading dose _____ mL. May repeat q _____ .
4. Test dose administered by _____ MD. Depth of epidural catheter insertion _____ cm.
   Specify medication/dose/time of test dose _____ .
5. After each loading dose & rate change, check: BP, HR, RR, LOS, & pain level 15 min after & q1hr × 4hr.
6. Monitor the following: BP, HR, RR, & LOS q1hr × 4hr, then q2hr.
   Postural BP before ambulating.
   Motor ability and sensation of lower extremities q4hr.
7. Pain assessment q4hr and PRN.
8. Check for urinary retention q4hr.
   If patient with indwelling catheter, check urine output q1hr.
9. Check epidural catheter site q4hr for signs of leakage &/or dislodgement.
10. Maintain IV access during epidural therapy & 24 hr after epidural discontinued.
11. Label catheter and PCEA pump with "EPIDURAL" labels.
12. Prochlorperazine (Compazine) _____ mg IV q6hr PRN for nausea/vomiting.
13. Diphenhydramine (Benadryl) _____ mg IV q4hr PRN for pruritus.
14. If respiratory rate ≤8 per minute and/or unable to arouse, STOP INFUSION, administer naloxone 0.2 mg IVp; may repeat q5min × 2. Call the anesthesia-pain management service immediately.
15. If #14 ineffective, start naloxone IV infusion of 1 mg/250 mL of normal saline at 5 mL/hr; titrate to patient responsiveness & RR >10/min at increments of 5 mL q10min to max of 50 mL/hr.
16. Call the aneesthesia-pain management service for the following:
    Inadequate analgesia (pain rating scale ≥6/10).
    Change in level of consciousness.
    Persistent headache unrelieved by medication.
    RR <10/min.
    Systolic BP < _____ mm Hg.
    Pulse <50/minor drop by 20 from baseline.
    Pruritus and/or nausea/vomiting refractory to ordered medications.
    Tingling, numbness of lower extremities, and/or inability to move legs.
    Urine output <30 mL/hr or inability to void.

BP, blood pressure; HR, heart rate; IV, intravenous; IVp, intravenous push; LOS, level of sedation; PCEA, patient-controlled epidural analgesia; PRN, as required.

Monitoring and Complications

Careful monitoring by trained personnel of any patient with an epidural infusion is imperative. Communication between the pain service and all other teams involved in the care of the patient is also essential. The parameters to be monitored and the personnel to be notified should any problems arise are detailed for each patient using standard preprinted orders (Table 18–4). These monitoring parameters include vital signs, level of sedation, pain score, epidural catheter site, urinary output, side effects, and neurologic examination of all extremities. Monitoring is directed at providing adequate analgesia and identifying side effects and complications, should they occur. Opioid side effects include sedation, nausea, vomiting, pruritus, urinary retention if no Foley catheter is in place, and respiratory depression. Local anesthetic side effects include hypotension, numbness, and weakness in the lower extremities. Infectious complications are extremely rare if the catheter is removed at 7 days. If continuation of epidural analgesia is necessary after 7 days, a new epidural catheter is inserted at a different site. Other complications include bleeding at the catheter site and migration of the epidural catheter into an epidural vein or into the subarachnoid space. If the catheter has migrated intravascularly, signs of local anesthetic toxicity will begin to appear. These include confusion, tinnitus, circumoral numbness, seizures, and cardiovascular collapse. If the catheter has migrated intrathecally, increasing sedation, respiratory depression, numbness, and inability to move the extremities will occur. Rarely, an epidural hematoma may develop if the patient is anticoagulated or develops a coagulopathy while the epidural catheter is in place. The incidence of this complication is reduced markedly by (1) paying careful attention to the patient's coagulation status and (2) not placing or manipulating the catheter in any patient who has a coagulation abnormality. The most common presentation of epidural hematoma is back pain or increasing numbness and difficulty moving the legs. This requires immediate evaluation and neurosurgical intervention to prevent permanent neurologic sequelae.

Conclusions

Epidural analgesia with opioids or local anesthetics or a combination of opioids and local anesthetics is an efficacious mode of therapy in trauma and critically ill patients. For patients with multiple rib fractures, flail chest, or severe chest wall trauma, improved outcomes and cost savings are realized as a result of decreased ventilator time and intensive care unit stays. In the absence of contraindications to the placement of a thoracic epidural catheter, this technique is now becoming the standard of care. The technique is safe when performed by trained anesthesia-pain practitioners in a setting where monitoring of the patients is carried out by trained nursing personnel. Communication between all practitioners involved in these patients' care is essential. Intensivists with an understanding of effective analgesia therapies will be able to improve their patients' outcomes even further.

Suggested Readings

1. Cicala RS, Voeller GR, Fox T, et al: Epidural analgesia in thoracic trauma: Effects of lumbar morphine and thoracic bupivacaine on pulmonary function. Crit Care Med 1990;18:229–231.
2. Heit JA, Horlocker TT: Neuraxial anesthesia and anticoagulation. Reg Anesth Pain Med 1998;23:129–177.
3. Mandabach MG: Intrathecal and epidural analgesia. Crit Care Clin 1999;15:105–118.
4. Morrow BC, Mawhinney IN, Elliott JR: Tibial compartment syndrome complicating closed femoral nailing: Diagnosis delayed by an epidural analgesic technique—case report. J Trauma 1994;37:867–868.
5. Nolan JP, Dow AA, Parr MJ, et al: Patient-controlled analgesia following post-traumatic pelvic reconstruction. A comparison with continuous epidural analgesia. Anaesthesia 1992;47:1037–1041.
6. Ullman DA, Fortune JB, Greenhouse BB, et al: The treatment of patients with multiple rib fractures using continuous thoracic epidural narcotic infusion. Reg Anesth 1989;14:43–47.
7. Ward AJ, Gillatt DA: Delayed diagnosis of traumatic rupture of the spleen—a warning of the use of thoracic epidural analgesia in chest trauma. Injury 1989;20:178–179.
8. Wisner DH: A stepwise logistic regression analysis of factors affecting morbidity and mortality after thoracic trauma: Effect of epidural analgesia. J Trauma 1990;30:799–804.
9. Yaksh TL: Spinal opiate analgesia: Characteristics and principles of action. Pain 1981;11:293–346.
10. Yaksh TL, Rudy TA: Analgesia mediated by a direct spinal action of narcotics. Science 1976;192:1357–1358.

19 Suprapubic Urinary Tube Placement

Marcus L. Quek and John P. Stein

One of the most common emergent calls in urologic practice involves the timely relief of lower urinary tract outlet obstruction. Urethral catheterization and bladder drainage with a straight rubber or latex catheter remain the first and ideal option in patients unable to void spontaneously, when diagnostic considerations require sterile sampling, or when strict monitoring of urinary output is required. If catheterization per urethra is unsuccessful, a number of alternative techniques may be employed to negotiate the urethra, including use of a coudé tip catheter, filiforms and followers, and cystoscopy-guided methods.

When urethral catheterization is unsuccessful or urethral access is contraindicated (e.g., with a history of blunt trauma with blood at the meatus), a percutaneous suprapubic cystostomy approach is desirable. The technique of suprapubic cystostomy is not difficult; however, if attention to surgical details is not maintained, complications can occur. Although a number of suprapubic catheters are currently available and the specific method of insertion differs slightly depending on the type, the basic principles are the same.

The following is a description of the two currently favored techniques practiced by the Urology Department at the Los Angeles County/University of Southern California Medical Center: (1) use of the Supra-Foley suprapubic introducer (Rüsch, Port Charlotte, Fla) and (2) use of the Stamey percutaneous suprapubic catheter set (Cook Urological, Spencer, Ind).

Technique

Rüsch SupraFoley Suprapubic Introducer

The following supplies should be readily available (Fig. 19–1):

1. Betadine (povidone-iodine) solution.
2. Razor.
3. Sterile drapes.
4. Sterile gloves.
5. Scalpel.
6. 23 G 3½ Spinal needle.
7. 10-mL Syringe.
8. 1% Lidocaine in 10-mL syringe with 21 G needle.
9. Package of 4 × 4 gauze sponges.
10. Rüsch Lawrence SupraFoley suprapubic catheter introducer (trocar and sheath).
11. 16 F Foley catheter.
12. 10-mL Syringe filled with sterile water.
13. Catheter drainage bag.
14. 2–0 Nonabsorbable suture (silk or nylon).
15. Needle driver.
16. Suture scissors.
17. 60-mL Catheter-tip syringe.
18. Normal saline solution for irrigation.
19. *Optional (if available):* ultrasound.

Periprocedural broad-spectrum antibiotics with gram-negative coverage should be administered, especially if urinary tract infection is suspected. The bladder should be percussed and should be palpable to prevent injury to bowel intervening between the anterior abdominal wall and the bladder. If the bladder is not palpable, one may consider administering a diuretic (if not medically contraindicated) to fill and distend the bladder. If there is a history or evidence of prior infraumbilical abdominal or pelvic surgery, suprapubic cystostomy should be attempted only with ultrasound guidance to avoid inadvertent injury to bowel or associated structures.

The patient is placed in the supine with slight Trendelenburg position, which helps displace the bowel contents in a cephalad direction. The suprapubic area is appropriately shaved, prepared with Betadine solution, and draped in a sterile fashion. A site approximately two fingerbreadths above the symphysis pubis in the midline overlying the distended bladder is identified. A subcutaneous wheal of 1% lidocaine is raised for local anesthesia. Deeper infiltration of the anterior rectus sheath should also be accomplished at this time. Adequate anesthesia is critical for patient comfort and to prevent the patient from making any excessive movements during cystostomy placement. A small nick incision is made in the skin and the subcutaneous tissue with the scalpel (Fig. 19–2). The spinal needle is attached to an empty 10-mL syringe and is directed at a 60-degree angle caudally through the skin incision toward the bladder and the pelvis (Fig. 19–3). Two

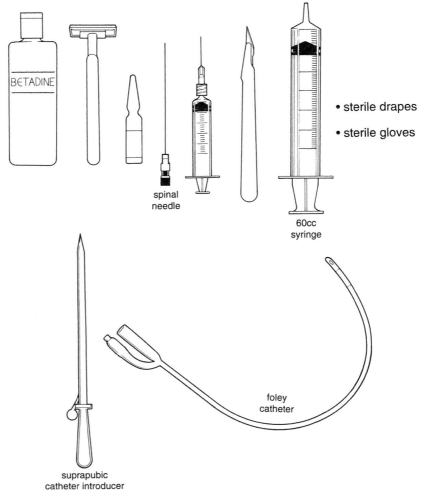

FIGURE 19–1. Rüsch suprapubic catheter placement set.

points of resistance are usually encountered: (1) the anterior rectus sheath and (2) the bladder wall.

As the spinal needle is advanced, the syringe is withdrawn under pressure to locate the urine and aspirate it from the bladder. Once urine has been aspirated, the spinal needle is left in place, and the depth and the angle at which the needle penetrated the bladder are measured. The pointed end of the Rüsch introducer (inside sheath) is then directed through the incision next to the spinal needle using steady downward pressure (Fig. 19–4). Again, two points of resistance will be encountered; these are better appreciated with the trocar than the spinal needle. When the bladder has been reached, it is critical to advance the trocar an additional 2 to 3 cm to ensure that the sheath portion of the introducer is also in the lumen of the bladder and not the detrusor wall. The trocar is then removed, leaving the sheath in place (Fig. 19–5A). If no urine returns through the sheath, the trocar should be replaced over the sheath, and the introducer should be advanced slightly or redirected to find the bladder.

Once urine return has been confirmed through the

sheath, the opening is covered with a finger so that the bladder will remain distended. The spinal needle may be removed at this point. A standard 16 Fr Foley catheter is inserted through the sheath until the hilt of the catheter is reached *and* urine is seen coming from the catheter port (Fig. 19–5B). The catheter balloon is inflated with 7 to 10 mL of sterile water to retain the catheter. The tab on the introducer is pulled, and the remaining portion of the sheath is peeled away from the catheter. A closed gravity drainage system is connected to the catheter, and a 2–0 nonabsorbable suture (such as silk or nylon) is used to secure the catheter at the skin level.

Stamey Percutaneous Suprapubic Cystostomy Set

The same general supplies should be readily available, with the exception of the Foley catheter and the Rüsch introducer (Fig. 19–6). The Stamey percutaneous cystostomy set contains a Malecot catheter with a needle obturator, which should be assembled before the start

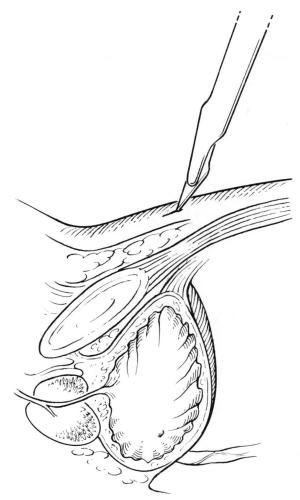

FIGURE 19–2. Incision in the skin.

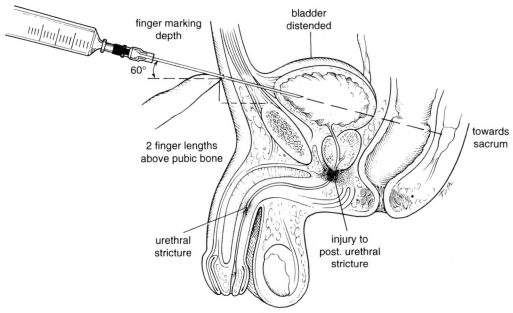

FIGURE 19–3. Insertion of spinal needle. post., posterior.

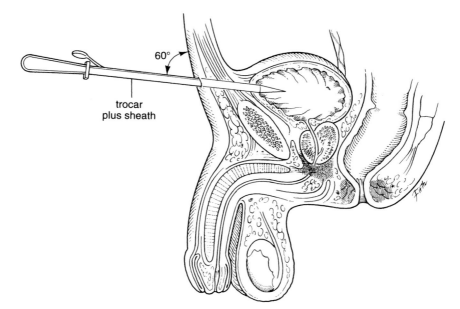

FIGURE 19–4. Insertion of trocar.

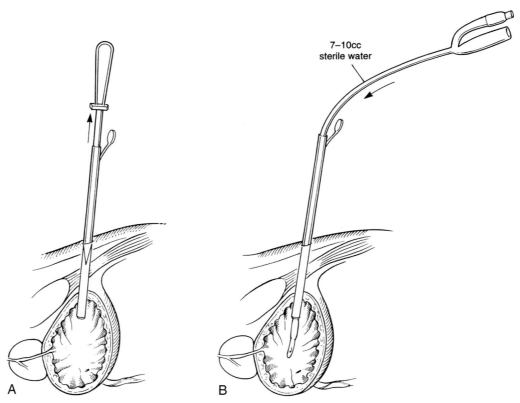

FIGURE 19–5. *A,* Removal of introducer. *B,* Insertion of Foley balloon.

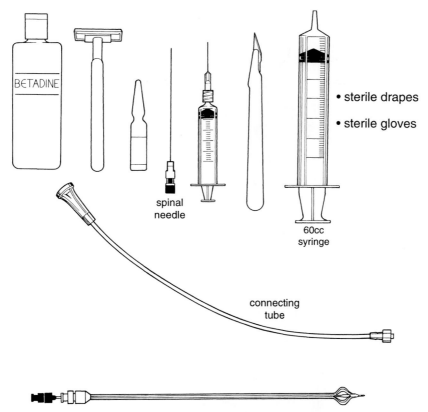

spinal
needle

• sterile drapes
• sterile gloves

60cc
syringe

connecting
tube

FIGURE 19–6. Stamey suprapubic catheter placement set.

of the procedure. The needle obturator is carefully guided into the Malecot catheter, thereby stretching and straightening the wings. The self-retaining obturator is locked in place by turning it clockwise relative to the catheter (Fig. 19–7). If the catheter is damaged while the needle obturator is being passed, the catheter should be discarded, and a new set should be used.

The patient is positioned as previously mentioned. Again, the skin (two fingerbreadths above the symphysis pubis) is shaved, prepared, and draped in the usual sterile fashion. A midline site is adequately anesthetized with injectable 1% lidocaine, and the spinal needle is used as a finder needle for the bladder. Once urine has been aspirated, the preassembled suprapubic catheter and the obturator are guided through the skin, the rectus sheath, and the bladder wall at the same angle and depth, adjacent to the spinal needle. A 10-mL syringe may then be connected to the proximal end of the obturator.

When urine is aspirated from the introducer, both the catheter and the obturator should be advanced another 2 cm to ensure that the Malecot wings open completely within the bladder lumen and not the detrusor wall. The obturator may then be removed from the catheter by turning the former counterclockwise against the catheter and stabilizing the Malecot as the obturator is pulled out. Removal of the obturator needle opens the wings of the Malecot and secures the catheter within the bladder (Fig. 19–8). Confirmation

of proper placement is made by aspirating urine from the catheter. The tubing is then connected to the catheter and a closed urinary drainage system. The catheter is secured to the skin with a nonabsorbable suture.

If no urine is aspirated from the catheter after removal of the obturator, the catheter should be removed. Under no circumstances should the obturator needle be guided back through the catheter while the distal end of the Malecot is in the body because so-called "blind" placement may inadvertently damage the catheter or the surrounding structures. Rather, the catheter should simply be removed in its entirety, and the obturator guide should be replaced under direct vision. The catheter and the obturator can then be redirected into the bladder as a single unit until adequate placement has been confirmed.

The methods of suprapubic cystostomy described herein can be performed with relative ease and safety so long as certain general principles are maintained. If suprapubic cystostomy is clearly indicated, all necessary supplies should first be obtained. Second, the bladder should be clearly palpable; on some occasions, one should have adequate ultrasound guidance to facilitate bladder visualization. Lastly, a small-gauge spinal needle should be used as a finder needle.

We prefer the Rüsch introducer method of catheter insertion to other forms of percutaneous suprapubic cystostomy because this technique allows the place-

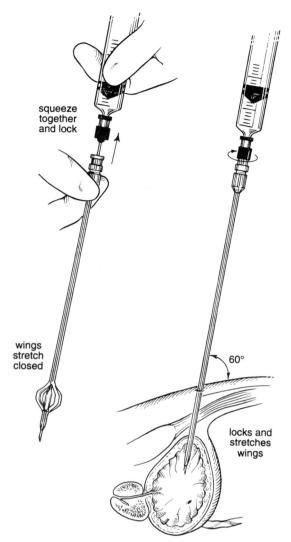

FIGURE 19–7. Insertion of obturator and Malecot catheter into the bladder.

ment of a standard 16 Fr Foley catheter, which is readily available, rather than a Malecot catheter, which has a tendency to become dislodged if not adequately secured. If properly performed, however, both techniques of bedside suprapubic cystostomy described here are simple and safe.

Indications

Indications include the inability to catheterize via the urethra, urethral stricture, traumatic urethral disruption, urethral false passage, periurethral abscess, and acute prostatitis.

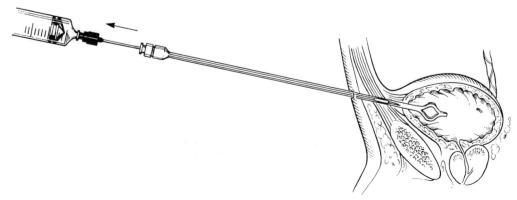

FIGURE 19–8. Removal of obturator. The wings of the Malecot catheter are open.

Contraindications

Contraindications include nondistended bladder, prior midline infraumbilical abdominal or pelvic surgery (without ultrasound guidance), coagulopathy, pregnancy, carcinoma of the bladder, and pelvic irradiation (relative contraindication).

Pitfalls and Complications

The most feared complication of percutaneous cystostomy is inadvertent bowel perforation. This is best prevented by assuring that the bladder is adequately distended and palpable in the lower abdomen. Use of ultrasound guidance when the bladder is not clearly palpable, and especially when prior surgery or pelvic irradiation may have led to bowel adhesions against the anterior abdominal wall, will significantly aid in the prevention of this complication.

If the spinal needle is inadvertently inserted into the bowel, the needle may be removed without significant adverse effects, and the procedure may be continued. Peritonitis is rare when the small-gauge spinal needle is used for localization.

Judicious use of diuretics, when not medically contraindicated, will facilitate bladder filling and distention. In addition, the bladder may be further distended by injecting saline solution through the spinal needle once an intravesical position has been confirmed. If urethral access is available during suprapubic cystostomy, saline solution may be flushed through the urethral catheter, and the tube is subsequently clamped. These measures may allow easier identification of the bladder in the lower abdomen before percutaneous puncture of the bladder.

Hematuria and blood clots may pose a significant problem in terms of the patency of the suprapubic catheter. The Rüsch introducer can accommodate only a 16 Fr catheter, whereas the Stamey set contains a 14 Fr Malecot. These are not optimal sizes for bladder irrigation of blood clots. If hematuria and clots are encountered, however, gentle catheter irrigation with a 60-mL catheter-tip syringe and normal saline solution can be successfully performed in most cases with resolution of the hematuria.

Interpretation of Data

If there is no urine output from the suprapubic catheter, one must first assess whether the catheter is correctly positioned. Catheter irrigation with a 60-mL catheter-tip syringe and normal saline solution should be attempted first. If the catheter irrigates (flushes and aspirates) easily, then the catheter is in the bladder, and another reason for anuria should be entertained: prerenal azotemia or supravesical obstruction. If the catheter flushes easily but does not aspirate, it usually suggests that the catheter is kinked or the distal opening of the catheter is against the wall of the bladder, therefore preventing free irrigation of the catheter. Simply change the catheter position or fill the bladder with at least 60 mL of saline solution and irrigate again. If these measures do not alleviate the problem, extravesical or peritoneal placement of the catheter must be excluded. A gravity cystogram through the suprapubic catheter may be performed with water-soluble contrast material (preferably under fluoroscopic guidance) to verify catheter placement. If the catheter neither flushes nor aspirates, the catheter is likely outside the bladder, and the suprapubic tube will need to be replaced.

Therapeutic Interventions

Especially in the setting of trauma, evaluation of the bladder and the lower urinary tract may be accomplished through the judicious use of contrast-enhanced radiography. A plain cystogram and computed tomographic cystograms through the suprapubic catheter allow evaluation of the bladder contour when urethral access is contraindicated (as in urethral disruptions).

Suprapubic cystostomy provides an excellent route for urinary diversion when disease or trauma prevents the natural flow of urine from the bladder through the urethra. The suprapubic tube can be maintained for long periods of time with only periodic catheter changes. After 1 month, the percutaneous tract is usually well-enough formed to allow the replacement of the catheter without difficulty.

In all patients requiring suprapubic tube placement, follow-up urologic evaluation is required to ascertain the cause and to provide treatment for the offending urethral obstruction, with the ultimate goal of providing natural urinary continuity.

Suggested Readings

1. Carter HB: Instrumentation and endoscopy. In Walsh PC, Retik AB, Vaughan ED, Wein AJ (eds): Campbell's Urology, 7th ed. Philadelphia, WB Saunders, 1998, pp 159–169.
2. Hilton P: Catheters and drains. In Stanton SL (ed): Principles of Gynaecological Surgery. New York, Springer-Verlag, 1987, pp 257–283.
3. Polascik TJ: Urologic procedures. In Chen H, Lillimoe KD, Sola JE (eds): Manual of Common Bedside Surgical Procedures. Baltimore, Williams & Wilkins, 1996, pp 199–206.
4. Zderic SA, Hanno PM: Suprapubic cystostomy and cutaneous vesicostomy. In Fowler JE (ed): Urologic Surgery. Boston, Little, Brown, 1992, pp 235–236.

Bedside Spinal Immobilization

William M. Costigan and Gordon L. Engler

Injury to the spinal column can be devastating. There is some degree of neurologic deficit in 10% to 15% of all spinal injuries (40% with injuries of the cervical spine and 15% to 20% at the thoracolumbar level).

The objectives of treatment of any spinal injury are (1) to prevent further neurologic damage, (2) to prevent further spinal deformity, (3) to reduce the existing deformity, and (4) to obtain a stable functional spinal column that will last for the remainder of the patient's life. At the acute stage, immobilization of the spine is of paramount importance. The development of neurologic deficit or the progression of an existing one due to inadequate spinal precautions has major consequences for the patient and the physician.

Bed Selection

Selection of a proper bed is important. The standard hospital bed, usually augmented with an egg crate mattress pad to prevent the formation of decubitus ulcers, can be used for most spinal injuries. Traction can be applied to both the cervical spine and one or all four extremities if necessary without interfering with the ability to care for the patient's spinal injury. The patient can be carefully logrolled on this type of bed if other injuries allow it.

The turning frame (e.g., Stryker) rotates the patient along the longitudinal axis from the supine to the prone position. This allows for skin care and is often effective in preventing decubitus ulcers. Traction can be applied in the longitudinal axis, but traction in other directions is difficult with this type of frame. This bed is rarely indicated and is used only in severely unstable spine injuries when logrolling is hazardous and relatively contraindicated.

The Roto-Rest bed allows for traction in multiple directions as well as decubitus ulcer care and prevention. This type of bed is very useful in multiply injured patients, especially those with severe pulmonary injuries for whom logrolling is difficult or contraindicated. This type of bed is expensive and often not available in many hospital facilities.

Bedside Immobilization for Specific Spinal Injuries

Cervical Injuries

The five most commonly used orthotic devices for the cervical spine include (1) the soft collar; (2) the Philadelphia collar; (3) the skull, occiput, mandibular immobilization (SOMI) brace; (4) the four-poster brace; and (5) the halo vest. The general consensus among treating physicians is that increasing the rigidity and the length of the orthosis results in a concomitant increase in the ability to limit the motion of the cervical spine. The soft collar provides the least amount of immobilization but provides comfort and security to the patient and is easily applied. Its use is limited to minor cervical sprains without osseous injuries.

The Philadelphia collar provides a circumferential grip on the neck and, when properly applied, limits some motion quite effectively (Fig. 20–1). In the acute setting, this type of brace is very useful. There is an anterior opening in most models to allow exposure of the neck and a tracheostomy, if necessary. A variation of the Philadelphia collar that provides a bit more rigidity, length, and immobilization is the Aspen collar (Fig. 20–2).

Four-poster braces place pressure on the occiput and the mandible through pads that connect to upright bars resting on the sternum anteriorly and the interscapular area posteriorly (Fig. 20–3). The effectiveness of the four-poster brace in restricting motion depends on the application of uniform and constant

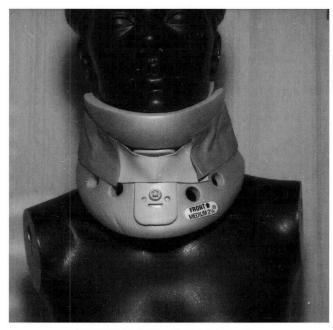

FIGURE 20–1. The Philadelphia collar.

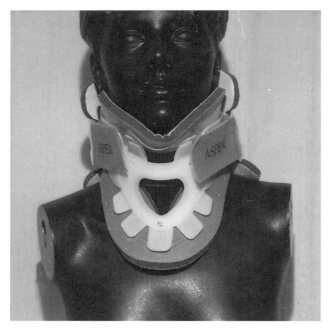

FIGURE 20–2. The Aspen collar.

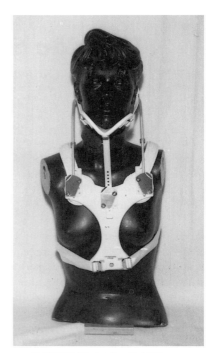

FIGURE 20–4. The SOMI brace.

pressure to the skull, the mandible, the chest, and the interscapular regions. This is often difficult to accomplish because frequent adjustments are needed. The use of this type of brace is limited because of these factors as well as patient complaints of discomfort and skin irritation.

The SOMI brace is designed to avoid the posterior thoracic pad and thus increase patient comfort (Fig. 20–4). It is easily applied with the patient in the supine position and may have an additional Minerva forehead band applied for further immobilization. It does allow some motion of the cervical vertebrae, however.

Extensive research has been published on the ability of the halo vest to limit motion of the unstable cervical spine (Fig. 20–5). Although the exact limitation of cervical motion that can be achieved is controversial, most authors agree that the halo vest is the best available orthosis for limitation of cervical motion and should be used in most unstable cervical spine injuries.

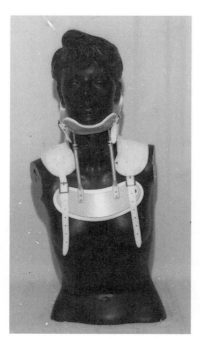

FIGURE 20–3. Four-poster brace.

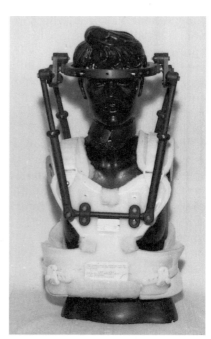

FIGURE 20–5. The halo vest.

When a patient is treated with cervical traction or a halo, pin care is important. The pin site in the skull should be cleaned on a regular basis, and an antibiotic ointment should be applied. The pin site is left without a dressing. If traction is applied to the cervical spine, daily examination for paralysis of the sixth cranial nerve (abducens) should be performed. Because this nerve exits the skull at an acute angle, it is the first to undergo neurapraxia, resulting in temporary paralysis of the lateral rectus eye muscle (cross-eyes). If this is noted, immediate reduction of the traction should be undertaken at a level that does not compromise overall cervical spine fixation.

Fractures of the Axis

Fractures of the axis (C1) are usually secondary to compressive forces that cause a centrifugal dissociation of the ring of C1. Because this spreading essentially decompresses the spinal canal without fragmentary implosion, these injuries are seldom accompanied by a neurologic injury. A minimally displaced burst fracture of C1 (Jefferson's fracture) can be treated initially with a Philadelphia or an Aspen collar at the bedside. Patients with significant displacement of the lateral masses on open-mouth radiography have unstable injuries. Treatment may be initiated in the emergency room or on the hospital ward with a Philadelphia or an Aspen collar, but the subsequent decision to apply a halo vest or to perform surgery should be made as soon as possible.

Odontoid Fractures

The severity of odontoid fractures varies greatly based on their location, as determined by radiographic examination. Type I fractures are relatively rare and involve avulsion of the tip of the odontoid. These are stable injuries if not associated with alar ligament disruption and can be treated with a soft, a Philadelphia, or an Aspen collar. Type II fractures occur at the base of the odontoid and can have variable displacement according to the ligamentous injuries. For acute, minimally displaced type II fractures, immediate immobilization with a Philadelphia or an Aspen collar is acceptable, with transfer to a halo vest as time and patient condition allow. This, then, allows for healing to occur with minimal motion. For significantly displaced type II fractures, cervical traction (Gardner-Wells tongs or halo) should be applied. Surgery is indicated if reduction is inadequate or delayed, or if nonunion becomes apparent.

Type III fractures of the odontoid occur through the body of C2. These fractures should be initially immobilized in a Philadelphia or an Aspen collar, with transfer to a halo vest after an appropriate period.

Traumatic Spondylolisthesis of the Axis

Traumatic spondylolisthesis of the axis (hangman's fracture) comprises fractures of the pars interarticularis of C2. Type I fractures typically demonstrate no angulation and have 3 mm or less of displacement. They are relatively stable and can be treated with a Philadelphia or an Aspen collar or a four-poster brace. Type II fractures have a similar fracture line through the pars interarticularis of C2 but have significant angulation, with displacement of C2 on C3 of 3 mm or greater. Fractures with displacement between 3 and 6 mm should be treated initially with halo traction followed by halo vest immobilization. A rolled towel may be judiciously placed beneath the neck to reduce translation with the patient in traction. This must be monitored with serial radiographic examinations. Fractures with greater than 6 mm of translation are best treated with cervical traction to accomplish reduction and with subsequent halo vest immobilization.

Cervical Ligamentous Injuries and Dislocations

The spectrum of posterior cervical disruptions ranges from minor subluxations to frank dislocations. These injuries may reduce spontaneously, or their facets remain "locked" unilaterally or bilaterally. The injuries that undergo spontaneous reduction can be treated with Philadelphia or Aspen collars, which can be changed to a soft collar after 6 to 8 weeks, depending on the severity of the initial injury, the subsequent radiographs, and the examination of the patient. The injuries that remain dislocated may be reduced by cervical traction, preferably a halo, which can also be used for long-term care. Nonreducible facet dislocations require open reduction and internal fixation followed by halo vest immobilization. If no attempt at reduction is undertaken, as in the case of concurrent intervertebral disc herniation, a Philadelphia or an Aspen collar may be used as temporary immobilization until surgery. Most often, however, halo traction is preferred. In patients with significant head trauma that prevents operative intervention, prolonged traction is acceptable. Anterior spontaneous fusion often occurs in these patients with resultant relative stability.

Thoracic Bracing

Braces are of little benefit for fractures of the thoracic spine from T1 to T7. It is extremely difficult to immo-

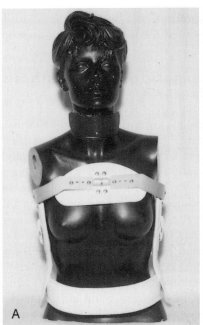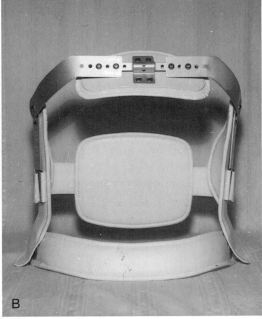

FIGURE 20–6. A, The Jewett brace. B, "Boomerang" bottom attachment.

bilize or support this level of the spine. Fortunately, the intact chest cage provides relative immobilization, and significant external bracing is not necessary. Although many orthotic devices have been used for treatment of thoracic spine injuries, most are difficult to fabricate, apply, and maintain. Furthermore, most are full contact and do not allow for adequate examination and treatment of other injuries involving the thorax or the abdomen. For these reasons, the authors have used the Jewett brace with a "boomerang" bottom attachment for essentially all thoracolumbar spine injuries (Fig. 20–6A and B). This device allows for easy access to chest tubes, thoracic and abdominal wounds, and gastrostomy sites as well as access for other nursing duties. It prevents inadvertent flexion of the thoracolumbar spine. It does not cause compression of the chest or limit respiration, as does the full-contact brace, which if properly applied does restrict chest expansion. The boomerang attachment to the Jewett brace applies inferior pressure to the anterior superior iliac spines bilaterally, thus avoiding pressure on the bladder and the symphysis pubis, which is a common complaint with the standard Jewett brace.

Upper and Middle Thoracic Injuries

The most common fracture of the thoracic spine is the simple compression fracture. Compressive forces can cause multilevel fractures in the thoracic spine. In the T1 to T6 region, immobilization is difficult to achieve. Most of these injuries are relatively stable, however, because of the intact rib cage and the sternum. An extended Philadelphia collar (Fig. 20–7), which incorporates the lower cervical and the upper thoracic spine, may be of some benefit. If fractures of the sternum or the ribs are present, great care must be exercised in the handling and the turning of the patient to avoid further injury and displacement of the spinal fracture.

Contiguous fractures of two or three spinal segments are not common and usually require early surgery for reduction and stabilization. For fractures between T7 and L2, a Jewett brace with a boomerang bottom may be used for initial immobilization and to allow careful

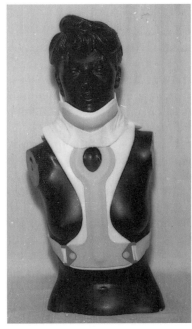

FIGURE 20–7. Extended Philadelphia collar.

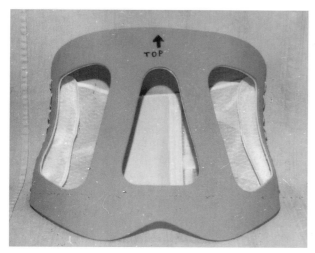

FIGURE 20–8. The Knight spinal brace.

transfer of the patient for radiographic, computed tomography, and magnetic resonance imaging studies with relative security. When excessive kyphosis has occurred as a result of the injury, operative reduction is usually required. The same Jewett brace may be used for postoperative management, if necessary.

Thoracolumbar Fractures

Fractures of the thoracolumbar junction account for the vast majority of spinal fractures between T1 and L5. In patients with isolated anterior column injuries, a brace that resists flexion is required. Again, the Jewett brace is appropriate. The initial bedside treatment is bed rest, with the head positioned for patient comfort. An overhead trapeze is not recommended because flexion forces would be generated in the spine if the patient used such a device to raise the upper body off the bed. For fractures that occur in the middle or the lower lumbar region, initial bedside care is the same. Eventually, a Knight spinal brace is used to provide patient comfort and to allow care and cautious transfer for computed tomography or magnetic resonance imaging studies (Fig. 20–8).

Injuries at the lumbosacral junction are often treated with bed rest and early surgical intervention. Braces with leg extensions, although recommended by many authors, are extremely difficult to fit, align, and manage. Because most have a variable hip-lock articulation, the benefit of lumbosacral immobilization is lost every time the lock is disengaged for sitting and toilet functions. A spica cast is sometimes used for constant immobilization after the initial phase of treatment.

Two-column injuries of the thoracolumbar junction are treated according to the amount of displacement of spinal fragments and the presence of neurologic deficit. Initial spinal precautions are exercised until a decision regarding bracing or surgery is made. Injuries to the transverse processes (avulsion fractures) or spinous process fractures can be treated symptomatically and require no specific bedside immobilization.

The Chance fracture (flexion-distraction) is unique to the lumbar area and is seen commonly after a motor vehicle accident with seat belt injury. These fractures are unstable, and the patient should lie supine under strict spinal precautions until bracing or surgery is accomplished. A trapeze is contraindicated. Chance fractures occur through bony elements and will heal if properly reduced. The Jewett brace with the boomerang bottom is often used. If surgery is required, the posterior tether of the disrupted elements is restored with a tension-band type of internal fixation, allowing healing to occur.

Burst fractures in the middle and the lower lumbar regions are usually three-column injuries. Strict spinal precautions are required initially followed by brace immobilization (Jewett). Early surgical intervention is indicated if the patient's conditions allows. Prolonged bed rest (greater than 1 week) is necessary only for patients with other injuries that prevent early bracing, mobilization, or surgery. Disused muscle atrophy and cardiorespiratory complications are increased in patients treated with prolonged bed rest. This should be avoided, and early mobilization and rehabilitative measures should be instituted as soon as possible.

Sacral Fractures

Isolated fractures of the sacrum occur predominantly in cases of direst trauma in patients with some degree of osteoporosis. Sacral fractures are also seen in conjunction with severe pelvic fractures. No immediate bedside immobilization is possible or indicated in these injuries, other than proper precautions similar to those exercised in patients with spinal injuries. An appropriate period of bed rest followed by early ambulation with crutches and limited weight-bearing is indicated.

Suggested Readings

1. Chapman JR, Anderson PA: Thoracolumbar spine fractures with neurologic deficit. Orthop Clin North Am 1994;25:595–612.
2. Delamarter RB, Coyle J: Acute management of spinal cord injury. J Am Acad Orthop Surg 1999;7:165–175.
3. Meyer PR: Acute injury retrieval and splinting techniques: On-site care. In Meyer PR (ed): Surgery of Spine Trauma. New York, Churchill Livingstone, 1989, pp 1–21.
4. Meyer PR: Emergency room assessment: Management of spinal cord and associated injuries, In Meyer PR (ed): Surgery of Spine Trauma. New York, Churchill Livingstone, 1989, pp 23–60.
5. Rizzolo SJ, Cotler JM: Unstable cervical spine injuries: specific treatment approaches. J Am Acad Orthop Surg 1993;1:57–66.
6. White AA, Panjabi MM, Posner I, et al: Spinal stability: Evaluation and treatment. J Am Acad Orthop Surg 1981;30:457–483.

Part II

MONITORING

21 Routine Clinical Monitoring in Acute Illnesses

William C. Shoemaker

All science is measurement.

HELMHOLTZ

This chapter summarizes routine or commonly used clinical monitoring methods. Invasive and noninvasive hemodynamic and oxygen transport monitoring methods are presented subsequently. The initial history-taking and the physical examination are essential but are not covered here. Commonly monitored variables are listed in Table 21–1.

Routine Noninvasive Clinical Monitoring

Vital Signs

Systolic, diastolic, and mean arterial pressures; heart rate; respiratory rate; and temperature—the so-called vital signs—are the simplest, the easiest, the most readily available, and the most commonly used noninvasively monitored variables. They are monitored routinely and are recorded graphically on the vital signs sheet during physical examination, daily nursing rou-

TABLE 21–1. Commonly Monitored Clinical Variables

Arterial blood pressure (systolic, diastolic, and mean)
Heart rate
Temperature
Hematocrit and hemoglobin concentration
Urine output
Electrocardiography
Serum electrolytes and blood chemistry
Central venous pressure
Arterial blood gases and pH
Gastric tonometry
Pulse oximetry
Transcutaneous oxygen and carbon dioxide tensions
Blood volume, plasma volume, and red cell mass
Plasma colloidal osmotic pressure
Plasma and urine osmolality, osmolar and free water clearances
Electroencephalography
Intracranial pressure
Pulmonary arterial and precapillary wedge pressures
Cardiac output and hemodynamic variables
Oxygen transport variables
Ventilatory monitoring

tines, hospital and intensive care unit admissions, and screening of acute illnesses in each hospitalized patient. This is done at each shift or at more frequent intervals during periods of circulatory instability, during initial resuscitation in emergency conditions, intraoperatively as part of the anesthetic record, and in special care units to give a running graphic record of events.[1]

Arterial Pressure

Manometric blood pressure measurements may be obtained with a sphygmomanometer cuff placed just above the elbow and a stethoscope over the brachial artery. The width of the cuff should be 40% of the circumference of the arm. The Korotkoff blood pressure sounds, heard through a stethoscope placed over the brachial artery distal to the occluding cuff, are used to identify the systolic pressure caused by the initial breakthrough of the pulse and the diastolic pressure caused by the lessening and then the disappearance of sounds as the pulse becomes unobstructed.

The normal arterial blood pressure is approximately 120/80 mm Hg for healthy young adults. The pressure may increase gradually with age, but the systolic pressure should not be more than 100 mm Hg plus the patient's age. Systolic pressures greater than 160 mm Hg and diastolic pressures greater than 90 mm Hg suggest hypertension. Young adults, especially teenaged girls, may normally have pressures as low as 90/60 mm Hg. It is important to know the patient's preillness pressures. Pressures should be measured in both arms early in the patient's hospital course, because unilateral arteriosclerotic or traumatic vascular lesions may result in 10 to 20 mm Hg differences between the left and the right sides. Normally, femoral arterial pressures are 5 to 10 mm Hg higher than brachial pressures. Aortic trauma or unilateral trauma to the femoral or the iliac arteries may produce appreciable pressure differences between the extremities.[1]

Mean arterial pressure (MAP) is defined as the sum of the diastolic pressure and one third of the pulse pressure. It may also be calculated as one third of the sum of the systolic pressure plus two times the diastolic pressure. It is more frequently measured directly as a dampened or "electrical mean" of the systolic and the diastolic pressures in various recording systems. The pulse pressure is the difference between the systolic and the diastolic pressures. Deceased pulse pressures may precede decreases in diastolic pressures in hypovolemic patients; this is a suggestive, but not a reliable, sign of shock.

The interactions of blood pressure, flow, and volume are extremely complex. Arterial pressures may reflect the overall circulatory status, or more particularly cardiac status, but lack diagnostic and physiologic specificity. Arterial pressures are useful for screening and surveillance to assess trends rapidly in acute conditions, such as hypovolemia from blood or fluid loss, high-risk surgery, acute myocardial infarction, cardiac failure, acute trauma, sepsis, anaphylaxis, vasovagal reactions, neurogenic shock, and terminal stages of most diseases. Hypotension does not directly reflect reduced blood flow and volume, however, but rather may reflect circulatory decompensation or therapeutic failures; increased pressures may indicate improved circulatory function, adrenal stress response, or vasopressor therapy.[1, 2]

Pressure and heart rate are useful as screening measures, but they are nonspecific changes that poorly reflect deficits of blood flow, blood volume, and cardiac function because compensatory adrenomedullary stress responses tend to maintain pressure in the face of falling blood flow. Wo and associates demonstrated these temporal patterns in the resuscitation of trauma patients in the emergency department.[2] Hypotension occurs after compensatory mechanisms are exhausted, which may be 40 minutes to 2 hours after significant hypovolemia.[1–4] On the other hand, arterial pressure may be restored by saline solutions before cardiac output and oxygen transport are corrected. This is particularly the case in hypertensive patients, who may spontaneously develop hypertension on sudden discontinuation of their low-salt diets.[5] Increased pressures may reflect acute hypertensive crisis, improved circulatory status, adrenomedullary stress response, anxiety, or excessive vasopressor therapy.

Continuous Noninvasive Blood Pressure Monitoring

Manometric blood pressure measurements obtained with sphygmomanometry using the Korotkoff sounds are routinely used to assess systolic and diastolic pressures. The Dinamap (GE Medical Systems, Milwaukee, Wis) was the first automatic noninvasive pressure monitor. With this instrument, an arm cuff is automatically inflated at frequent intervals, and the sound recording is used to derive and display systolic, mean, and dia-

stolic pressures. Motion artifacts may be a problem, however. Initially, Dinamap measured only MAP, but current models display systolic, mean, and diastolic pressures.

Early systems were developed to measure blood pressure by oscillometric sensing of variations in pressure on a blood pressure cuff; by use of crystal microphones; and by use of ultrasonic blood flow detectors positioned over the bronchial artery. The Accutorr (Datascope, Montvale, NJ) also uses mechanical oscillometry to inflate and deflate the pressure cuff automatically. The Infrasonde device (Puritan-Bennett, Carlsbad, Calif) employs an auscultatory method to determine systolic and diastolic pressures. The Roche (Cranbury, NJ) Ateriosonde, an electromechanical device, used a piezoelectric crystal to detect the point at which vessel walls begin to move as blood flow passes the occluding pressure cuff.

Heart Rate

Heart rate is a nonspecific hemodynamic variable with the same clinical indications as for arterial pressure. Heart rates are usually determined by manual palpation of the radial artery just above the wrist for at least 30 seconds. Heart rates may be measured electronically from the electrocardiogram (ECG) or the arterial pulse wave. Heart rates of more than 100 beats per minute are regarded as tachycardia. When premature ventricular contractions or other rhythm abnormalities are present, the true heart rate may be determined by auscultation at the apex; the difference between the apical and the radial rates represents the number of dropped beats. Increased heart rate is part of an early neurohormonal stress response that tends to increase cardiac output even in the presence of falling pressure. Its increase suggests blood volume and blood flow deficits; the faster the heart rate, the greater the hypovolemia or the cardiac impairment. Heart rate also increases with infection, anxiety, fear, fever, exercise, pain, discomfiture, and other nonspecific stresses, however.[1]

Bradycardia, defined as a heart rate of less than 50 beats per minute, may occur with various types of arteriosclerotic heart disease and, on occasion, in cervical cord injuries and other neurologic trauma. It may occur with inferior myocardial infarction when right coronary artery occlusion produces ischemia that blocks the sinoatrial node. Bradycardia during low cardiac output is an ominous sign suggesting markedly reduced coronary blood flow that compromises myocardial performance.

Temperature

Body temperature measurement is a useful but nonspecific screening test; it is measured routinely with the blood pressure, pulse, and respiratory rate. Usually, it is measured either orally, when significant elevations are not expected, or rectally, in ill patients. The central core temperature may be measured at the tympanic membrane or at the midesophagus for greater accuracy. Pulmonary arterial temperature, which also reflects core temperature, is routinely and continually measured with the pulmonary artery thermodilution catheter.

Temperature elevations are most often associated with infection, the septic syndrome or systemic inflammatory response syndrome (SIRS), tissue necrosis, late-stage carcinomatosis, Hodgkin disease, leukemia, hyperthyroidism, malignant hyperthermia, heat exhaustion, strenuous exercise, and other hypermetabolic states. Low-grade fever is also present after accidental or surgical trauma, particularly when hematomas, foreign bodies, fistulas, urinary extravasation, or stasis of urinary or bronchial secretions is present. Hypothermia may occur in some patients with septic shock, reduced metabolism associated with hypothyroidism, malnutrition, severe anemia, or cold exposure.

Urine Output Rate

Urine output rates, usually obtained routinely via Foley catheterization in a closed sterile system, are measured and recorded hourly. Minimal to acceptable values within the normal range are 0.5 to 1.0 mL/kg/hour. In the absence of renal disorders, urine output may reflect fluid status. The catheter must be flushed with aseptic solution at regular intervals because the most common cause of low urine output or anuria in the hospitalized patient is a plugged catheter.

Hourly urine output obtained via an indwelling urethral catheter is a rough approximation of renal perfusion, provided that the patient has an adequate blood volume and no preexisting renal disease. In resuscitation from acute injury, decreased urine flow may reflect low blood volume, low cardiac output, poor perfusion of the kidney, or the onset of acute oliguric renal failure. Urine output is not an adequate reflection of tissue perfusion in shock states, however, especially in septic shock; satisfactory urine output rates until 1 hour before death have been documented in patients with severe septic shock. Creatinine, osmolar, and free water clearance rates are better measures of renal function.

Plasma and Urine Osmolarity and Osmolar and Free Water Clearance Rates

Concentration of the urine is the kidney's most sensitive and important function. This capacity, which con-ventionally has been inferred from urine output rates and specific gravity, is best evaluated by measuring the ratio of the osmolalities of urine and plasma (UOsm/POsm) or by measuring osmolar and free water clearances. Osmolality of both plasma and urine is easily measured by the freezing point depression method or the vapor pressure method. UOsm/POsm is readily calculated as the ratio of these two measurements. A UOsm/POsm ratio of greater than 1.7 suggests good concentrative ability, but in the presence of oliguria, this ratio may be normal even when osmolar clearance is low.

Renal function is better evaluated by determination of osmolar clearances, which express the rate of solute removal from the plasma. If urinary output is also measured at the same time, the osmolar clearance may be calculated as follows:

$$COsm = UOsm/POsm \times V$$

where V is the urinary output and COsm is the osmolar clearance. Normally, the osmolar clearance is 120 mL/hour, but it decreases in acute renal failure.

Free water clearance, which more explicitly considers osmotic clearance with respect to the rate of urinary output, is a sensitive indicator that may be used to predict the early onset of postoperative acute renal failure. The free water clearance can be calculated as follows:

$$CH_2O = V - COsm$$

Normally, it is strongly negative, ranging from -25 to -100 mL/hour. Transient positive values followed by values close to zero precede the development of acute renal failure. For example, a patient with urine osmolality of 330 mOsm/L, plasma osmolality of 300 mOsm/L, and urine output of 100 mL/hour has a relatively normal osmolar clearance (110 mL/hour); however, the high free water clearance (10 mL/hour) indicates high-output renal failure.

Electrocardiographic Monitoring

The ECG evaluates the electrical events of cardiac contraction by sensing voltages at the body surface. Early studies assumed the body to be a homogenous volume conductor with uniform geometry, similar to a tank of saline solution, to accommodate the body's complex three-dimensional character, in which there are varying distances between the heart and the recording electrodes. The Dutch physiologist Einthoven represented the heart with two charged electrodes: a dipole with one positive pole and one negative pole. This dipole is surrounded by a hypothetical equilateral triangle. The electrical activity of the heart, repre-

TABLE 21–2. Glasgow Coma Score*

Score	Eye Movement	Verbal Function	Motor Response
1	None	None	Flaccid, unresponsive
2	To painful stimuli	Incomprehensible sounds	Abnormal extension
3	To voice	Inappropriate responses	Abnormal flexion
4	Spontaneous	Disoriented	Withdraws from pain
5		Oriented and conversant	Localizes stimuli
6			Obeys commands

*The score is calculated by adding together the best response in each of the three categories.

sented by the equivalent dipole, changes its magnitude and orientation during the cardiac cycle. The sides of the triangle, which represent the axes of the three standard limb leads, provide a triaxial frame of reference for spatial orientation of magnitudes and directions of cardiac electrical activity. The model was combined with the chest (V lead) readings and was further refined to frontal, sagittal, and horizontal components; this has greatly expanded understanding of cardiac electrophysiology.

The routine three-lead ECG is recorded from the right arm (RA), the left arm (LA), and the left leg (LL). The standard limb leads are defined as lead I (LA-RA), lead II (LL-RA), and lead III (LL-LA), and differences in electrical potential produced by the heart are measured across the designated limbs. Small electrodes corresponding to each lead are attached to the chest after application of a conductive salt paste to the skin. These electrodes pick up ECG waveforms, which are continuously displayed and, when desired, recorded on a permanent record at the patient's bedside. A 12-lead ECG is diagnostic for cardiac conditions and is useful to rule out cardiac complications in acutely injured patients, postoperative patients, and patients with sepsis. Lead II or other individual leads may be continuously monitored for early detection of arrhythmias, which may be associated with disorders of the cardiac muscle.

Continuous ECG monitoring is essential in acute myocardial infarction because arrhythmias are the most common life-threatening complication. Although done routinely, continuous ECG monitoring of the postoperative general surgical patient is infrequently useful because the incidence of significant arrhythmias is rather low; the authors have discovered three acute myocardial infarctions during and shortly after 8000 operations in a county hospital setting. The ECG is overemphasized in the noncardiac patient after elective surgery who has no risk factors.[6] In hypovolemic and traumatic shock, however, arrhythmias, subendocardial ischemia, and bradycardia may occur with inadequate oxygen delivery to the myocardium and may suggest precardiac arrest conditions.

Level of Consciousness

The level of consciousness may be assessed in postoperative and post-traumatic patients by the Glasgow Coma Scale (Table 21–2); this provides a semiquantitative clinical measure of the degree of unconsciousness or coma.[7]

Biochemical and Minimally Invasive Monitoring Methods

Serum Electrolytes

Measurements of serum electrolyte levels are useful in acutely ill patients. Hypokalemia is associated with alkalosis as a result of gastric outlet obstruction and other gastrointestinal conditions that produce severe vomiting. Hyperkalemia is associated with acidosis; hyperglycemia is associated with diabetes, stress, trauma, and head injury; hypoglycemia is associated with insulin reactions, insulinoma, or nutritional deficiencies; and increasing levels of blood urea nitrogen and creatinine are associated with renal failure.

Blood Chemical Measurements in Shock and Tissue Hypoxia

Five laboratory values indicate tissue hypoxia with anaerobic metabolism due to inadequate tissue perfusion or unevenly distributed microcirculatory flow: (1) acidosis (pH of less than 7.2), (2) base deficit of greater than 5 mEq and bicarbonate less than 20 mEq/L, (3) anion gap greater than 8 mEq/L, (4) blood lactate levels of more than 2 mEq/dL, and (5) gastric mucosal pH of less than 7.2 or gastric-arterial CO_2 gap of more than 40 mm Hg.[1] These are not direct measures of tissue perfusion and oxygenation but are reflections of anaerobic tissue metabolism. They are not sufficiently sensitive to evaluate the small changes in circulatory function that are needed to titrate therapy. More important, they may reflect relatively advanced circulatory changes that have already affected body metabolism. Finally, they have not been shown to be quantitatively related to the degree of oxygen debt.

Prothrombin time, partial thromboplastin time, fibrinogen determination, fibrin split product, and platelet counts are used to monitor acute bleeding and clotting problems associated with shock, sepsis, trauma, and hemorrhage. In acute illnesses, routine measurements of serum sodium, potassium, chloride, blood glucose, lactate, blood urea nitrogen, and creatinine are also taken. These chemical indicators are used to confirm or rule out other diagnoses, monitor progress, and assess therapeutic effectiveness.

Arterial Blood Gases and pH

Measurement of arterial blood gases and pH is used to screen for pulmonary function in the following: critical or respiratory illness (e.g., tachypnea, dyspnea, chronic obstructive pulmonary disease, adult respiratory distress syndrome), fluid and electrolyte problems, accidental trauma, acute emergency, extensive surgery, burns with smoke inhalation, and drug overdose. They are also measured in patients who are suspected of developing respiratory complications, patients who fail to respond appropriately after anesthesia, and patients who are suspected to have circulatory dysfunction or shock (suggested by restlessness, anxiety, mental confusion, and altered mental status) and other potential respiratory conditions. In addition, they are used in the monitoring of patients on controlled or assisted mechanical ventilation or oxygen therapy, in preoperative evaluation, and in postanesthesia surveillance.

The first laboratory signs of early lung problems are usually arterial blood gas abnormalities, such as an arterial partial pressure of oxygen (PaO_2) value of less than 70 torr or an arterial hemoglobin saturation (SaO_2) value of less than 96% in patients breathing room air (fractional inspired oxygen [FIO_2] = 0.21); an arterial partial pressure of carbon dioxide ($PaCO_2$) value of more than 45 torr; and a pH value of less than 7.3 or more than 7.5. Respiratory failure is suggested by PaO_2 values of less than 50 mm Hg in a patient breathing room air or a PaO_2/FIO_2 ratio of less than 250. Usually, the acutely ill patient is given supplementary oxygen by mask or nasal prongs and chest therapy prophylactically. If these measures do not improve the blood gas values, endotracheal intubation and mechanical ventilation should be considered before PaO_2 decreases to less than 60 torr. Patients with chronic respiratory insufficiency may tolerate low blood gas values but not require mechanical ventilation.

Hematocrit

The hematocrit—the percentage of red blood cells in a sample of venous blood—has been widely used to assess blood loss after covert hemorrhage, trauma, or surgery. In general, hematocrit values decrease with hemorrhage, fluid administration, and hypovolemia;

they increase with dehydration and whole blood or packed red cell transfusions. The hematocrit is measured in the following situations: routine admission; emergency conditions, including trauma and hemorrhage or suspected hemorrhage; fever, dehydration, or other water losses; suspected overtransfusion or overhydration; hemolysis, cell aggregation, or sludging after trauma and burns; destruction of red blood cells after fresh water drowning, envenomation, consumption coagulopathies, and disseminated intravascular coagulation; acute illnesses, circulatory shock, or sepsis; and postoperatively in high-risk patients, especially when intraperitoneal bleeding is present.

To measure hematocrit, blood samples are drawn from a peripheral vein or an artery, are immediately injected into four or more heparinized capillary tubes, and are promptly spun for 4 minutes in a microcentrifuge. The results of repeated samples should agree to within 1%. Alternatively, 4 mL of blood is drawn into a syringe containing 0.1 mL of heparin (1000 U/mL) and is immediately placed into a Wintrobe tube; the latter is centrifuged at 2000 g for 30 minutes.

Errors can be minimized when the hematocrit tubes are filled immediately after the blood is drawn. When blood is allowed to stand for even brief periods, the red blood cells begin to settle or aggregate, leaving the top half of the syringe with considerably fewer cells than the bottom half; shaking the sample does not eliminate this problem because cell aggregates are not completely broken up by simple shaking, and they rapidly reform.

A decrease in hematocrit is an indirect effect of blood loss produced by the compensatory transcapillary refilling of plasma volume by interstitial water. This compensation takes appreciable time. If a patient rapidly exsanguinates within a few minutes, the first and the last drops of blood have nearly the same hematocrit.[8] A blood loss of 600 mL in human volunteers is replaced by interstitial water in about 18 hours.[8, 9] Plasma volume replacement under these conditions occurs at about 1 mL/min for the first few hours and at successively decreasing rates thereafter. In the severely bled anesthetized dog, replacement occurs at a rate of 2.5 mL/min.[10] When blood loss is suspected, such as in trauma or postoperative shock, serial hematocrit values are usually recorded at 2- to 4-hour intervals.

Decreases in serial hematocrit values in postoperative and post-traumatic patients can signal the possibility of intra-abdominal hemorrhage. Serial hematocrit values are a reasonably good screening test for assessing gross changes in the early stages of hemorrhage but do not reliably reflect blood volume status.[11] Hematocrit values are not specific and have major limitations. The hematocrit represents static measurement of the venous red blood cell concentration; it is affected by gains or losses of plasma water as well as by gains or losses of red blood cells. For example, the hematocrit does not distinguish between the effects of hemorrhage and the loss of red blood cells from the circulation via cell aggregation, microthrombosis, or fluid retention. Moreover, the hematocrit does not distinguish between transfused red blood cells and newly synthesized red cells and may not be greatly affected by intravenous fluids that equilibrate or leak from the plasma into the interstitial space. After a patient has been given large volumes of crystalloids and transfusions, hematocrit changes may be uninterpretable.

Central Venous Pressure

Central venous pressure (CVP) and right atrial pressure monitoring are used to guide volume replacement for both medical and surgical patients. Because it is simple and available, CVP monitoring is routinely used to guide fluid therapy after hemorrhage, surgery, accidental trauma, sepsis, and other emergency conditions with suspected blood volume deficits or excesses, particularly when large amounts of fluids are needed. Measurement errors are caused by catheter obstruction, motion artifacts, or failure to establish consistent baseline values in patients who must be frequently repositioned or whose bed must be lowered or elevated; in the latter instance, it is absolutely necessary to make corresponding transducer changes.

The catheters are simple to place, and the pressures are easy to read. The most important problem in accurately measuring CVP is the establishment of a consistent "zero" point that permits measurement of meaningful changes by individual attendants on different shifts. When the patient is in the supine position, the point of entrance of the vena cava into the right atrium is about 10 cm above the lowest surface of the back or 10 cm below the sternum in the sixth interspace. The point selected may be marked on the patient's side with a felt-tip pen, and the pressure transducer is adjusted to this level as the bed is raised or lowered; alternatively, changes in body position or height of the bed may be corrected electronically.

Central venous pressure values in healthy persons range from -2 to $+6$ mm Hg during normal inspiration and expiration, respectively. On assuming the supine position, healthy, ambulatory individuals have CVP values that average about 6 to 8 mm Hg, but the values decrease gradually as vascular wall tone accommodates. A value of 10 mm Hg is commonly used as the upper limit of normal for acutely ill patients. Critically ill patients receiving mechanical ventilation and positive end-expiratory pressure who require fluid to maintain arterial pressure may develop a CVP value of 20 mm Hg, however. When CVP values exceed 15 to 18 mm Hg, a pulmonary arterial balloon flotation catheter may be used to measure the pulmonary artery occlusion (wedge) pressure (PAOP) for more precise titration of fluids.[1, 12, 13]

Central venous pressure is increased by blood volume, impaired cardiac function, increased intrathoracic or intra-abdominal pressure, vasopressors, and fluid therapy. It is lowered by improved cardiac function, reduced intrathoracic pressure, vasodilators, hypovolemia, and sudden blood or fluid losses; however, CVP values and changes after therapy also depend on venous wall compliance. Large fluid infusions may produce only small, transient CVP changes in hypovolemic patients, but even small fluid volumes may appreciably elevate CVP in patients with stress, chronic congestive cardiac failure, fluid overload, overtransfusion, or hypervolemia. Patients with chronic renal and cardiac failure are particularly vulnerable to either fluid overload or more fluid than they can handle; by contrast, acutely ill hypovolemic patients are particularly vulnerable to delayed or inadequate fluid therapy. This problem is overcome by careful titration of fluids.

Although reduced CVP occurs during and immediately after acute hemorrhage, the blood volume and the CVP correlate poorly after the patient has stayed in the intensive care unit a day or so, despite major blood volume deficits or excesses. This is because venous wall compliance rapidly accommodates to wide variations in blood volume. CVP and PAOP usually remain at about 8 to 12 mm Hg in patients in the intensive care unit despite carefully measured blood volume ranging from a deficit of 1 L/m² to an excess of 2 L/m² (Fig. 21–1).[11] It is seriously misleading to assess blood volume status based on CVP or PAOP.

Patients with right heart failure classically have distention of the neck veins, which reflects increased CVP. In many instances, right heart failure is secondary to left heart failure; in such cases, left atrial pressure, end-diastolic pressure, and PAOP rise; pulmonary artery pressure elevations increase the work of the right heart. If the pulmonary artery systolic pressure is less than 40 mm Hg in chronic conditions, the right ventricle usually maintains normal flow. With prolonged elevation of PA pressure, the right ventricle may fail, and the CVP may increase. Less commonly, right heart failure occurs with right myocardial infarction and without left heart failure, particularly in patients with pulmonary hypertension. Also, right heart failure may occur in the presence of high pulmonary vascular resistance due to pulmonary emboli, chronic obstructive lung disease, adult respiratory distress syndrome, aspiration pneumonia, and other types of respiratory failure. Wide variations in the CVP may occur (1) if the central line slips into the right ventricle, (2) in severe right heart failure with dilatation of the atrioventricular ring, and (3) in tricuspid insufficiency.

Central venous pressure measurements are most useful during early resuscitation from acute injury with

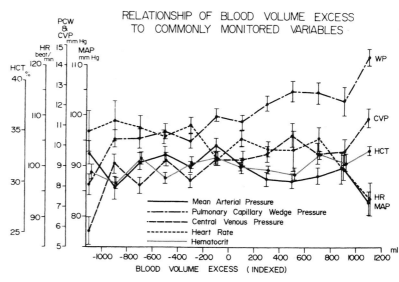

FIGURE 21–1. Mean (± standard error of the mean) of the commonly monitored variables on the y-axis plotted against their corresponding indexed blood volume excess (+) or deficit (−). Note the poor capacity of the monitored variables to predict blood volume. CVP, central venous pressure; HCT, hematocrit; HR, heart rate; MAP, mean arterial pressure; PCW, pulmonary capillary wedge; WP, wedge pressure. (From Shippy CR, Appel PL, Shoemaker WC: Reliability of clinical monitoring to assess blood volume in critically ill patients. Crit Care Med 1984;12:107.)

hypotension. Initially, hypovolemia occurs with low CVP. A CVP in excess of 20 to 25 mm Hg usually indicates that (1) too much fluid has been given, (2) fluids were given too rapidly, or (3) an exaggerated stress response has occurred. Knowledge of CVP is most helpful with failure of only one organ system, such as cardiac failure, or with uncomplicated blood loss. Increased CVP or PAOP in response to administration of a standardized volume load over a prescribed time period provides valuable information on the compliance of the venous tree; tolerance to volume loads indicates adequate cardiac reserve capacity.

High peripheral venous pressure reflects CVP, but measurements of these pressures diverge in the low ranges. The central venous system, including the right atrium, the vena cava, and its major branches, acts as a unicameral system with nearly equal pressures. In hypovolemia, the extent of this unicameral behavior is limited, and the peripheral venous pressures largely reflect local influences upstream from their site of measurement. By contrast, in hypervolemia and right heart failure, the venous tree is distended by the accumulation of blood behind the right ventricle; as this venous engorgement increases, the dimensions of the unicameral central venous pool increase along with peripheral venous pressures. Then high peripheral venous pressure values are similar to CVP values.

Intra-arterial Blood Pressure

Intra-arterial blood pressure, measured via the axillary, the radial, the ulnar, or the femoral artery, provides continuous display of the arterial waveform along with measurements of MAP and systolic and diastolic pressures. Intra-arterial catheters with pressure transducers and a continuous recording apparatus that has been zeroed and calibrated are more accurate than cuff

measurement. Under normal conditions, pressures obtained from intra-arterial catheters are about 2 to 8 mm Hg greater than cuff-measured pressures.[1] In critically ill patients, intra-arterial pressures may be 10 to 30 mm Hg greater than cuff-measured pressures. Furthermore, cuff-measured pressures may be inaccurate in patients with severe vasoconstriction and low stroke volume. Differences of 50 mm Hg between intra-arterial catheter-measured and cuff-measured pressures have been reported.

The indications for continuous intra-arterial pressure recording are shock, critical illness, peripheral vasoconstriction, and intraoperative and postoperative monitoring in high-risk patients undergoing life-threatening operations. In these cases, accurate continuous display of arterial pressure is needed to observe trends and to titrate therapy. Arterial catheters also allow frequent blood gas measurements.

Gastric Tonometry

Gastric tonometry measures gastric and intestinal wall CO_2 by equilibration of CO_2 partial pressure between a saline-filled balloon on the end of a nasogastric tube and the gut wall layers. After 40 to 60 minutes have been allowed for equilibration, the balloon's saline solution is sampled and is analyzed for P_{CO_2} in a blood gas analyzer; at the same time, an arterial blood sample is obtained to assess blood bicarbonate levels, and the pH is calculated from the Henderson-Hasselbalch equation.[14, 15] The balloon CO_2 values are in equilibration with tissue CO_2 so that increases in the balloon CO_2 reflect increased tissue CO_2 production and indirectly reflect the degree of anaerobic metabolism. In shock, anaerobic metabolism generates hydrogen ions (H^+), which are then buffered by tissue bicarbonate and result in CO_2 production.[16–18] Normal tonometric measurement of gastric CO_2 establishes the adequacy of gastric circulation, whereas cellular accumulation of CO_2 reflects tissue hypoxia and acidosis.

Recent improvements include an automated system that pumps air into the tonometer's balloon and then measures and records CO_2 by infrared analysis every 10 to 15 minutes.[18] An alternative method being developed is balloonless fiberoptic CO_2 sensors situated directly in the gastric bubble; their usefulness and reliability are being evaluated in clinical trials.

Blood Volume

Blood volume measurement, cardiac functional capacity, and colloidal osmotic pressure are of major importance in fluid therapy.[5, 8–11, 19–22] Hypovolemic patients with normal cardiac reserve can readily tolerate a volume load (fluid challenge). Those with low colloidal osmotic pressure, diminished cardiac reserve, or chronic respiratory conditions are less able to tolerate infusion of large volumes of fluids, particularly crystalloids, without developing pulmonary edema. Blood volume is often inferred indirectly from measurements of arterial pressure, heart rate, CVP, urinary output, hematocrit, and PAOP. These are useful during resuscitation, but they are unreliable indicators of blood volume, especially in patients who are critically ill or in shock (see Fig. 21–1). Blood volume measurements provide definitive therapeutic answers to hypovolemia and hypervolemia but have largely been replaced by PAOP measurements because of the hazards of radioactivity, the time required for measurement, and the associated cost.

Blood volume may be measured by the indicator dilution concept. A known amount of dye or indicator that mixes uniformly with the plasma or the blood is injected intravenously, and its concentration or radioactivity is measured in blood samples obtained at timed intervals after injection of the indicator.[11, 19] The indicator's concentration is inversely proportional to its volume of dilution; the latter is calculated by the dilution formula:

$$C1V1 = C2V2$$

where C1 and V1 are the concentration and volume, respectively (i.e., mass of the injected indicator), and C2 and V2 are the indicator's concentration and volume of distribution at the time of sampling.

Initially, plasma volume was measured by photometric assay of injected dyes, such as Evans blue or indocyanine green.[20–22] After intravenous injection, the distribution of the indicator is measured in the plasma volume (PV), and the blood volume (BV) is calculated as

$$BV = PV/(1\text{-}Hct)$$

where Hct is hematocrit. The dye methods were replaced by radioassay of injected iodine-labeled human serum albumin and, to a lesser extent, by ^{55}Cr- or ^{32}P-labeled erythrocytes. The ^{125}I- or ^{131}I-tagged albumin is more convenient, whereas red cell labels are more technically demanding. Starch has also been used as an indicator.[23] In the labeled albumin method, two or more preinjection control serum samples are radioassayed in duplicate. After injection of a measured dose of the labeled albumin, three to six timed postinjection samples are similarly assayed; 4% corrections in the hematocrit values are made for the packing fraction of plasma, and 6% corrections are made for the difference between venous hematocrit and total body hematocrit.[11, 22] Radioactive-labeled indicators are rarely used at present because of potential biohazards. Recently, blood volume has been measured using carbon monoxide as the indicator and a ventilator-driven closed breathing system for administration of the carbon monoxide[24]; arterial samples were taken from an indwelling catheter, and carboxyhemoglobin values were measured. When red cell labels are used, red cell mass (RCM) is measured and blood volume is (BV) calculated as

$$BV = RCM/Hct$$

Normal blood volume is 2.74 L/m^2, or 7.5 mL/kg, for males and 2.37 L/m^2, or 7 mL/kg, for females. The patient in shock due to hemorrhage, trauma, and sepsis has been found empirically to do better with about 500 mL in excess of the expected norm (i.e., 3.2 L/m^2 for males and 2.9 L/m^2 for females). This extra volume compensates for uneven distributions of blood volume, pooling of blood in the splanchnic area, red blood cell aggregation in the microcirculation, and formation of red blood cell microthrombi. Measurements require meticulous technique for reproducibility within an 8% to 10% error.

Colloidal Osmotic Pressure

Plasma and interstitial fluid are two aqueous solutions separated by capillary basement membranes. The capillary membrane is semipermeable: freely permeable to water and electrolytes but barely permeable to macromolecules, such as plasma proteins. In an analogous manner, cell membranes separate the intracellular water from the extracellular water. Water migrates through each membrane to equalize the concentrations of the solutions on either side by the process of osmosis. The colloidal osmotic pressure, or oncotic pressure, is the osmotic force exerted on a membrane by macromolecules. It is a measure of the hydrostatic pressure applied to a solution of greater concentration that is just able to prevent the net movement of water across the membrane. Colloidal osmotic pressure is determined solely by the number of molecules in solution on each side of the membrane.

The distribution of water between the intravascular and the interstitial compartments of the systemic circulation depends on the balance of Starling forces. Plasma water escapes from the vascular space at the arterial end of the capillary, where hydrostatic pressure is greatest. Water returns at the venous end because venous colloid osmotic pressure is greater than that of interstitial water. The equivalent of the plasma volume (i.e., 3000 mL in the healthy 70-kg man) leaves and returns to the vascular space each minute. By contrast, about 1% of the plasma proteins also leave the vascular space per minute; most of these proteins are returned by way of the lymphatics. About one fifth of the plasma water may be outside the anatomic confines of the vasculature at any given time. The hydrostatic pressures at the arterial end of the capillary are about 25 to 35 mm Hg, the tissue pressures are -2 to $+2$ mm Hg, the capillary venous pressures are 10 to 15 mm Hg, the venous oncotic pressures are 24 to 28 mm Hg, and the interstitial oncotic pressures are about 15 to 20 mm Hg. Normally, the forces that determine net water movement across a capillary are close to zero or are slightly negative; excess water driven into the tissues by this low net pressure is returned to the vascular space by the lymphatics. Two to four liters of lymph are returned to the circulation via the thoracic duct each day. After hemorrhage, capillary refilling of the plasma volume occurs primarily as a result of osmotic forces.[22]

Tissue Perfusion/Oxygenation Monitoring

Pulse Oximetry

Microprocessors and light-emitting diodes have made continuous noninvasive monitoring of arterial oxygenation a routine standard of care. In this technique, a red diode and an infrared diode are rapidly pulsed in sequence, and the amounts of light transmitted by each throughout successive heartbeats are used to calculate a running average of arterial hemoglobin saturation (SaO_2), which may be displayed continuously. The pulse oximeter is designed to measure oxygen saturation differences in the pulse waveform; it does not distinguish the oxyhemoglobin level from that of carboxyhemoglobin or methemoglobin. (The latter is needed in patients exposed to carbon monoxide.) Without satisfactory waveforms, the instrument does not function accurately. The accuracy of pulse oximetry decreases progressively below 92% and becomes unreliable at values of less than 85%. Early recognition of respiratory problems is more important than SaO_2 accuracy at these low values, however.

Pulse oximeters are useful during initial resuscitation in acute emergencies, intraoperative and postoperative high-risk surgery, and anesthesia induction and in critically ill patients with unstable hemodynamics or suspected respiratory problems. Pulse oximetry is particularly useful for titration of FIO_2 during mechanical ventilation and for weaning patients from mechanical ventilation. The frequency of arterial blood gas measurement may be reduced with pulse oximetry. This is important in children and in those with acute, rapidly changing illnesses. Disposable probes are used in patients with infectious conditions.

Transcutaneous Oxygen and Carbon Dioxide Monitoring of Tissue Perfusion

The Clark polarographic oxygen electrode is the standard blood gas analyzer.[25] Hüch and associates and Eberhard and colleagues used heated Clark electrodes for continuous noninvasive transcutaneous oxygen tension ($PtcO_2$) measurement.[26, 27] With the assumption that PaO_2 and $PtcO_2$ were nearly identical, the latter was used for more than 25 years as a surrogate for PaO_2 values in neonates and infants to reduce the need for arterial blood sampling. When differences between PaO_2 and $PtcO_2$ occurred, they were usually attributed to failure of the instrument measuring $PtcO_2$. Although $PtcO_2$ usually reflects PaO_2 when the neonate is hemodynamically stable, it is appreciably lower than PaO_2 in the seriously ill neonate with circulatory problems that produce poor tissue perfusion.

In adults, $PtcO_2$ is about 80% of the value for PaO_2 during normal hemodynamic conditions; however, when blood flow limits body metabolism, $PtcO_2$ tracks flow. In both normal and low-flow states, $PtcO_2$ was used to track oxygen delivery (DO_2). In essence, $PtcO_2$ is only indirectly related to PaO_2; it is directly related to local tissue perfusion and tissue oxygenation.[28-31] Heating of the skin by the transcutaneous electrode changes the structure of the lipoproteins in the stratum corneum from the gel to the sol state and allows rapid diffusion of oxygen from subcutaneous tissues to the surface electrode. An electrode temperature of 44°C to 45°C increases oxygen diffusion across the stratum corneum and reduces local vasoconstriction of the skin.[30] This allows the $PtcO_2$ to become closer to PaO_2 in hemodynamically stable patients. This degree of heating, however, decreases oxygen solubility, shifts the oxyhemoglobin dissociation curve to the right, and dilates local metarterioles.

In adults, $PtcO_2$ measures tissue O_2 tension in a local segment of heated skin, which explicitly and quantitatively reflects the oxygenation of this skin segment.[28-30] This is not necessarily the same in all skin segments or in other peripheral tissues; however, the skin is very sensitive to peripheral vasoconstriction from the adrenomedullary stress response and therefore provides an earlier warning than SvO_2 and VO_2. $PtcO_2$ has been shown to reflect the delivery of oxygen to the local area of skin, and it parallels the mixed venous oxygen tension (SvO_2) except under terminal conditions, when peripheral shunting leads to high SvO_2 values.[29] Because $PtcO_2$ values are dependent on both PaO_2 and local blood flow, $PtcO_2$ may track PaO_2 when flow is adequate and may track flow (or local DO_2) when PaO_2 is adequate. In either case, $PtcO_2$ reflects local DO_2. From a practical clinical viewpoint, the $PtcO_2$ pattern is a useful screening tool that reflects tissue perfusion and oxygenation. On room air, $PtcO_2$ values greater than 65 torr suggest satisfactory perfusion; values from 40 to 65 torr suggest marginal perfusion; values from 25 to 40 torr indicate impaired tissue perfusion; and values less than 25 torr indicate severe shock.[31-34] Oxygen consumption (VO_2) was compared with simultaneous transcutaneous oxygen tension ($PtcO_2$) at the initial baseline period, the nadir, and the postresuscitation period in 32 patients (Fig. 21–2). Although the changes were significant ($P < .05$), they were frequently not synchronous; the $PtcO_2$ nadir occurred 12 minutes ($P > .05$) before the VO_2 nadir.[32]

Limitations of $PtcO_2$ are the following: artifacts from patient movements, need to change the electrode site every 4 to 6 hours to avoid first-degree skin burns, need to calibrate the membranes before each use and each change in skin site, and need for a reasonably constant thermal environment (i.e., free from cold drafts). The membrane also must be changed when readings become unstable.

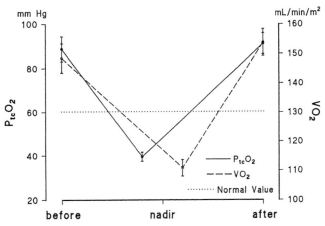

FIGURE 21–2. Comparison of oxygen consumption (VO_2) with simultaneous transcutaneous oxygen tension ($PtcO_2$) at the initial baseline period (before), the nadir, and the postresuscitation period (after). (From Shoemaker WC, Belzberg H, Wo CCJ, et al: Multicenter study of noninvasive monitoring systems as alternatives to invasive monitoring of acutely ill emergency patients. Chest 1998;113:1643–1652.)

Transcutaneous carbon dioxide tension ($PtcCO_2$) measurement using the Stowe-Severinghaus carbon dioxide electrode was initially used in neonates to approximate $PaCO_2$ values. $PtcCO_2$ values parallel but consistently overestimate by about 10 to 15 torr the $PaCO_2$ values in both hemodynamically stable neonates and adults. In shock, $PtcCO_2$ may be greatly elevated to values of more than 100 torr; it is inversely related to cardiac output.[31] Differences between the values of $PaCO_2$ and $PtcCO_2$ reflect accumulation of tissue CO_2 from inadequate tissue perfusion, especially in shock states.[32-34]

Ventilatory Monitoring

In the intubated mechanically ventilated patient, airway pressures and flow and volume measurements can be obtained from modern ventilators. Ventilation, the movement of gas into and out of the lungs, is assessed by the mean tidal volume (VT), which is the volume of gas inspired with each breath (normally 65 to 75 mL/kg); the minute volume (MV), the mean volume of inspired gas per minute; and the respiratory rate, the mean number of breaths taken per minute (normally 10 to 15). Timed measurement of VT (e.g., FEV_1, the volume of air forcibly expired in 1 minute) is a more explicit measure of obstructive airway disease; however, this is not often used in critically ill patients who are usually unable to give the effort needed. Airway pressures are continuously displayed by mechanical ventilators, and from this display, the mean airway pressure, the plateau pressure, and the peak pressure may be derived. FIO_2 is the fractional inspired oxygen concentration; this varies from 21% at room air to 1.0 at 100% oxygen concentration.

The elasticity of the lungs and the thoracic wall taken together is evaluated physiologically as compliance, the change in volume for a given change in the distending transthoracic pressure. The effective static thoracic compliance is estimated as VT changes in airway pressure at a time of zero gas flow using an "inspiratory hold" or by occluding the expiratory port long enough (1 or 2 seconds) to allow airway pressure to reach a relatively constant plateau. Dynamic pulmonary compliance curves are derived from continuous measurements of airway pressure and volume curves.

Positive end-expiratory pressure (PEEP) and continuous positive airway pressure (CPAP) are automatically measured and adjusted by ventilator settings. The I-to-E ratio measures inspiratory/expiratory time.

Expiratory capnograms measure the breath-by-breath pattern of the patient's expired CO_2 tension by means of infrared sensors or mass spectrometry. Infrared sensors are easier and cheaper to use and have response times of about 150 to 200 milliseconds. Mass spectrometry has faster response times (about 100 milliseconds) and the ability to measure other gases simultaneously, including anesthetic agents, but is expensive and requires costly maintenance. Expired gas may be measured by including mainstream sensors as part of the ventilator circuit or by employing a sidestream method, in which a remote analyzer measures gas sampled through a small tube placed on the side wall of the external ventilatory circuit. Three phases of CO_2 concentration in expired gas are recognized: (1) near zero, which represents the dead space of the mechanical device plus the patient's upper airway; (2) increasing CO_2 concentrations, from progressive emptying of the alveolar gas; and (3) relatively flat plateau at the end of expiration, which may have a slightly positive slope. The highest value, or end-tidal carbon dioxide tension (PET_{CO_2}), represents alveolar gas; this usually corresponds to the arterial CO_2 (Pa_{CO_2}). When near-zero CO_2 concentrations occur throughout the respiratory cycle, the endotracheal tube has not been properly positioned and is most likely in the esophagus.

The rate of carbon dioxide production (VCO_2) may be measured directly by means of spirometry or may be calculated from the PET_{CO_2} and the minute volume.

The respiratory quotient, VCO_2/VO_2, is the ratio of carbon dioxide production to oxygen consumption. It is normally 0.8 but may increase with glucose loads, sepsis, or some hypermetabolic states and may decrease with starvation, diabetes, or high fat intake.

The dead space (Vd/Vt) is calculated as a percentage of the tidal volume as follows:

$$Vd = VT(Pa_{CO_2} - PE_{CO_2}/Pa_{CO_2})$$

where Vd is dead space, VT is tidal volume, Pa_{CO_2} is arterial CO_2 tension, and PE_{CO_2} is mixed expired CO_2 tension.

Maximal inspiratory strength is measured by calculating the maximal negative pressure against the closed airway. It normally is between -40 and -100 cm of water, but it is between 0 and -40 cm in adult respiratory distress syndrome that requires mechanical ventilation.

Conclusions

Routine clinical monitoring attempts to organize early parameters of circulatory failure and failure of other systems or organs (1) to screen patients who might be more ill than initially realized and (2) for surveillance of patients who might deteriorate while being diagnosed or treated for more benign disorders. The occurrence of hypotension and tachycardia, which are nonspecific vital signs, is frequently used in clinical situations to warn of circulatory dysfunction or shock. They represent decompensation or failure to sustain protective circulatory mechanisms, however, not the primary pathophysiologic defect of shock, which is inadequate tissue oxygenation from inadequate perfusion. Nevertheless, these and other clinical parameters are routinely used to identify problems for early diagnosis and management.

References

1. Shoemaker WC, Parsa MH: Invasive and physiologic monitoring. In Grenvik A, Ayres SM, Holbrook PR, Shoemaker WC (eds): Textbook of Critical Care, 4th ed. Philadelphia, WB Saunders, 2000, pp 74–91.
2. Wo CJ, Shoemaker WC, Appel PL, et al: Unreliability of blood pressure and heart rate to evaluate cardiac output in emergency resuscitation and critical illness. Crit Care Med 1993;21:218–223.
3. Shoemaker WC, Kram HB, Appel PL, et al: The efficacy of central venous and pulmonary artery catheters and therapy based upon them in reducing mortality and morbidity. Arch Surg 1990;125:1332–1338.
4. Monson DO, Shoemaker WC: Sequence of hemodynamic events after various types of hemorrhage. Surgery 1968;63:738–749.
5. Shoemaker WC, Kram HB: Effects of crystalloids and colloids on hemodynamics, oxygen transport, and outcome in high-risk patients. In Simmons RC, Udeko AS (eds): Debates in Clinical Surgery. Chicago, Year Book, 1990, pp 263–316.
6. Lewis FJ, Quinn ML: Continuous electrocardiogram monitoring in a surgical intensive care unit. Crit Care Med 1977;5:73–75.
7. Teasdale G, Jennett B: Assessment of coma and impaired consciousness. A practical scale. Lancet 1974;2:81–84.
8. Skillman JJ, Awwad HK, Moore FD: Plasma kinetics of the early transcapillary refill after hemorrhage in man. Surg Gynecol Obstet 1967;123:983–996.
9. Moore FD: Effects of hemorrhage on body composition. N Engl J Med 1965;273:567–577.
10. Wiggers CJ: Physiology of Shock. New York, Commonwealth Fund, 1950.
11. Shippy CR, Appel PL, Shoemaker WC: Reliability of clinical monitoring to assess blood volume in critically ill patients. Crit Care Med 1984;12:107–112.
12. Guyton AC, Hall JE: Textbook of Medical Physiology, 9th ed. Philadelphia, WB Saunders, 1996.
13. Wilson JN, Grow JB, Demong CV, et al: Central venous pressure in optimal blood volume maintenance. Arch Surg 1962;83:563.
14. Fiddian-Green RG, Pittenger G, Whitehouse WM: Back diffusion of CO_2 and its influence on the intramural pH in gastric mucosa. J Surg Res 1982;33:39–48.
15. Gutierrez G, Palizas F, Doglio G, et al: Gastric intermucosal pH as a therapeutic index of tissue oxygenation in critically ill patients. Lancet 1992;339:195–199.
16. Clark CH, Gutierrez G: Gastric intramucosal pH: A noninvasive method for indirect measurement of tissue oxygenation. Am J Crit Care 1992;1:53–60.
17. Schlichtig R, Bowles SA: Distinguishing between aerobic and anaerobic appearance of dissolved CO_2 in intestine during low flow. J Appl Physiol 1994;76:2443–2451.
18. Gutierrez G, Brown SD: Gastrointestinal tonometry: A monitor of regional dysoxia. New Horiz 1996;4:413–419.
19. Shoemaker WC, Monson DO: Effect of whole blood and plasma expanders on volume-flow relationships in critically ill patients. Surg Gynecol Obstet 1973;137:453–457.
20. Davis HA: Blood Volume Dynamics. Springfield, IL, Charles C Thomas, 1962.
21. Albert SN: Blood Volume. Springfield, IL, Charles C Thomas, 1963.
22. Moore FD: The body cell mass and its supporting environment: Body composition in health and disease. Philadelphia, WB Saunders, 1963.
23. Tschaikowsky K, Meisner M, Durst R, et al: Blood volume determination using hydroxyethyl starch: A rapid and simple method. Crit Care Med 1997;25:599–606.
24. Dingley J, Foex BA, Swart M, et al: Blood volume determination

by carbon monoxide method using a new delivery system. Crit Care Med 1999;27:2435–2441.

25. Clark LC Jr: Monitor and control of blood and tissue oxygen tensions. Trans Am Soc Artif Intern Organs 1956;2:41–49.

26. Hŭch A, Hŭch R, Meinzer K, et al: Eine schnelle behizte Proberflach-electrode zur kontinuierlichen Uberwachung des PO2 beim Menschen. In Electrodenaufbau und Eigenschaften. Stuttgart, Proc Medizin-Technik, 1972.

27. Eberhard P, Mindt W, Hammacher K: Perkutane Messung des Sauerstoff-partialdruckes. In Methodik und Anwendungen. Stuttgart, Medizin-Technik, 1972.

28. Tremper KK, Shoemaker WC: Transcutaneous oxygen monitoring of critically ill adults with and without low flow shock. Crit Care Med 1981;9:706–709.

29. Tremper KK, Waxman K, Shoemaker WC: Effects of hypoxia and shock in transcutaneous PO$_2$ values in dogs. Crit Care Med 1979;7:526–531.

30. Tremper KK, Huxtable RF: Dermal heat transport analysis for transcutaneous O$_2$ measurements. Acta Anesth Scand 1978;(suppl 68):4–7.

31. Tremper KK, Shoemaker WC, Shippy CR, Nolan LS al: Transcutaneous PCO$_2$ monitoring on adult patients in the ICU and the operating room. Crit Care Med 1981;9:752–755.

32. Shoemaker WC, Belzberg H, Wo CCJ, et al: Multicenter study of noninvasive monitoring systems as alternatives to invasive monitoring of acutely ill emergency patients. Chest 1998;114:1643–1652.

33. Shoemaker WC, Appel PL, Kram HB, et al: Multicomponent noninvasive physiologic monitoring of circulatory function. Crit Care Med 1988;16:482–490.

34. Shoemaker WC, Wo CCJ, Demetriades D, et al: Early physiologic patterns in acute illness and accidents. New Horiz 1996;4:395–412.

22 Invasive Hemodynamic Monitoring

William C. Shoemaker and Charles C.J. Wo

Cardiac catheterization and, subsequently, the balloon-tipped pulmonary artery (PA) catheter with thermodilution cardiac output computer have made hemodynamic and oxygen transport values available at the bedside and have changed our understanding of shock and the way we treat life-threatening circulatory problems. Cardiac output measurements reflect overall circulatory function and its capacity to increase to compensate for the increased metabolic needs of exercise, fever, and acute severe illness, which may be limited by cardiac insufficiency or hypovolemia. The partial pressure of oxygen in blood (PaO_2), the ratio of PaO_2 to the fraction of inspired oxygen (FIO_2), oxygen delivery (DO_2), the volume of oxygen consumption (VO_2), and pulmonary venous admixture, or shunt (Qs/Qt), reflect pulmonary function and tissue perfusion. The principal overall function of the circulation is to support body metabolism with sufficient amounts of oxygenated blood and nutrients in normal conditions as well as in the rapidly changing metabolic activity of exercise, stress, and acute illness. Invasive hemodynamic and oxygen transport monitoring may be useful in suspected acute circulatory problems in patients with high surgical risk (Table 22–1) and in trauma patients with overt or covert blood loss, major trauma, head injury, blunt injury to the chest or the abdomen, shock, or circulatory dysfunction from potentially life-threatening conditions. Invasive monitoring is done (1) to identify circulatory deficiencies, (2) to evaluate underlying physiologic problems, (3) to define criteria for therapeutic goals, and (4) to titrate therapy to achieve these optimal goals. Surveillance monitoring is used less precisely to show the general status and the direction of monitored patterns.

Pulmonary Artery and Pulmonary Artery Occlusion Pressure

The PA catheter is commonly used to measure PA pressure and PA occlusion (wedge) pressure (PAOP) to assess left ventricular filling pressure; this is similar to the use of central venous pressure (CVP) values to assess right ventricular filling pressure. The PA catheter is used to diagnose circulatory deficiencies and to differentiate acute cardiac failure from hypovolemic or hypervolemic problems. It is also used with cardiac output and oxygen transport measurements to monitor the progress of therapy in patients with acute myocardial infarction or other types of cardiac problems, shock, trauma, high-risk surgery, or other acute critical illnesses in which the fluid status is uncertain.

The expected hemodynamic pattern in acute myocardial infarction is hypotension, low cardiac output, and increased ventricular filling pressure (PAOP), often with decreased ventricular contractility and compliance. Monitoring PA pressure and PAOP may be used with thermodilution to observe the progress of the disease and to titrate various therapeutic interventions.

In normal conditions, left atrial pressure is within 2 or 3 mm Hg of the PAOP but may be slightly higher than the right atrial pressure or the CVP. There are significant differences between CVP and PAOP in valvular heart disorders, in unilateral ventricular disease, and when pulmonary vascular resistance is elevated with acute postoperative respiratory failure.

Pulmonary artery hypotension is often seen in hypovolemic shock, but PA hypertension may occur after rapid fluid resuscitation for hypovolemic or traumatic shock as well as in patients with congenital intra-atrial or intraventricular defects, chronic obstructive lung disease, or primary pulmonary hypertension. Transiently increased PA pressure may accompany fluid and transfusion therapy, particularly in shock syndromes.

The PAOP closely parallels left atrial and left ventricular end-diastolic pressures unless significant mitral valve stenosis or pulmonary venous resistance exists (as may be seen in chronic obstructive pulmonary disease). In mitral stenosis, high PAOP does not mean that left ventricular filling is adequate, because increased pressure gradients across the mitral valve also increase PAOP. The latter is affected by the same factors that influence CVP (i.e., blood volume, ventricular contractility, intrathoracic and intra-abdominal pressures, vasopressors, vasodilators, and fluid therapy) as well as by conditions that increase cardiac afterload.

Pulmonary artery occlusion pressure, similar to CVP, is not a reliable measure of blood volume because in time pulmonary and systemic venous wall tone accommodates to blood volume deficits or excesses. With fluid therapy, sudden increases in the PAOP to greater than 20 mm Hg may be due to infusion of too much intravenous fluid too rapidly, inadequate left ventricular contractility, high positive end-expiratory pressure, or high intrathoracic pressure.

TABLE 22–1. Monitoring Criteria for High-Risk Surgical Patients

Preoperative
1. Previous severe cardiorespiratory illness (e.g., acute MI, COPD, stroke)
2. Extensive ablative surgery planned for carcinoma (e.g., esophagectomy and total gastrectomy or prolonged surgery [>6 hr])
3. Severe multiple trauma (e.g., involving more than three organs or more than two systems; opening of two body cavities [left side of chest and abdomen]; multiple long bone and pelvic fractures)
4. Massive blood loss (>8 units): BV > 1.5 L/m² and Hct > 20 mL/dL within 48 hr of admission
5. Age of more than 70 yr and evidence of limited physiologic reserve of one or more vital organs
6. Shock: MAP < 60 mm Hg; CVP < 5 mm Hg; UO < 20 mL/hr; cold, clammy skin
7. Septicemia: positive blood culture, WBC count > 12,000/mm³, spiking fever > 101°F for 48 hr, chills
8. Evidence of septic shock (temperature > 101°F, WBC count > 12,000/mm³) plus hypotension (MAP < 70 mm Hg)
9. Severe nutritional problems associated with a surgical illness: weight loss > 20 lb, albumin concentration < 3 g/dL, osmolarity < 280 mOsm/L
10. Respiratory failure (e.g., PaO₂, < 60 mm Hg or FIO₂ > 0.4, Qsp/Qt > 30%, patient on mechanical ventilation)
11. Acute abdominal catastrophe (e.g., pancreatitis, gangrenous bowel, peritonitis, perforated viscus, or internal gastrointestinal bleeding)
12. CVP > 15 mm Hg after fluid resuscitation
13. Acute renal failure: blood urea nitrogen > 50 mg/dL, creatinine > 3 mg/dL, C_H2O > 10 mL/hr
14. Acute hepatic failure (bilirubin > 3 mg/dL, albumin concentration < 3 g/dL, LDH > 200 U/mL, alkaline phosphatase > 100 U/mL, ammonia > 120 µg/mL)
15. Acute agitation, depressed nervous system, or coma

Postoperative
1. Acute catastrophic change, suggesting fresh MI, pulmonary embolus, or postoperative bleeding
2. Hypotension: MAP < 70 mm Hg or unstable vital signs
3. Operative misadventure (e.g., use of > 8 units of WB or PRBCs for estimated 4000-mL blood loss in the operating room)
4. Severe sepsis, perforated viscus, gangrenous bowel, peritonitis, pneumonia, positive blood culture, aspiration pneumonia, temperature elevation >101°F for > 2 days
5. Any vital organ failure (e.g., the same as 9 to 15 of the list of preoperative conditions)
6. Postoperative fluid or electrolyte problem requiring more than 5000 mL of fluids per day
7. Failure to respond to adequate volume therapy, which is replacement of blood losses estimated from sponge and lab counts and as judged by clinical criteria, such as arterial pressure, UO, Hct, level of consciousness, and motor responses

BV, blood volume; C_H2O water clearance; COPD, chronic obstructive pulmonary disease; CVP, central venous pressure; Hct, hematocrit; LDH, lactate dehydrogenase; MAP, mean arterial pressure; MI, myocardial infarction; PaO₂, partial pressure of oxygen in arterial blood; PRBC, packed red blood cells; Qsp/Qt, pulmonary venous admixture (shunt) as the ratio of shunt flow to cardiac output; UO, urinary output; WB, whole blood; WBC, white blood cells.

Although blood volume should not be inferred from the absolute or "static" CVP or PAOP values, these pressure measurements may reflect the capacitance of the vascular tree for additional fluids. For example, after a standardized volume of 500 mL of colloids or 1000 mL of crystalloids is given over a 1-hour period, the increase in CVP or PAOP and the duration of this increase indicate tolerance to additional fluid therapy.

An increase in CVP or PAOP from 10 to 14 mm Hg that finally settles at 11 mm Hg 30 minutes after fluid infusion suggests that more fluids may be safely given if needed to achieve physiologic goals. Increases from 10 to 17 mm Hg that persist suggest limited tolerance for additional fluids, however.

Cardiac Output: Methods and Concepts

The important hemodynamic variables are blood pressure, blood volume, and blood flow. Cardiac output is the rate of blood flow pumped by the heart per minute; measurements are easy to make, readily automated, simple in concept, and relatively straightforward, and with appropriate quality control, they may be obtained by residents, nurses, and medical technologists. Although cardiac output may not be considered very useful because of its wide variations, the patterns of changes can be very helpful when allowance is made for confounding factors, including age, comorbid conditions, time in the course of the acute illness, previous cardiac conditions that limit reserve capacities, and indexing to body surface area in square meters to account for differences in body size. The value obtained by dividing volume and flow measurements by the patient's body surface area or body weight is the cardiac index. This standardization allows comparison of hemodynamic values among patients with widely varying size and body habitus. The various hemodynamic variables are calculated from pressure and flow data using standard formulas (Table 22–2).

Early studies in humans by Cournand and associates and by others documented increased cardiac output after surgery, trauma, and sepsis, but there was reduced flow when hypovolemia intervened.[1–22] When severe shock occurred after trauma, the average blood volume deficit was found to be 1330 mL.[1] Variable changes in cardiac output after surgery were reported in early studies, but most found increased cardiac output. Clowes and coworkers found slight increases in cardiac output in postoperative patients but marked increases when peritonitis was also present.[2] Del Guercio and colleagues documented increased cardiac output in patients with advanced cirrhosis; they termed this the "hyperdynamic state."[3]

Studies of cardiac output were greatly facilitated by the development of the balloon-tipped, flow-directed PA catheter 30 years ago.[4, 5] High-risk surgery, sepsis, and trauma were found to be associated with higher-than-normal cardiac index, DO₂, and VO₂; moreover, these values were higher in those who survived than in those who died later during hospitalization.[6–21] These changes were more apparent when the data were described by diagnostic categories and placed in a temporal sequence.[22]

TABLE 22–2. Normal Values for Hemodynamic and Oxygen Transport Variables

Variable	Formula	Normal Value	Units
Cardiac index (CI)	CI = Cardiac output/BSA	3.2 ± 0.2	L/min•m^2
Systemic vascular resistance index (SVRI)	SVRI = 79.92 × (MAP − CVP)/CI	2180 ± 210	Dyne s/cm^5 m^2
Pulmonary vascular resistance index (PVRI)	PVRI = 79.92 × (MPAP − PAOP)/CI	270 ± 15	Dyne s/cm^5 m^2
Mean transit time (MTT)	Direct measurement	15 ± 1.4	Seconds
Central blood volume (CBV)	CBV = MTT × CI × 16.7	830 ± 86	mL/m^2
Stroke index (SI)	SI = CI/HR	46 ± 5	mL/m^2
Left ventricular stroke work (LVSW)	LVSW = SI × MAP × .0144	56 ± 6	g•m/m^2
Right ventricular stroke work (RVSW)	RVSW = SI × MPAP × .0144	8.8 ± 0.9	g•m/m^2
Left cardiac work (LCW)	LCW = CI × MAP × .0144	3.8 ± 0.4	kg•m/m^2
Right cardiac work (RCW)	RCW = CI × MPAP × .0144	0.6 ± 0.06	kg•m/m^2
Arterial Hgb O$_2$ saturation	Direct measurement	96 ± 1	%
Mixed venous Hgb saturation	Direct measurement	75 ± 1	%
Arterial oxygen content (CaO$_2$)	CaO$_2$ = SaO$_2$ × 1.36 × Hgb + (.0031 × PaO$_2$)	19 ± 1	mL/dL
Mixed venous O$_2$ content (CvO$_2$)	CvO$_2$ = SvO$_2$ × 1.36 Hgb + (.0031 × PvO$_2$)	14 ± 1	mL/dL
Oxygen delivery (DO$_2$)	DO$_2$ = CI × (CaO$_2$)	520 ± 16	mL/min m^2
Oxygen consumption (VO$_2$)	VO$_2$ = CI(CaO$_2$ − CvO$_2$)	131 ± 2	mL/min m^2
Oxygen extraction	O$_2$ ext = VO$_2$/DO$_2$	26 ± 1	%

.0144 and 79.92 are conversion terms.

BSA, body surface area; CVP, central venous pressure; Hgb, hemoglobin; HR, heart rate; MAP, mean arterial pressure; MPAP, mean pulmonary artery pressure; PAOP, pulmonary artery occlusion pressure; PaO$_2$, partial pressure of oxygen in arterial blood; PvO$_2$, partial pressure of oxygen in mixed venous blood; SaO$_2$, oxygen saturation in arterial blood; SvO$_2$, venous oxygen saturation.

Direct Fick Method

More than a century ago, Fick postulated that if the oxygen content of arterial (CaO$_2$) and mixed venous (CvO$_2$) blood, as well as VO$_2$, were known, then blood flow could be calculated by dividing the VO$_2$ by the arteriovenous O$_2$ content difference. The direct Fick method of estimation of cardiac output has become the gold standard against which other methods are evaluated. VO$_2$ is now calculated by metabolic carts that measure inspired and expired oxygen concentrations and tidal volume.[23–29] These measurements and calculations require meticulous standardization and calibration as well as steady state conditions. In general, the direct Fick method is applicable when the FIO$_2$ is less than 0.6 and when the system is well calibrated and free of air leaks. It is not applicable in unstable physiologic states, severe trauma, and critically ill patients, particularly in early nonsteady conditions.

Thermodilution Method

The thermodilution method is an application of the indicator dilution principle. In thermodilution, the indicator is a measured quantity of either room temperature or iced saline or 5% glucose solution; dilution of this injectate in the bloodstream is measured by a calibrated thermocouple positioned about 10 cm downstream from the point of injection. The small amount of solution injected into the PA does not measurably affect the temperature of venous blood returning to the right side of the heart and therefore does not produce errors caused by recirculation of the indicator, as do dyes (e.g., indocyanine green and Ev-

an's blue) or radioactive labels of albumin (^{125}I) and red cells (^{55}Cr). This obviates the need to separate the primary washout curve from the recirculating indicator, simplifies cardiac output calculations, allows frequently repeated measurements, and does not require removal of blood for photometric or radioactivity analysis. Thermodilution in conjunction with use of the PA balloon flotation catheter to obtain simultaneous PAOPs has become the clinical standard for hemodynamic evaluation, particularly in acute critical illness.

Comparison of Cardiac Output by Direct Fick and Thermodilution Methods

The direct Fick method measures oxygen consumption of all tissues from outside the capillary-alveolar membrane, including the lung parenchyma, whereas the indirect Fick method measures cardiac output via thermodilution together with arterial and mixed venous blood gas analysis and then calculates VO$_2$ as the product of cardiac output and the arteriovenous O$_2$ content difference. This VO$_2$ includes the metabolism of all tissues inside the capillary-alveolar membrane but excludes the lung parenchyma. When careful simultaneous measurements of the VO$_2$ were made by both the direct and the indirect Fick method under ideal steady state conditions, results of the two methods were considered to be in good agreement.[24–29] Davies and coworkers found the correlation (r) between Fick cardiac output and thermodilution cardiac output to be 0.86.[25] Nanas and associates reported a mean difference between the direct Fick method and the dye method of 0.214 ± 0.922 (standard deviation) L/minute in 1022 patients; 74.7% were within 20% of the line of identity.[28] Confirmation of the validity of these two approaches was also reported by Keinanen and colleagues, Hankeln and associates, and others.[26, 29]

Hemodynamic and Oxygen Transport Measurements with Pulmonary Artery Catheters

Hemodynamic variables can be measured repeatedly with a systemic arterial catheter and the balloon-tipped PA catheter with thermodilution cardiac output computer, together with measurement of arterial and venous pressures of the systemic and pulmonary circulations, cardiac output, arterial and mixed venous gases, and hemoglobin or hematocrit.[6–9, 11–20] Table 22–2 lists the calculated hemodynamic and oxygen transport variables, their formulas, and normal values. All flow and volume measurements should be indexed to body surface area or body weight to standardize values among patients with differing sizes and body habitus.

Clinical Significance of Cardiac Index Patterns

Many internists and cardiologists find that cardiac output is not useful because the values vary widely. Hemodynamic and oxygen transport patterns begin to emerge, however, with careful sorting of patients by specific cause of shock or acute illness, age, severity and time course of the illness, comorbid conditions, and therapeutic responses. Normative standards have been developed for cardiac index in normal volunteers and preoperative patients of various ages.[22]

Low cardiac index is characteristic of hemorrhage, myocardial infarction, cardiac tamponade, and other forms of central pump failure. Characteristically, patients with septic, postoperative, or traumatic shock have patterns of high blood flow unless they are severely dehydrated, hypovolemic, elderly, or bedridden or have associated cardiac problems. Patients with severe sepsis or burn shock may have more than twice the normal cardiac index. Similarly, stroke index, both left and right ventricular stroke work indexes, left cardiac work index, and right cardiac work index are reduced in hypovolemic and cardiogenic shock but are usually increased in septic, postoperative, and traumatic shock. Increased cardiac index, stroke work, and myocardial performance in the latter conditions may be the body's response to increased circulatory and metabolic requirements, wound healing, tissue repair, immunochemical mediators, and restored body metabolism after oxygen debt, inadequate tissue perfusion, severe stress, and failure to keep up with blood or fluid losses. In essence, values that are normal for the unstressed volunteer are not appropriate as goals for the critically ill patient or the patient in shock.

Increased vascular resistance resulting from the neurohumoral adrenal stress response is a very early transient compensatory response to hypotensive low cardiac output from hypovolemia and cardiogenic shock. This stress response maintains arterial pressures in the face of decreasing blood flow, at least for a limited time. Hypotension occurs when compensatory responses that increase blood pressure and systemic vascular resistance index values are overwhelmed, exhausted, or attenuated by acidosis and metabolic vasodilatory mechanisms. Pulmonary vascular resistance may increase with trauma, hemorrhage, lung hypoxia, altitude sickness, adult respiratory distress syndrome, and other forms of stress. An increased pulmonary vascular resistance index, which is initiated by neural and other mechanisms, precedes the increased pulmonary venous admixture or shunting that occurs in postoperative and post-traumatic adult respiratory distress syndrome.

Oxygen Transport Variables as Measures of Tissue Perfusion

Major circulatory problems involve changes in one or more of the three major components of the circulation: cardiac, respiratory, and tissue perfusion. Simultaneous monitoring of all three of these circulatory components provides a more comprehensive hemodynamic evaluation. The primary function of the circulation is to perfuse (oxygenate) peripheral tissues. Tissue perfusion has conventionally been inferred from the subjective signs and symptoms of shock but not specifically measured. Quantitative evaluation of tissue oxygenation according to the temporal patterns of DO_2, VO_2, and O_2 extraction is a useful application of invasive monitoring in acute illness.

Even though reduced tissue oxygenation is the major early hemodynamic deficiency of shock, oxygen transport is monitored infrequently, largely because of the inconvenience and the cost of blood gas analysis for both systemic and pulmonary arterial samples.

DO_2 as a Measure of Overall Circulatory Function

The bulk movement of oxygen is a useful measure of tissue perfusion because (1) oxygen is easily measured in arterial and mixed venous blood, (2) it has the largest arteriovenous gradient of any blood constituent, (3) it is related to overall tissue perfusion and outcome, and (4) oxygen cannot be stored—therefore, the amount taken up by the cells is a measure of overall body metabolism. Oxygen transport is not frequently monitored, however, despite the fact that reduced tissue oxygenation is the major functional impairment in hemorrhagic, traumatic, septic, and postoperative shock.

Overall measurement of the peripheral circulation and tissue perfusion may be calculated using DO_2, which is the product of cardiac output and arterial content. Similarly, overall body metabolism may be evaluated by VO_2, which is the product of cardiac output and the arteriovenous content difference, $C(a\text{-}v)O_2$. The oxygen content of arterial and mixed venous blood is the product of hemoglobin concentration, percent hemoglobin saturation, and a constant, which represents the volume of oxygen carried by each gram of saturated hemoglobin plus a small amount of oxygen dissolved in plasma ($0.0031 \times PaO_2$).

Oxygen delivery (i.e., the amount of oxygen delivered to the tissues per minute) is the overall function of the circulation. Spontaneous increases in DO_2 over the normal range in the face of trauma, infection, and other forms of stress represent compensatory responses to inadequate tissue oxygenation. The temporal pattern of changes in DO_2 is more informative than a single set of measurements because the sequential pattern of changes provides a history of physiologic events that lead to circulatory dysfunction, shock, organ failure, and death.

The amount of increase in cardiac index and DO_2 in response to a standard fluid volume load is also an indirect measure of the capacity of the circulation to compensate. Limited circulatory reserve capacity may be revealed by failure of the DO_2 to increase after fluid challenge with 500 mL of colloids or 1000 mL of crystalloids or after stimulation with an inotropic agent, such as dobutamine, 5 to 10 µg/kg/minute (Fig. 22–1).

VO_2 as a Measure of Body Metabolism

The rate of oxygen consumption, VO_2, represents the total of all oxidative metabolic reactions and reflects the overall status of body metabolism. It represents the actual amount of oxygen consumed at the time of the measurement, not the real need, which may be more than the amount burned. At some point, VO_2 may be limited by decreasing DO_2.

Oxygen Supply Dependency Evaluated by DO_2 and VO_2 Relationships

Oxygen consumption may be plotted against the corresponding DO_2 values to visualize their relationships. Experimentally, when DO_2 is progressively decreased by hemorrhage in normal dogs, the VO_2 temporarily

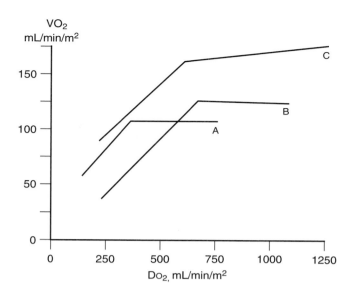

FIGURE 22–1. Three published series of volume of oxygen consumption (VO_2) values plotted against their corresponding oxygen delivery (DO_2) values. *Line A,* Anesthetized cardiac patients coming off cardiopulmonary bypass intraoperatively, showing a plateau beginning at about 330 mL/min/m². *Line B,* Medical patients with sepsis, showing a plateau at about 720 mL/min/m². *Line C,* Critically ill postoperative patients. (From Shoemaker WC: Oxygen transport and oxygen metabolism in shock and critical illness. Crit Care Clin 1996;12:939–969.)

remains at normal baseline values; that is, the supply-independent VO_2 phase forms a relatively horizontal plateau. When a critically low DO_2 value is reached, the VO_2 and the DO_2 decrease together; then the VO_2 is said to be supply dependent because the rate of oxygen consumed is limited by the rate of oxygen delivered to the tissues.[30] Although DO_2/VO_2 relationships were demonstrated in experimental laboratory conditions, the patterns are not as obvious in clinical situations, when many other associated problems may obscure them. In three clinical series, widely scattered DO_2 and VO_2 relationships suggested both a plateau above a critical DO_2 value (supply-independent VO_2) and a sloping line below the critical DO_2, indicating supply-dependent VO_2 increases concurrent with increased DO_2 (Fig. 22–1). In practice, supply-dependent VO_2 is indicated by increased VO_2 after fluid challenge.[30]

Operational Efficiency of the Pulmonary Artery Catheter

Risk-benefit considerations require timely and accurate collection of data and use of this information for maximal advantage. Because the potential risks of PA monitoring are appreciable, it is important to obtain important information relative to tissue perfusion. The opportunity to identify and correct a life-threatening circulatory problem may be lost if DO_2 and VO_2 patterns are not measured in the early stages of illness, but identification is delayed until after organ failure has developed.

Oxygen Transport Variables

Cardiac output and PAOP are important hemodynamic variables that reflect cardiac function in relation to inflow; however, the primary function of the circulation is to provide for body metabolism by microcirculatory tissue perfusion. This is reflected by the bulk delivery of oxygen and nutrients and by the removal of carbon dioxide and other end products of metabolism (e.g., lactate and pyruvate) that will be recycled through hepatic intracellular metabolic pathways. Oxygen has the highest percentage of extraction of all blood components, is the most flow-dependent blood constituent, and is the constituent whose arteriovenous gradient is easiest to measure. Moreover, oxygen is essential to body metabolism; hypoxic brain death or permanent neurologic deficit occurs when cardiac arrest lasts more than 5 minutes. For many reasons, it is useful to monitor oxygen metabolism as early as possible to observe the complete patterns of circulatory dysfunction and shock.

At present, it is not possible to measure tissue perfusion directly. The functional circulatory status is evaluated by observing changes in the temporal patterns of VO_2 in relation to the patterns of the cardiac index and DO_2 (Fig. 22–2 and Table 22–2). A decrease in VO_2 indicates a reduction in the overall rate of oxidative metabolism. It may be due to (1) inadequate delivery of oxygen to the tissues as a result of low flow (i.e., DO_2); (2) low hemoglobin concentration (e.g., anemia); (3) low arterial blood oxygen (e.g., hypoxemia); (4) inadequate tissue perfusion resulting from uneven or maldistributed microcirculatory flow; or (5) decreased metabolic rates resulting from specific disease states (e.g., hypothyroidism, malnutrition, vitamin deficiencies), cancericidal drug therapy, drug overdose or other metabolic poisoning, hypothermia, or terminal states.

An increase in VO_2 indicates an increase in tissue metabolism as a result of (1) increased metabolic demand as a result of sepsis, hyperthermia, post-traumatic states, burns, vigorous exercise, or hyperthyroidism; (2) compensatory increases in metabolism after tissue hypoxia due to low blood flow or uneven flow, tissue injury, hypothermia, or cardiac event; (3) the use of various drugs, anesthetics, adrenergic agonists that stimulate metabolism, or poisons that dissociate oxidative phosphorylation.

Greater-than-normal VO_2 does not mean that the circulation is adequate, because increased metabolic requirements associated with tissue repair or previous oxygen debt may require greater-than-normal metabolism to restore normal function. Patients with major trauma, sepsis, or burns require appreciable increases in VO_2. If VO_2 is greater than normal before therapy but does not increase with therapy, then (1) tissue perfusion is already adequate, (2) therapy is ineffective, or (3) the circulatory defect is irreversible, as in the late stage of shock or after multiple vital organ failures. Infrequent or random measurements of VO_2 give only a limited snapshot view of the situation. When therapeutic agents are given one at a time and VO_2 is monitored before, during, and after each treatment, changes in VO_2 may reflect changes in metabolism or tissue perfusion produced by the therapy.[30] A low or normal VO_2 before and after therapy suggests that the therapy is ineffective or that the defect is irreversible. When VO_2 is low before therapy and increases afterward, either the patient's condition has spontaneously improved or the administered agent has improved tissue perfusion and oxygen metabolism.[30]

Effectiveness of the Pulmonary Artery Catheter

The effectiveness of the PA thermodilution catheter in critically ill patients has recently been challenged; however, randomized trials in surgical patients performed early showed improved outcome.[6, 8–13, 19] These differences in outcome may be due to differences in the definition of the term *early* as well as to differences in the nature of circulatory problems in medical and surgical patients and the use of well-defined treatment plans. Improved outcome should not be expected if therapy is not changed. In a meta-analysis, Boyd and coworkers reviewed six prospective randomized series of patients who entered the intensive care unit after organ failure or sepsis had occurred and who had no improvement in outcome with therapy.[21] They compared these with five other prospective randomized series with control mortality rates of greater than 10%, which showed significant improvement in outcome when therapy was given early in the first 8 to 12 hours postoperatively or prophylactically. Clearly, time is of the essence.

Conclusions

1. The aim of invasive physiologic monitoring is (1) to describe the functional basis of acute circulatory problems; (2) to evaluate cardiac function in terms of inflow pressure; (3) to evaluate pulmonary function in terms of arterial blood gases or pulse oximetry; (4) to evaluate tissue perfusion in terms of DO_2 and VO_2 or in terms of transcutaneous oxygen tension ($PtcO_2$) and the $PtcO_2/FIO_2$ index; (5) to evaluate the relative effectiveness of alternative therapies on these interacting circulatory functions; and

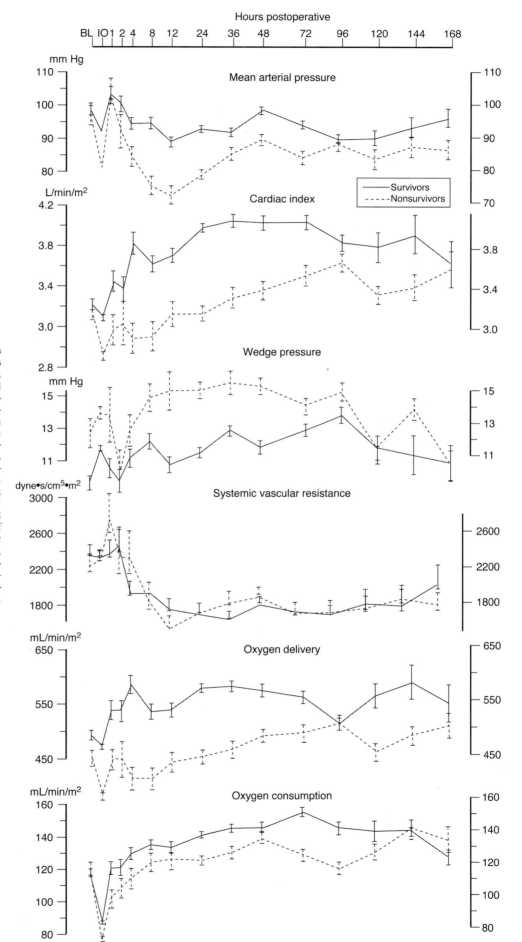

FIGURE 22–2. Temporal patterns of selected monitored variables before, during, and after high-risk elective surgery. Mean arterial pressure, cardiac index, pulmonary artery wedge pressure, systemic vascular resistance, oxygen delivery, and oxygen consumption are shown before operation (baseline, BL), intraoperatively (IO), and at successive periods designated in hours postoperatively. *Solid lines* show survivors' data; *dashed lines* show nonsurvivors' data. *Dots* are mean values, and *vertical bars* are standard error of the mean. Note higher values for cardiac index, oxygen delivery, and oxygen consumption in survivors. (From Shoemaker WC: Oxygen transport and oxygen metabolism in shock and critical illness. Crit Care Clin 1996;12:939–969.)

(6) to titrate therapy to achieve optimal physiologic goals that effect the best outcome.

2. The PA (Swan-Ganz) catheter has enabled catheterization laboratory data to be obtained at the bedside of intensive care unit patients and has changed the way we treat these patients.

3. Invasive monitoring with PA catheters has become the gold standard for critically ill patients in the intensive care unit.

4. Initial studies in high-risk surgical patients, gunshot victims, and acutely ill patients with blunt trauma, septic shock, gastrointestinal bleeding, acute myocardial infarction, chronic congestive heart failure with an acute exacerbation, drug overdose, adult respiratory distress syndrome, or other acute illness have shown higher cardiac index, transcutaneous oxygen tension, DO_2, and VO_2 in survivors before the onset of hypotension.

5. The interactions of heart, lung, and tissue perfusion and associated compensations are easiest to evaluate early.

6. It is easier and more effective to observe, analyze, and treat mild circulatory changes at their earliest appearance, when they are more responsive to therapy.

7. It is important to understand insufficiency or failure of each circulatory component. It is inappropriate to treat perfusion failure with the concepts and the therapy designed for cardiac failure, or to treat cardiac failure as though it were pulmonary failure. Similarly, it may be disastrous to block increased cardiac function with beta-blockers if the increased cardiac output is a compensation for pulmonary or tissue perfusion failure.

References

1. Cournand A, Riley RL, Bradley SE, et al: Studies of the circulation in clinical shock. Surgery 1943;13:964–995.
2. Clowes GHA, DelGuercio LRM: Circulatory response to trauma of surgical operations. Metabolism 1960;9:67–81.
3. Del Guercio LRM, Commarswamy RF, Feins NR, et al: Pulmonary arteriovenous admixture and the hyperdynamic state. Surgery 1964;56:57–65.
4. Swan HJ: The role of hemodynamic monitoring in the management of the critically Ill. Crit Care Med 1975;3:83–89.
5. Forrester JS, Diamond G, Chatterjee J, et al: Medical therapy of acute myocardial infarction by application of hemodynamic subsets. N Engl J Med 1976;295:1356–1404.
6. Shoemaker WC, Appel PL, Kram HB, et al: Prospective trial of supranormal values of survivors as therapeutic goals in high-risk surgical patients. Chest 1988;94:1176–1186.
7. Bishop MW, Shoemaker WC, Appel PL, et al: Relationship between supranormal values, time delays and outcome in severely traumatized patients. Crit Care Med 1993;21:56–62.
8. Boyd O, Grounds M, Bennett D: Preoperative increase of oxygen delivery reduces mortality in high-risk surgical patients. JAMA 1993;270:2699–2704.
9. Berlauk JF, Abrams JH, Gilmour IJ, et al: Preoperative optimization of cardiovascular hemodynamics improves outcome in peripheral vascular surgery. Ann Surg 1991;214:289–297.
10. Schulz RJ, Whitfield GF, La Mura JJ, et al: The role of physiologic monitoring in patients with fractures of hip. J Trauma 1985;25:309–316.
11. Fleming AW, Bishop MH, Shoemaker WC, et al: Prospective trial of supranormal values as goals of resuscitation in severe trauma. Arch Surg 1992;127:1175–1181.
12. Bishop MH, Shoemaker WC, Kram HB, et al: Prospective randomized trial of survivor values of cardiac index, oxygen delivery, and oxygen consumption as resuscitation endpoints in severe trauma. J Trauma 1995;38:780–787.
13. Shoemaker WC, Kram HB, Appel PL, et al: The efficacy of central venous and pulmonary artery catheters and therapy based upon them in reducing mortality and morbidity. Arch Surg 1990;125:1332–1338.
14. Scalea TM, Simon HM, Duncan AO, et al: Geriatric blunt multiple trauma: Improved survival with early invasive monitoring. J Trauma 1990;30:129–136.
15. Moore FA, Haenel JB, Moore EE, Whitehill TA: Incommensurate oxygen consumption in response to maximal oxygen availability predicts postinjury organ failure. J Trauma 1992;33:58–65.
16. Hankeln KB, Senker R, Schwarten JU, et al: Evaluation of prognostic indices based on hemodynamic and oxygen transport variables in shock patients with adult respiratory distress syndrome. Crit Care Med 1987;15:1–7.
17. Tuchschmidt J, Fried J, Astiz M, Rackow E: Evaluation of cardiac output and oxygen delivery improves outcome in septic shock. Chest 1992;102:216–220.
18. Creamer JE, Edwards JD, Nightingale P: Hemodynamic and oxygen transport variables in cardiogenic shock secondary to acute myocardial infarction, and response to treatment. Am J Cardiol 1990;65:1297–1300.
19. Yu M, Levy MM, Smith P, et al: Effect of maximizing oxygen delivery on morbidity and mortality rates in critically ill patients: A prospective, randomized, controlled study. Crit Care Med 1993;21:830–838.
20. Rady MY, Edwards JD, Rivers EP, Alexander M: Measurement of oxygen consumption after uncomplicated acute myocardial infarction. Chest 1993;104:930–934.
21. Boyd O, Hayes M: The oxygen trail: The goal. Br Med Bull 1999;55:125–139.
22. Shoemaker WC, Appel PL, Kram HB: Hemodynamic and oxygen transport responses in survivors and nonsurvivors of high risk surgery. Crit Care Med 1993;21:977–990.
23. Guyton AC: A continuous cardiac output recorder employing the Fick principle. Circ Res 1959;7:661–669.
24. Westenskow DR, Culter CA, Wallace WD: Instrumentation for monitoring gas exchange and metabolic rate in critically ill patients. Crit Care Med 1984;12:183–187.
25. Davies GG, Jebsen PJR, Glasgow BM, et al: Continuous Fick cardiac output compared to thermodilution cardiac output. Crit Care Med 1986;14:881–885.
26. Keinanen O, Takala J, Kari A: Continued measurement of cardiac output by the Fick principle: Clinical validation in intensive care. Crit Care Med 1992;20:360–365.
27. Levison MR, Groeger JS, Miodownick S, et al: Indirect calorimetry in mechanically ventilated patients. Crit Care Med 1987;15:144–147.
28. Nanas JN, Anastasiou-Nana MI, Sutton RB, et al: Comparison of Fick and dye cardiac outputs during rest and exercise in 1,022 patients. Can J Cardiol 1986;2:195–199.
29. Hankeln KB, Michelsen H, Kubiak V, et al: Continuous on-line, real-time measurement of cardiac output and derived cardiorespiratory variables in the critically ill. Crit Care Med 1985;13:1071–1073.
30. Shoemaker WC, Appel PL, Kram HB: Oxygen transport measurements to evaluate tissue perfusion and titrate therapy. Crit Care Med 1991;19:672–688.

23 Noninvasive Cardiac Output Monitoring:

Bioimpedance and Partial CO$_2$ Rebreathing Methods

William C. Shoemaker and Charles C.J. Wo

> Whatever practical people may say, this world is, after all, absolutely governed by ideas, and very often by the wildest and most hypothetical ideas.
>
> THOMAS HUXLEY, "On the Study of Biology"

The specific aims of monitoring are (1) to provide prompt recognition of circulatory problems at the earliest possible time, beginning with admission to the emergency department (ED) or the onset of the causative event; (2) to describe the temporal patterns of hemodynamic and oxygen transport leading to inadequate oxygen transport, reduced tissue perfusion, tissue hypoxia, hypotension, organ failure, and death in various types of life-threatening stress, including hemorrhagic, surgical, traumatic, septic, and cardiogenic shock; (3) to provide, or reinforce clinical opinions with, physiologic analyses that provide a rationale for therapeutic decisions; (4) to describe and evaluate circulatory complications; (5) to provide baseline values and objective criteria to evaluate effectiveness of alternative therapies; and (6) to predict outcome based on documented hemodynamic and oxygen transport patterns that occur in survivors and nonsurvivors of each etiologic category. Surveillance monitoring is used less precisely to indicate the general direction for appropriate therapy.

Circulatory measurements obtained with the invasive pulmonary artery (PA) balloon-tipped thermodilution (Swan-Ganz) catheter have been the gold standard for evaluation of circulatory function. This technology is expensive, time consuming, and personnel intensive. Noninvasive alternatives to the thermodilution technique in cardiac output estimation are the use of thoracic electric bioimpedance, transthoracic echocardiography and transesophageal echocardiography, and partial CO$_2$ rebreathing. Noninvasive monitoring allows calculation of the net cumulative deficits or excesses of each variable by integrating the area between continuously monitored variables and normal or optimal values.

Thoracic Electric Bioimpedance Monitoring

In the impedance method, electrodes inject a small-amplitude (0.2 to 4.0 mA) alternating current at 40 to 100 kHz to produce an electrical field across the thorax from the base of the neck to the level of the xiphisternal junction; the electrical signals travel predominantly down the aorta rather than through aerated alveoli. The changes in aortic flow throughout the cardiac cycle are correlated with changes in impedance (i.e., the apparent changes in resistance).[1-4] Bernstein evaluated the advantages and the limitations of bioimpedance and Doppler cardiac output systems.[4] The ideal cardiac output monitoring method should produce a continuous display as well as being noninvasive, reproducible, inexpensive, user friendly, in reasonable agreement with thermodilution results, and acceptable to patients.

Background

Application of electric bioimpedance to the thorax was initiated by Nyboer, and a medical instrument (Minnesota Impedance Cardiograph; Surcom, Minneapolis, Minn) incorporating the technique was developed by Kubicek and colleagues in the 1970s.[1,2] Subsequently, several improvements were made, including diastolic clamping of the electrical signal. The BoMed noninvasive continuous cardiac output monitor was marketed in 1982; it used an analog-based processing technique in which cardiac output was calculated from the observed heart rate and empirical equations largely based on healthy volunteers. This instrument has been improved and has been replaced by the BioZ (CardioDynamics, San Diego, Calif). Bernstein mathematically represented the thorax as a truncated cone rather than as a cylinder; he also corrected for changes in body habitus.[3] Sorba Medical Systems (Brookfield, Wis) modified the Minnesota software by ensemble averaging of the impedance waveforms.

The impedance (dZ/dt) waveform should be inspected carefully to verify acceptability. Early impedance systems had simple threshold detection, "lookup" tables, ensemble averaging, and complicated user interfaces. They often lost transient information and generated a significant amount of "jitters" in the local frequency and amplitude determination processes. The r values (correlation coefficients) in several series were usually 0.7 to 0.9.[6-15] When the waveform is not displayed and inspected, the r values may be as low as 0.5. Low correlation values were also reported in coronary bypass patients by Sageman and Amundson.[5] In cardiac failure with significant amounts of pulmonary edema, differences between thermodilution and simultaneous impedance measurements often exceeded 40% of the thermodilution measurement and were considered unacceptable disparities that obviated the usefulness of impedance as a reliable clinical measure of cardiac function. Fuller found a "moderately good" correlation ($r^2 = 0.66$) in an extensive meta-analysis of impedance studies.[6] In a review of 154 studies over 30 years, Raaijmakers and associates showed pooled coefficients of correlation (r^2 values) of 0.67; the correlation was better in animals or normal subjects and worse in patients with severe cardiac illnesses.[7]

Methodologic Advances in Noninvasive Monitoring

An improved impedance system was developed by Wang and colleagues at Drexel University and was marketed as the IQ System (Wantagh, Bristol, Pa).[8-10] Using noninvasive disposable prewired hydrogen electrodes positioned on the skin and three electrocardiographic (ECG) leads placed across the precordium and the left shoulder, they passed a 100-kHz, 4-mA alternating current through the patient's thorax from the outer pairs of electrodes. The voltage is sensed by the inner pairs of electrodes, which capture the baseline impedance (Z_0), the first derivative of the impedance waveform (dZ/dt), and the ECG output.[8-14] The ECG and the bioimpedance signals are filtered with an all-integer-coefficient technology that simplifies computations and decreases signal processing time.

The signal processing technique is based on time-frequency distribution technology, which provides high signal-to-noise ratios that precisely time and measure mechanical functions of the heart. The two-dimensional raw dZ/dt waveform (Fig. 23–1) is converted into a three-dimensional generalized Wigner distribution, which in turn converts the dZ/dt signal into time, frequency, and power of the signal for each mechanical event in the cardiac cycle. This increases the speed of signal processing and allows near real-time operation without deterioration in accuracy.[8] It is, therefore, powerful because it shows the relationship among time, frequency, and power of the signal, which would otherwise be unobtainable from the standard fast Fourier analysis.

This is particularly important in the identification of the opening and closing of the aortic valve (B and C points), which are often buried in artifacts that make them difficult to identify. Because these points have a distinct frequency range (30 to 40 Hz) that clearly distinguishes them from other events or artifacts, they can be extracted from the Wigner distribution by integrating the power at every point in time over the frequency range of interest. This process extracts only the power contributed by those frequencies of interest;

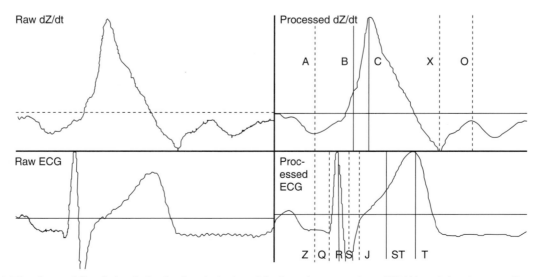

FIGURE 23–1. The observed "raw" signals for the first derivative of the impedance waveform (dZ/dt) and the electrocardiogram (ECG) are shown on the *left*, and the reconstructed "processed" waveforms are shown on the *right*. Also noted are the standard components of the impedance waveform (A, Z, B, C, X, and O) and the ECG waveform (Q, R, S, T, and J). (From Shoemaker WC, Ub CC, Bishop MH, et al: Multicenter trial of a new thoracic electrical bioimpedance device for cardiac output estimation. Crit Care Med 1994;22:1907–1912.)

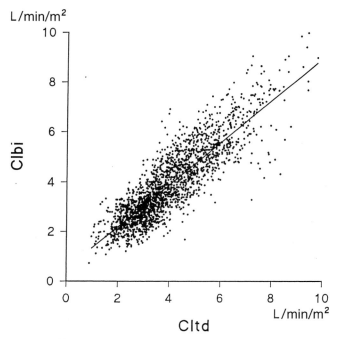

FIGURE 23–2. Regression analysis of 2192 bioimpedance cardiac index values (CIbi) plotted against simultaneously measured thermodilution cardiac index (CItd) values. The regression equation was y = 0.85x + 0.50; r = 0.85; r^2 = 0.73; $P < 0.001$.

it therefore provides relatively high signal-to-noise ratio because each of the points is obtained by moving averaging of frequency sections inside of sliding windows. As a result, the contribution from a single noise spoke is reduced to its minimum.[8–10]

The points of interest are A (beginning of electromechanical systole), B (opening of aortic valve), C (maximal mechanical contraction; dZ/dt max), X (closing of aortic valve), and O (mitral valve opening). Because the ECG and the impedance waveform are on the same time scale, opening and closing times of the aortic valve can be determined by aligning the ECG and the waveform.[8–10]

Comparisons of Bioimpedance and Thermodilution Measurements

In two large multicenter studies, the IQ impedance device provided stable signals and reliable cardiac output estimations, even under extenuating emergency conditions.[11, 12] Two thousand eighty-one simultaneous bioimpedance and thermodilution cardiac output measurements were obtained from 860 critically ill patients in the ED, the operating room, and the intensive care unit. The correlation coefficient, r, was 0.85, r^2 was 0.73, and $P < .001$; the precision and bias were $-0.124 + 0.75$ L/min/m² (Figs. 23–2 and 23–3). No instances of spurious impedance values that would have led to incorrect or harmful therapy were observed.[12]

When there is extensive pulmonary edema, pleural effusion, hemothorax, massive chest wall edema, or chest tubes parallel to the aorta, electrical signals may travel through these electrolyte solutions preferentially to the aorta and may thereby reduce the impedance signal-to-noise ratio. When these conditions interfere with accuracy, they can be identified by reductions in the baseline impedance (Z_0) of less than 15 ohms and by the height of the impedance waveform (<0.3

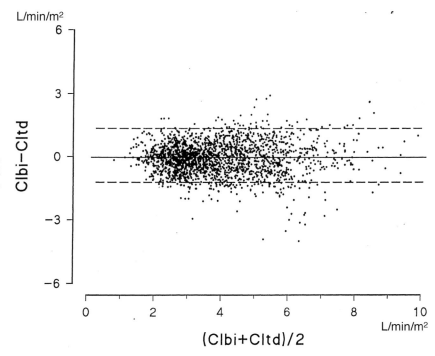

FIGURE 23–3. The differences between the two cardiac index values (CIbi − CItd) plotted against their average values ([CIbi + CItd]/2). The bias and precision analysis was − 0.124 + 0.85 L/min/m².

ohms). When these values were used as criteria in a prospective evaluation of 213 data pairs in 46 patients, r was 0.93, and r^2 was 0.87; bias and precision were $-0.14 + 0.54$ L/min/m^2 (Table 23–1). The average difference between thermodilution and impedance measurements was $9.8\% \pm 6.7\%$; this was similar to the differences between successive thermodilution measurements ($9.4\% \pm 6.2\%$) under similar conditions and is consistent with previous studies, in which thermodilution decreased an average of 15% with expiration and increased 12% to 15% with inspiration.[12] When Z_0 and dZ/dt values were less than 15 ohms and 0.3 ohms, respectively, impedance estimates were observed to track thermodilution values but were not regarded sufficiently reliable to be taken at face value. This is a major limitation of the method.

Noninvasive monitoring compared favorably with invasive thermodilution catheter monitoring in postoperative patients and in patients with blunt trauma, gunshot wound, head injury, sepsis, stroke, drug overdose, hypertensive crisis, acute myocardial infarction (AMI), or acute gastrointestinal bleeding. There was appreciable disparity in the presence of pulmonary edema, advanced adult respiratory distress syndrome, congestive heart failure, and late-stage septic shock with capillary leak. The comparison was considered sufficiently accurate, however, to be useful clinically in making therapeutic decisions in more than 90% of acute, critically ill patients. Moreover, the continuous online display of the data, which allows calculation of net cumulative deficits or excesses, more than makes up for relatively minor differences in cardiac output estimations obtained via the invasive thermodilution method. Absolute accuracy is not as essential as the direction and the patterns of changes in hemorrhagic, traumatic, septic, and postoperative shock, because preinjury or preillness baseline values are rarely available and there are considerable variations in optimal therapeutic goals. Nevertheless, the trends in cardiac output detected via bioimpedance closely track the changes in cardiac output detected by means of the thermodilution method.[12]

The correlations between cardiac output measured via bioimpedance and output measured via thermodilution were equivalent to the correlations seen between pulse oximetry and standard blood gas analysis performed in the same clinical series.[12] The differences between thermodilution and impedance estimations were more than offset by the continuous online display of data, which allowed instant recognition of changes in the course of the illness, calculation of the deficit for each monitored variable, and evaluation of therapeutic responses.[12–23]

Limitations of Bioimpedance Measurements

In all monitoring and imaging techniques, motion, anxiety, restlessness, shivering, agitation, and hyperventilation may interfere with measurements and may increase physiologic responses. It is less important in emergency conditions to have the same accuracy required in stable intensive care unit conditions, however, because the patient's own baseline measurements are often unknown and optimal values for each patient may vary according to comorbid conditions. In practice, a 15% difference between invasive and noninvasive cardiac output estimations would be acceptable when greater than 50% changes from the normal range are present. Thermodilution also has appreciable inaccuracies in both high and low cardiac output ranges, however, especially when the patient has hypothermia, dysrhythmias, Valsalva effects, motion artifacts, shivering, anxiety, or errors from injectate temperature calibration. Direct Fick oxygen consumption (VO_2) measurements, the physiologists' gold standard, are often precluded by the nonsteady states of emergency conditions, when monitoring is most often needed.

Increased lung fluid, which permits electrical signals to bypass aortic flow during cardiac systole, may result in erroneous values owing to low signal-to-noise ratios. Appreciable differences between bioimpedance and thermodilution calculations were seen with pleural effusions, pulmonary edema, severe congestive heart failure, severe pneumonia, hemothorax, and open thoracotomy with metal retractors. In each of these conditions, the electrical field distortions produced by fluid and electrolyte abnormalities allowed the electri-

TABLE 23–1. Correlations of Simultaneous Thermodilution and Bioimpedance Measurements in the Emergency Department, Operating Room, and Intensive Care Unit

Site	Data Pairs	r	r^2	Formula	Bias and Precision, L/min/m^2
ED	990	0.83	0.68	Y = 0.81X + 0.63	-0.058 ± 0.78
OR	407	0.88	0.77	Y = 0.84X + 0.48	-0.027 ± 0.46
ICU	795	0.85	0.73	Y = 0.92X + 0.23	-0.17 ± 0.68
Total	2192	0.85	0.73	Y = 0.85X + 0.50	-0.124 ± 0.75
Recent series*	213	0.93	0.87	Y = 0.82X + 0.67	-0.14 ± 0.54

*$Z_0 > 15$, dZ/dt > 0.3 ohms.
dZ/dt, impedance waveform; ED, emergency department; ICU, intensive care unit; OR, operating room; Z_0, baseline impedance.

cal signal to bypass aortic blood flow, which is the source of impedance changes.

Finally, there is a group of clinical conditions (e.g., late-stage cirrhosis, hyperdynamic states, tachycardia, and cardiac dysrhythmias) in which cardiac output measurements obtained by means of bioimpedance underestimate the thermodilution values. In heart rates of more than 140 beats per minute, the percentage of total aortic blood flow occurring in systole is appreciably less than that associated with normal heart rates. In these conditions, the estimation of cardiac output by impedance methods may be less than that calculated by thermodilution.

Partial Carbon Dioxide Rebreathing Method

Carbon dioxide can be used instead of oxygen in the direct Fick method of cardiac output measurement during mechanical ventilation.[24–27] The calculated cardiac output is actually the pulmonary capillary blood flow, so that the formula becomes:

$$\text{Cardiac output} = V_{CO_2}/CvCO_2 - CaCO_2$$

where V_{CO_2} is the rate of CO_2 production, $CvCO_2$ is the mixed venous CO_2 content, and $CaCO_2$ is the arterial CO_2 content. In this technique, after a 60-second baseline control period, an additional dead space is automatically activated, and the patient rebreathes the expired gas over 50 seconds. The expired CO_2 is measured continuously by conventional end-tidal infrared methods until a plateau is reached. When this occurs, the alveolar CO_2 is in equilibrium with the CO_2 in pulmonary arterial blood and is a measure of mixed venous carbon dioxide pressure (PCO_2). The partial pressure of carbon dioxide in arterial blood ($PaCO_2$) is calculated from the hemoglobin concentration and the hemoglobin-CO_2 dissociation curve. The arterial PCO_2 is approximately equal to the alveolar CO_2 and is estimated by the end-expiratory CO_2 value; this obviates the need to sample and measure pulmonary arterial blood. The CO_2 production or V_{CO_2} is obtained by measuring the timed volume and the CO_2 content of the expired gas, because the inspired CO_2 concentration is essentially zero. This system has now been fully automated (Niko; Novemetrics Medical Systems, Wallingford, Conn). De Abreu and colleagues reported good correlation of the partial CO_2 rebreathing method with nonshunted pulmonary blood flow in sheep; $r^2 = 0.73$, and the bias and the precision were 0.25 ± 0.83 L/minute.[26]

Limitations and Problems of the Carbon Dioxide Rebreathing Methods

The CO_2 rebreathing approach requires mechanically ventilated, intubated patients. Because the difference between mixed venous and arterial CO_2 is only about 6 torr under resting conditions, small errors in the analysis of CO_2 concentrations may have large effects on the cardiac measurements. For example, a 1-torr error in either analysis may result in about a 15% error in cardiac output estimation. In carefully controlled and automated systems, this is less of a problem. The Niko device has the added advantage of quantifying the stability of the measurements by employing a rating system of one to five stars. Four or five stars indicates stable, reproducible values. This approach is more accurate in low cardiac outputs because the (a-v)CO_2 differences are greater than normal.

Future Role of Multiple Noninvasive Monitoring Systems

It is feasible to use multiple noninvasive physiologic monitoring systems as initial screening or as the "front end" of invasive monitoring during the resuscitation of acutely ill patients shortly after ED admission. The temporal patterns of cardiac function, pulmonary function, and tissue perfusion obtained from noninvasive monitoring compared reasonably well with the patterns from invasive monitoring. These noninvasive monitoring systems display early small changes that can be treated before they progress to life-threatening proportions. Early deficits are usually easily and effectively corrected, whereas late effects of shock and hypovolemia may be irreversible. These systems have been evaluated clinically in widely varying circumstances and severity in a large series of severely ill patients to identify clinical conditions in which the impedance methodology is appropriate.[19–21]

Early Noninvasively Monitored Circulatory Events Beginning in the Emergency Department

The ED is the primary entry point into medical care for many acutely ill patients, and this early period provides a crucial opportunity for early assessment and rapid therapeutic interventions that may affect outcome. A major dilemma is that shock is easily diagnosed in late stages when therapy is ineffective, but early diagnosis is difficult because shock is first recognized by imprecise signs and subjective symptoms. Noninvasive monitoring of circulatory dysfunction is an alternative approach that allows very early application in the ED or the operating room and on hospital floors. The continuous online graphic displays of data allow prompt recognition of circulatory abnormalities and early therapeutic intervention and titration of therapy to optimal physiologic goals in acutely ill emergency patients, for whom time is crucial.[10, 17, 18, 20, 21] Monitoring provides objective circulatory criteria that can replace clinical suspicion and guesswork with physiologic criteria related to outcome.

Clinical evaluations under worst-case scenarios (emergency trauma in an inner-city county hospital) have shown stable impedance signals and satisfactory agreement with simultaneous thermodilution cardiac output measurements. Simultaneous noninvasive measurements may be used to evaluate: (1) cardiac function via blood pressure and noninvasive impedance methods, Doppler echocardiography, or partial CO_2 rebreathing cardiac output systems; (2) pulmonary function via pulse oximetry estimation of arterial hemoglobin saturation; and (3) tissue perfusion by means of transcutaneous oxygen tension ($PtcO_2$), $PtcO_2/PaO_2$ (partial pressure of oxygen in arterial blood) index, and transcutaneous partial pressure of carbon dioxide ($PtcCO_2$). These may be supplemented by invasively measured cardiac index (CI), oxygen delivery (DO_2), and VO_2, when available, to validate noninvasive methods and to provide additional information for physiologic interpretation. Baseline data sets, the low point (nadir) of the event, and the period of recovery immediately afterward describe the patterns of the interacting circulatory components: heart, lungs, and peripheral tissue perfusion and oxygenation. A microcomputer-based data acquisition system was developed to measure and record up to eight channels of data simultaneously and to display any two of them.[15–17, 20, 21]

Procedures For Early Application of Noninvasive Monitoring

Shortly after admission to the ED, patients suspected of having acute circulatory problems were evaluated for circulatory instability by assessment of routine clinical findings, such as hypotension, tachycardia, altered mental status, cold wet skin, oliguria, and pallor. In patients identified as having circulatory instability, the bioimpedance electrodes, the pulse oximeter, and the transcutaneous O_2 sensors were attached as soon as possible, and the values of each were observed and recorded. When required on clinical grounds for fluid management, a central venous catheter was placed. Measurements were also made before initiation of therapeutic interventions and at various periods after therapy to evaluate improvement and to titrate therapy to physiologic and clinical goals.

Monitoring of Selected Diagnostic Groups

Early Noninvasive Monitoring in High-Risk Postoperative Patients

The patient who has undergone elective surgery without complications may be easily monitored with routine screening, which includes assessment of vital signs, ECG, and central venous pressure monitoring. More comprehensive hemodynamic and oxygen transport monitoring is needed in high-risk surgical patients during and after major surgery. The mortality rates after major surgical procedures usually range from 1% to 2%, but for many high-risk patients in the surgical intensive care unit, the mortality rate may be as high as 20% to 30%. To reduce this rate, it is advisable to monitor all potentially fatal cases (i.e., preoperative patients with high-risk factors as well as critically ill, medical, septic, and postoperative patients). It may be necessary to monitor at least four or five times the number of patients who die to be sure that the optimal therapy is given to patients with potentially fatal results. Invasive PA monitoring may be indicated when screening with noninvasive monitoring suggests the presence of more extensive hemodynamic problems not responding to therapy.[15–23]

Evaluation of Early Monitored Circulatory Events

In the aforementioned studies, early monitored circulatory changes in cardiac, pulmonary, and tissue perfusion in patients with trauma, high-risk surgery, sepsis, late-stage cirrhosis, or cardiogenic shock were usually abnormal. These patterns of monitored changes were arbitrarily defined as (1) decrease of more than 20% in CI, $PtcO_2$, or $PtcO_2/PaO_2$ index or (2) reduction of CI to less than 2.5 L/min/m², decreased oxygen saturation in arterial blood (SaO_2) by pulse oximetry to less than 90%, $PtcO_2$ to less than 30 torr on room air, and $PtcO_2/FIO_2$ (fraction of inspired oxygen) to less than 100 torr.[18–22] There were 636 postoperative monitored events observed in 247 patients during and after high-risk surgical operations.[16] Tables 23–2 and 23–3 show the percentage of patients with abnormal values and the mean of these abnormalities at their nadir. The frequency and the extent of these abnormalities suggest that low flow, hypotension, and poor tissue perfusion are common circulatory problems in these patients. Flow tends to increase to compensate for deterioration of respiratory function or perfusion, and vice versa. The capacity of the heart to compensate is much greater than that of the lungs and the peripheral tissues, however.[18–20]

TABLE 23–2. Percentage of Patients with Abnormal Values and Mean of Abnormal Values at Their Nadirs

Variable	Units	Normal Values	Abnormal Values	Percent Abnormal	Mean ± SD at Nadir
CI	L/min/m²	2.8–3.6	<2.6	52	1.78 + 0.69
MAP	mm Hg	80–95	<70	41	57.5 + 1.8
SapO₂	%	95–97	<90	18	84.8 + 1.4
PtcO₂	torr	50–80	<45	55	19.2 + 2.6
PtcCO₂	torr	45–55	>60	45	70.5 + 1.8
VO₂	mL/min/m²	130 ± 10	<110	50	91.6 + 3.8

CI, cardiac index; MAP, mean arterial pressure, PtcCO₂, transcutaneous carbon dioxide tension; PtcO₂, transcutaneous oxygen tension; SapO₂, pulse oximetry; SD, standard deviation; VO₂, oxygen consumption.

Early Hemodynamic and Oxygen Transport Patterns after Trauma

Evaluation of circulatory dysfunction is often essential in deciding whether to perform an immediate operation in patients with blunt trauma. The timing of surgery may depend on clinical evaluation of the circulation as well as the temporal progression of clinical signs and symptoms. In the standard advanced trauma life support course, the degree of shock and the amount of blood loss are estimated by assessing the following: systolic and diastolic blood pressure, pulse pressure, pallor, skin (cold and clammy), pulse rate, capillary refill, temperature, respiratory rate, and mental status. Unfortunately, neither blood pressure nor other signs and symptoms correlate well with blood flow or outcome.[7]

For survivors and nonsurvivors of 139 consecutive cases of severe blunt trauma, mean arterial pressure (MAP), CI, arterial saturation by pulse oximeter (SapO₂), and tissue perfusion measured by PtcO₂/FIO₂ during the first 8 hours after ED admission are shown (Figs. 23–4 and 23–5). The circle diagrams represent the changing patterns of cardiac, pulmonary, and tissue perfusion. In survivors, there is slight hypertension, high CI that almost reaches optimal goals, and relatively normal SapO₂ and PtcO₂/FIO₂ during resuscitation in the first 8 hours after admission. In contrast, nonsurvivors had pronounced hypertension in the first hour, relatively normal CI, reduced SapO₂ (corrected by intubation, mechanical ventilation, and high FIO₂ values), and marked reduction in PtcO₂/FIO₂ values.

Calculation of Net Cumulative Excess or Deficit of Monitored Variables in Trauma Patients

Multiple noninvasive hemodynamic monitoring systems were used to evaluate circulatory patterns prospectively in 151 consecutively monitored, severely injured patients, beginning with admission to the ED in a university-run county hospital (Table 23–4). The net cumulative deficit or excess of each monitored parameter was calculated from the area between normal values and the curve produced by the continuously monitored values for each variable in each patient (Figs. 23–6 and 23–7). The deficits in cardiac, pulmonary, and tissue perfusion were analyzed in relation to survival by discriminant analysis and were cross-validated. The mean (± standard error of the mean) net cumulative excesses (+) or deficits (−) in surviving versus nonsurviving patients, respectively, were +81+52 versus −232+138 L/m² ($P < .037$) for CI; −10+13 versus −57+24 mm Hg/hour ($P < .078$) for MAP; −1+0.3 versus −8+2.6 percent/hour ($P < .006$) for arterial saturation; and +313+88 versus −793+175 torr/hour ($P < .001$) for tissue perfusion. Discriminant analysis classified 95% of the survivors and 62.5% of the nonsurvivors shortly after initial resuscitation (Table 23–5).[21] Survival was predicted by discriminant analysis models based on quantitative assessment of the net cumulative deficits of flow, arterial hypoxemia, and poor tissue perfusion.

The data illustrate how relatively small changes tolerated over short periods may accumulate into apprecia-

TABLE 23–3. Incidence and Mean of Abnormal Values in Survivors and Nonsurvivors at Their Nadir or Maximum Change

Variable	Survivors Incidence, %	Survivors Value ± SEM	Nonsurvivors Incidence, %	Nonsurvivors Value ± SEM
CI	48	1.93 ± 0.12	75	1.64 ± 0.27
MAP	43	58 ± 2	33	58 ± 4
SapO₂	16	85.2 ± 1.7	17	83 ± 0.7
PtcO₂	52	20.9 ± 2.8	50	9.5 ± 6
PtcCO₂	46	69 ± 1.5	42	78 ± 7
VO₂	63	93 ± 3.6	50	89 ± 9

CI, cardiac index; MAP, mean arterial pressure; PtcCO₂, transcutaneous carbon dioxide tension; PtcO₂, transcutaneous oxygen tension; SapO₂, pulse oximetry; SEM, standard error of the mean; VO₂, oxygen consumption.

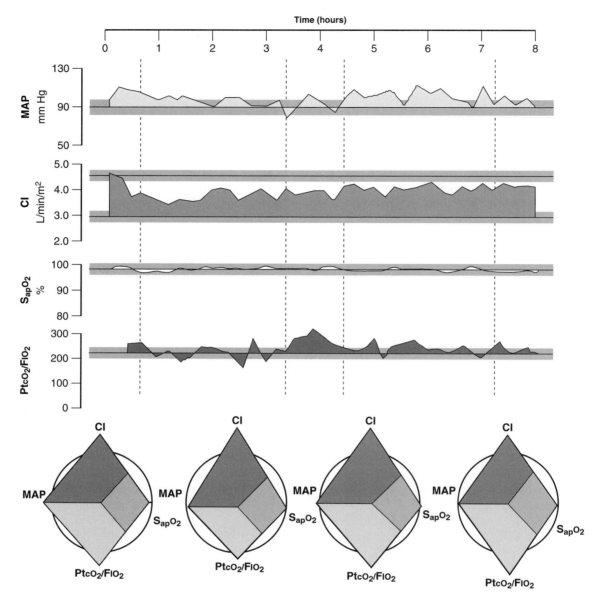

FIGURE 23–4. Hemodynamic data from 82 consecutively monitored survivors of severe blunt trauma during resuscitation in the first 8 hours after admission to the emergency department (ED). *Top line*, Time from ED admission. Mean arterial pressure (MAP), cardiac index (CI), arterial hemoglobin saturation by pulse oximetry (SapO$_2$), and transcutaneous oxygen tension indexed to the fractional inspired oxygen concentration (PtcO$_2$/FIO$_2$) are shown. All values are keyed to the time of admission to the ED. The *circle diagrams* at the bottom represent interacting cardiac, pulmonary, and tissue perfusion functions at the time indicated by the *vertical dashed lines*.

TABLE 23–4. Mean Noninvasive Hemodynamic Values for Survivors and Nonsurvivors

Variable, Unit	Optimal Value	Survivors (N = 103), Mean ± SEM	Nonsurvivors (N = 48), Mean ± SEM	P value
CI, L/min/m²	4	4.14 ± 0.02	3.87 ± 0.03	0.001
MAP, mm Hg	85	88 ± 0.37	80 ± 0.69	0.066
SapO$_2$, %	98	99 ± 0.05	96 ± 0.26	0.001
PtcO$_2$/FIO$_2$, torr	200	206 ± 2.9	93 ± 2.6	0.001

CI, cardiac index; MAP, mean arterial pressure; PtcO$_2$/FIO$_2$, transcutaneous oxygen tension indexed to FIO$_2$; SapO$_2$, arterial hemoglobin saturation by pulse oximetry; SEM, standard error of the mean.

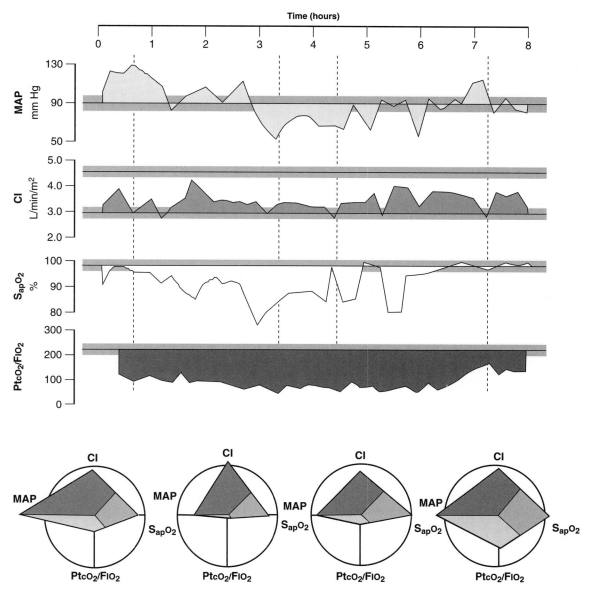

FIGURE 23–5. Hemodynamic data from 27 consecutively monitored nonsurvivors of severe blunt trauma during resuscitation in the first 8 hours after admission to the emergency department (ED). *Top line,* Time from ED admission. Mean arterial pressure (MAP), cardiac index (CI), arterial hemoglobin saturation by pulse oximetry (SapO2), and transcutaneous oxygen tension indexed to the fractional inspired oxygen concentration (PtcO2/FIO2) are shown. All values are keyed to the time of admission to the ED. The *circle diagrams* at the bottom represent interacting cardiac, pulmonary, and tissue perfusion functions at the time indicated by the *vertical dashed lines.*

TABLE 23–5. Classification Summary for the Series

	Predicted to Die		Predicted to Live		Total	
	N	*(Row%)*	*N*	*(Row%)*	*N*	*(Col%)*
Died	30	62.5	18	37.5	48	31.8
Lived	5	4.9	98	95.1	103	68.2
Total	35	23.2	116	76.8	151	100.0

Misclassification: 23/151 = 15.2%.

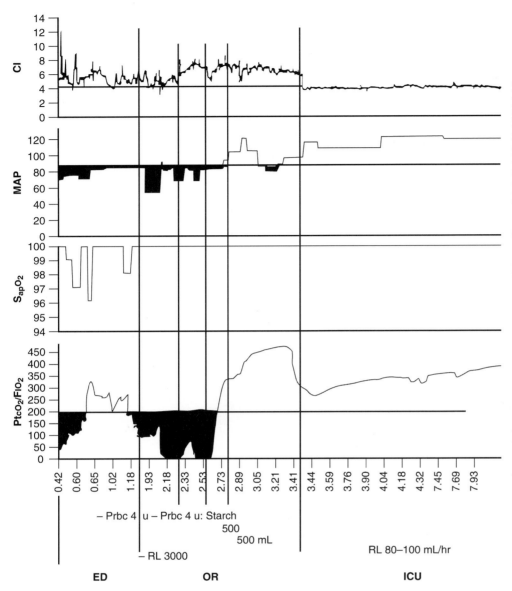

FIGURE 23–6. Data from a 27-year-old female who sustained a stab wound of the right chest with lacerations of a branch of the pulmonary artery and an intercostal artery resulting in a 1500-mL hemopnuemothorax. The graft shows continuous values for cardiac index (CI) mean arterial pressure (MAP), arterial hemoglobin saturation by pulse oximetry ($SapO_2$), and transcutaneous oxygen tension indexed to the fractional inspired oxygen concentration ($PtcO_2/FIO_2$), reflecting tissue perfusion. The time in hours after emergency department (ED) admission is shown immediately below the monitored values. Below this are the therapeutic interventions. In the ED, the initial decrease in tissue perfusion was corrected by 4 units of packed red cells (Prbc); in the operating room (OR), bleeding recurred, and the patient was given 4 more units of Prbc, 3000 mL of Ringer's lactate (RL) solution, and 1000 mL of 6% hydroxyethyl starch with correction of all monitored variables. The patient made an uneventful recovery. ICU, intensive care unit. (From Shoemaker WC: Invasive and noninvasive hemodynamic monitoring of high-risk patients to improve outcome. Semin Anesth 1999;18:63–70.)

ble losses over time. Furthermore, these net cumulative changes demonstrate major differences in survivor and nonsurvivor patterns. Monitoring in the ED can document low flow states and poor tissue perfusion and can provide the means for titrating therapy to achieve the desired end point and to maintain those parameters until the patient is satisfactorily recovering.

Dehydration and Hypovolemia

Hypovolemia from dehydration, poor fluid intake, blood loss, diarrhea, vomiting, or excessive diuretic therapy may be easy to recognize and straightforward to treat in most instances. Hemodynamic monitoring is particularly useful when there are associated comorbid conditions, such as history of cardiac infarction, early cardiac failure, dysrhythmias, chronic pulmonary dis-

orders, or other complex conditions, or age of greater than 65 years.

Blood pressure may be mediated by the production of catecholamines and other vasoactive substances, which are elements of the stress response. Other researchers showed that increased flow is critical to survival in high-risk critically ill patients.[11–23] The vasoconstrictive response leads to "peripheral shunting" from uneven microcirculatory flow within the vascular bed. The low or uneven flow to the skin, which is often the first organ affected, is directly reflected by low $PtcO_2$, which was often the first abnormality observed. The compensatory stress response may be inadequate when the stress response becomes either overwhelmed or exhausted. The transient nature of the blood pressure response may be due to overwhelming injury, hypovolemia, or exhaustion of the stress response. The smaller initial transient fall in CI in survivors and the subsequent rise in flow and DO_2 are compensatory

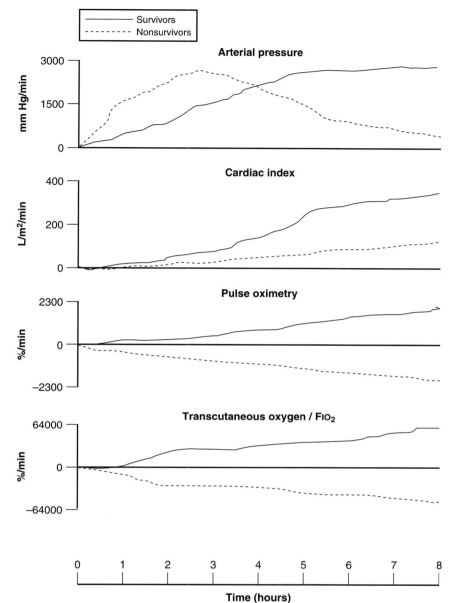

FIGURE 23–7. Net cumulative deficit (less than zero) or excess (more than zero) for shown henodynamic values from survivors and nonsurvivors of severe blunt trauma for the first 8 hours after admission. These data illustrate the deficit or the excess of flow, arterial oxygenation, and tissue perfusion in quantitative terms for those who survive and those who fail to survive their current hospitalization. Survivors had a net cumulative excess over normal values of +81 L/hour for cardiac index. The data illustrate how relatively small changes that may be easily tolerated over short periods may accumulate into appreciable losses over time. Furthermore, these net cumulative changes during the initial resuscitation period characterize survivor and nonsurvivor patterns in this type of circulatory dysfunction.

responses to the initial low-flow state.[15–19, 23] This is affected by the amount of injury, hypovolemia, preload, therapy, and increased metabolic demand produced by the trauma itself. The combination of increased demand and abnormal perfusion leads to oxygen debt, multiorgan failure, and death.[20, 23]

Sequential Hemodynamic Patterns in Hemorrhagic Shock

Table 23–6 shows the immediate direct effects of sudden hemorrhage (more than 4 units of blood) evaluated by noninvasive methods in the ED. For survivors and nonsurvivors, the initial baseline values on admission to the ED, the values at the nadir (or lowest recorded value) for variables that fell or the highest

recorded value for $PtcCO_2$ (the only variable that rose), and the value after initial resuscitation are shown. There was reduced flow, MAP, and $PtcO_2$ with increased $PtcCO_2$; these effects were more pronounced in nonsurvivors. Initial $SapO_2$ and PaO_2 were usually close to normal, whereas tissue perfusion (reflected by reduced $PtcO_2$ and increased $PtcCO_2$) rapidly deteriorated, with moderate degrees of hypovolemia. With severe hypovolemia, hyperpnea and tachypnea occurred, usually with slightly reduced PaO_2 and pH. With prolonged shock, poor tissue perfusion led to acidosis, base deficits, and increased lactate levels.

Rapid hemorrhage in the intensive care unit, studied by invasive and noninvasive monitoring, demonstrated a reduction in MAP, CI, central venous pressure, PA occlusion pressure, stroke index, stroke work, mixed venous oxygen saturation (SvO_2), pH, hematocrit, DO_2,

TABLE 23–6. Noninvasive Hemodynamic Patterns in Acute Emergencies

Variables,* Units	Survivors			Nonsurvivors		
	Baseline	*Nadir*	*Resuscitation*	*Baseline*	*Nadir*	*Resuscitation*
Hemorrhage						
CI, L/min/m²	3.91 ± .78	2.15 ± .57	3.85 ± .83	4.42 ± 1.35	1.24 ± .30	2.30 ± .10
MAP, mm Hg	98 ± 29	65 ± 8	97 ± 13	71 ± 17	52 ± 23	88 ± 3
SaO₂, %	93 ± 4	89 ± 1	95 ± 3	91 ± 4	88 ± 6	94 ± 4
PtcO₂, torr	54 ± 7	32 ± 14	60 ± 15	82 ± 38	17 ± 14	58 ± 34
PtcCO₂, torr†	59 ± 7	65 ± 8*	55 ± 3	83 ± 43	121 ± 61*	34 ± 23
Cardiogenic Shock						
CI, L/min/m²	2.93 ± .76	2.30 ± .68	3.15 ± .72	1.82 ± .66	1.41 ± .57	2.37 ± .41
MAP, mm Hg	87 ± 14	74 ± 18	92 ± 16	73 ± 18	51 ± 13	79 ± 16
SaO₂, %	97 ± 4	92 ± 6	96 ± 3	95 ± 5	91 ± 1	94 ± 4
PtcO₂, torr	43 ± 18	26 ± 9	43 ± 10	28 ± 18	19 ± 13	42 ± 24
PtcCO₂, torr†	56 ± 8	65 ± 9	58 ± 9	107 ± 46	113 ± 44	109 ± 42
Hypertension						
CI, L/min/m²	2.85 ± .50	2.32 ± .63	3.26 ± .57	1.83 ± .48	1.52 ± .54	2.55 ± .79
MAP, mm Hg	120 ± 14	134 ± 13*	119 ± 11	122 ± 19	138 ± 12*	127 ± 2
SaO₂, %	96 ± 3	95 ± 2	96 ± 3	94 ± 3	93 ± 4	95 ± 2
PtcO₂, torr	45 ± 14	27 ± 9	41 ± 8	74 ± 9	20 ± 15	38 ± 14
PtcCO₂, torr†	61 ± 15	73 ± 17	64 ± 12	42 ± 6	64 ± 4	40 ± 6
Early Sepsis						
CI, L/min/m²	3.88 ± 1.03	3.03 ± 1.10	3.84 ± 1.38	3.23 ± 1.11	2.51 ± 1.11	3.72 ± 1.31
MAP, mm Hg	80 ± 5	65 ± 12	86 ± 16	79 ± 15	59 ± 13	87 ± 8
SaO₂, %	96 ± 2	90 ± 9	95 ± 3	95 ± 3	84 ± 12	94 ± 3
PtcO₂, torr	55 ± 19	23 ± 16	56 ± 25	39 ± 17	16 ± 14	43 ± 21
PtcCO₂, torr†	67 ± 16	69 ± 21	61 ± 10	88 ± 5	174 ± 6	51 ± 6
Drug Overdose						
CI, L/min/m²	3.52 ± .90	3.30 ± .76	3.97 ± .95	2.36 ± 1.84	1.19 ± .76	3.14 ± .75
MAP, mm Hg	87 ± 6	80 ± 7	85 ± 9	55 ± 3	43 ± 12	68 ± 22
SaO₂, %	95 ± 3	94 ± 4	95 ± 3	93 ± 4	68 ± 18	92 ± 7
PtcO₂, torr	34 ± 6	29 ± 5	37 ± 5	9 ± 2	1 ± 3	10 ± 11
PtcCO₂, torr†	56 ± 6	60 ± 6	56 ± 3	85 ± 21	87 ± 31	73 ± 28
Stroke						
CI, L/min/m²	2.66 ± .51	2.16 ± .55	3.01 ± .61	2.14 ± .95	1.84 ± .77	2.80 ± 1.90
MAP, mm Hg	84 ± 23	68 ± 20	86 ± 11	68 ± 24	29 ± 5	57 ± 24
SaO₂, %	95 ± 3	92 ± 3	95 ± 4	96 ± 4	88 ± 6	95 ± 4
PtcO₂, torr	40 ± 3	29 ± 4	43 ± 7	25 ± 14	19 ± 13	35 ± 30
PtcCO₂, torr†	55 ± 5	62 ± 2	55 ± 5	61 ± 13	65 ± 10	55 ± 12

*Values are mean ± standard error of the mean. CI, cardiac index; MAP, mean arterial pressure; PtcCO₂, transcutaneous carbon dioxide tension; PtcO₂, transcutaneous oxygen tension; SaO₂, arterial oxygen saturation.
†The highest recorded value for PtcCO₂ and MAP in hypertension.

and VO₂ concomitant with an increase in systemic vascular resistance index and oxygen extraction ratio.[20] The initial compensatory responses included increased heart rate, which increased CI by neural and neurohormonal mechanisms; increased systemic vascular resistance index, which tended to maintain arterial pressures in the face of decreasing flow; and increased oxygen extraction ratios, which improved tissue oxygenation when blood flow had been reduced.

With slow prolonged hemorrhage, the shock pattern showed greater reductions in hematocrit and lesser reductions in MAP, CI, DO₂, and VO₂; the reduction in VO₂ was lower quantitatively but more prolonged than after rapid losses of comparable quantities of blood. After bleeding was stopped and blood volume was restored with appropriate fluids, the survivors' recovery pattern usually consisted of normal or elevated values for CI, DO₂, and VO₂.[20] The smaller initial transient decrease in CI in survivors and the subsequent increase in flow and DO₂ are compensation for the initial low-flow state.[15-20] This is affected by the amount of injury, hypovolemia, preload, therapy, and increased metabolic demand from the trauma itself. The combination of increased demand and abnormal tissue perfusion leads to oxygen debt, multiorgan failure, and death.[20-23]

Acute Myocardial Infarction

Invasive and noninvasive monitoring of central hemodynamics and of peripheral perfusion was used to describe the sequence of circulatory events in 12 patients with AMI who entered the ED with unstable angina,

ECG evidence of AMI, and positive enzyme (CK-MB) values. Invasive clinical monitoring was also employed via a radial artery catheter and a thermodilution PA catheter. Survivors had higher mean arterial pressure, CI, oxygen delivery, oxygen consumption, and transcutaneous oxygen levels than did nonsurvivors; they also had lower heart rates and transcutaneous carbon dioxide levels. Pulse oximetry values for the two groups were maintained in the normal range by means of supplemental oxygen administration and were not significantly different. Satisfactory correlation was noted between the thermodilution and the bioimpedance methods of estimating cardiac output in these patients with early AMI who did not have pulmonary edema. After thrombolytic therapy, noninvasive hemodynamic monitoring of patients with AMI provided early warning of outcome and was used to guide therapy.[28]

Heart Failure

Heart failure occurs in 400,000 Americans annually and is the primary diagnosis for more than 900,000 hospitalizations per year. It is associated with exercise intolerance, hemodynamic abnormalities, and activation of the sympathetic nervous system and the renin-angiotensin-aldosterone system. Cardiac problems may be complicated by hypovolemia, hypoxemia, acidosis, anemia, dysrhythmias, inadequate tissue perfusion, and activation of the adrenomedullary stress response as well as by associated medical conditions such as hypertension, sepsis, diabetes, and pulmonary and renal disorders. The median survival after diagnosis is 1.7 years in men and 3.2 years in women; the 5-year survival rate is less than 50%.[28]

Therapy is generally aimed at reducing cardiac work, controlling fluid retention, and enhancing myocardial contractility. Vasodilators, diuretics, oxygen, and inotropes are often given starting in the ED to relieve circulatory congestion. Real-time noninvasive monitoring of patients with early heart failure in the ED identifies circulatory deficiencies and provides criteria to titrate therapy to meet specific hemodynamic end points related to survival. Cardiac index values measured invasively and noninvasively were higher in survivors, and DO_2 and VO_2 were noted to be significantly higher ($P < .001$). Transcutaneous measurements of oxygen (PaO_2/FIO_2 ratio) and carbon dioxide showed higher levels of oxygen tension and lower levels of carbon dioxide in survivors compared with nonsurvivors. MAP, heart rate, and pulse oximetry and oxygen extraction ratios were not significantly different in the two groups.[28]

Septic Shock

Septic shock was redefined as sepsis, in which infection is present (now called the systemic inflammatory response syndrome)—and the septic syndrome, in which infection is not present or documentable. The sequential hemodynamic and oxygen transport patterns of various septic shock syndromes have been described previously in medical and surgical patients.[29] In an effort to obtain earlier values, 45 patients with septic shock were studied on admission to the ED.[28, 29] Table 23–6 contrasts the patterns for survivors and for nonsurvivors of septic shock in regard to MAP, heart rate, pulse oximetry, PaO_2, SaO_2, $PtcO_2$, and CI beginning with the time of admission. In general, the survivors had significantly higher values for MAP, CI, SaO_2, and $PtcO_2$ than did the nonsurvivors at comparable time periods after admission. In the first 12 hours, the initial heart rate was higher in nonsurvivors, whereas the initial values for CI, central venous pressure, PA wedge pressure, DO_2, and VO_2 were lower than those of the survivors. The nonsurvivors' values increased appreciably over the subsequent period as they developed organ failure and septic complications, however. The other variables had fluctuating values without clearly defined patterns.

Other Cardiovascular Emergencies

Cardiovascular emergencies present with a wide range of signs and symptoms. The initial history and the physical examination may not differentiate between a life-threatening condition and the slow progression of an underlying disease. Similarly, two acute life-threatening situations—AMI and dissecting aortic aneurysm—may be indistinguishable on initial presentation. Mistaking one for the other may lead to increased morbidity and mortality; thrombolytic therapy for an aortic dissection or surgical intervention for an AMI may lead to avoidable death. A range of cardiovascular diseases may share common manifestations that make differentiation by means of routine assessment and monitoring difficult. Intermittent arrhythmias, congestive heart failure, and pulmonary embolism can all present with a chief complaint of shortness of breath. Late in the course of disease, physiologic compensatory mechanisms may fail and may unmask the underlying pathologic processes.

The ED may be used for patients at risk of an ischemic cardiac event because of history or risk factors who have an unremarkable physical examination and ECG. Current practice is to order cardiac enzyme evaluation to monitor for release of intracellular cardiac myocytes signaling cell death. Cardiac enzymes take several hours to peak, and the test must be repeated to increase specificity. Regional wall motion abnormalities noted on echocardiography in the ED may indicate cardiac ischemia. Noninvasive hemodynamic monitoring is a useful approach to measure the physiologic deficiencies and to plan therapy. Unmonitored interventions targeted at supporting circulatory function may not be effective. For in-hospital cardiac arrest, unsuccessful resuscitation was associated with the use of epinephrine, atropine, bicarbonate, calcium, and lidocaine.

Table 23–6 reviews our experience with cardiogenic shock in 39 patients with complicated cardiac failure and in 6 patients with AMI. Treatment is often aimed at reducing cardiac work, controlling fluid retention, and enhancing myocardial contractility by means of vasodilators, diuretics, and inotropes. Intervention is initially based on clinical assessment, vital signs, and radiographic findings; however, overly vigorous diuresis can decrease preload and thereby reduce contractility. Because both overtreatment and undertreatment are dangerous, it is appropriate to titrate therapy to attain predetermined physiologic goals assessed by hemodynamic monitoring. In the absence of invasive monitoring, therapeutic interventions may be suboptimal and may lead to increased mortality, but it is not usually feasible to place PA catheters in the busy ED. The new bioimpedance system provides similar information without the attendant risks of invasive procedures. Accurate assessment, effective treatment, and meaningful hemodynamic variables can be obtained quickly and accurately and can be used to titrate appropriate pharmacologic interventions.

Other Medical Emergencies in the Emergency Department

Table 23–6 describes changes in hemodynamic patterns in 23 patients with hypertensive crisis, 45 patients with sepsis or septic shock, 15 patients who experienced a drug overdose, and 21 patients with acute stroke. This table summarizes the initial baseline values on admission to the ED, the nadir of variables that fell or the highest value of MAP or $PtcCO_2$ (the variables that rose at their worst), and the values after initial resuscitation. In general, the common circulatory pattern was low pressure, low flow, and low tissue perfusion, usually associated with evidence of hypovolemia; these abnormalities were worse in the patients who subsequently died during the same hospitalization.

Summary of Early Responses to Acute Illness

An appropriate basic assumption is that low flow, poor tissue perfusion, shock, and other forms of circulatory dysfunction can be recognized early from objective noninvasive criteria and that more promptly delivered therapy might be more efficacious. Noninvasively monitored data may be used to titrate early fluid and inotropic therapy to achieve optimal physiologic crite-

ria to prevent development of lethal organ failure. To a large extent, the circulatory findings in acute illnesses may be explained by well-documented physiologic responses to trauma. Tissue injury, hemorrhage, pain, fear, and hypovolemia activate the sympathoadrenal axis, releasing epinephrine and norepinephrine from the adrenal medulla and the sympathetic effector neurons.[14, 20, 21] The continued stress of hypovolemia, hypotension, tissue injury, and the sympathoadrenal response activate the hypothalamic-hypophyseal-adrenal axis via afferent neural signals. This activation causes corticotropin-releasing hormone to be released by the hypothalamus and elaboration of adrenocorticotropic hormone by the adenohypophysis. Adrenocorticotropic hormone stimulates the adrenals to secrete cortisol, which increases cardiac output and in part mediates the post-traumatic hypermetabolic state. The hypermetabolic state, which requires increased blood flow, makes tissues more susceptible to local ischemic events.[20]

Cardiopulmonary catecholamine effects immediately after trauma include increases in blood pressure, heart rate, cardiac contractility, minute ventilation, and peripheral vasomotor tone. Although these adaptive effects are often beneficial, especially in minor insults, exaggerated but uneven peripheral vasoconstriction in severe trauma or hemorrhage leads to increased but maldistributed microcirculatory flow with localized areas of hypoperfusion, tissue hypoxemia, and localized intravascular hypovolemia.[15] The hypoxic acidotic endothelium of poorly perfused capillaries activates macrophages and leukocytes and produces cytokines, platelet-activating factor, eicosanoids, intravascular coagulation, and many other known and unknown immunochemical cascades; the activated macrophages and the white blood cells produce oxygen free radicals and local tissue destruction, which mark the systemic inflammatory response syndrome.

With resuscitation and reperfusion of hypoxic capillaries, these activated cellular and immunochemical cascades are washed into the venous circulation and lead to the systemic inflammatory response syndrome, end-organ dysfunction, multiple vital organ failures, and death. The survivors have greater physiologic reserve capacity and the ability to generate increased flow and tissue perfusion to provide adequate tissue oxygenation in the presence of increased metabolic need. Differences between hemodynamic patterns in survivors and in nonsurvivors have motivated investigators to suggest that aggressive fluid therapy, titrated to reach optimal physiologic goals (defined by the patterns in survivors), can be a strategy to improve patient outcome. Fluid therapy is titrated to maintain intravascular volume, improve tissue perfusion, and overcome regional circulatory deficiencies caused by uneven, maldistributed vasoconstriction.

Conclusions

1. The goal of multicomponent noninvasive monitoring is to obtain information comparable to that obtained by invasive monitoring but continuously and in real time.

2. The feasibility of a multicomponent noninvasive monitoring system was demonstrated in the immediate postadmission period. Impedance cardiography devices can be applied like ECG electrodes in the ED, the operating room, or the intensive care unit; on hospital floors; or in doctors' offices and other prehospital settings. They are less labor intensive, easier to operate, simpler, cheaper, and safer for both the patient and the staff.

3. The multicomponent noninvasive monitoring system allowed description of the time course of the major components of the circulation: total body blood flow, reflecting cardiac function; arterial oxygenation obtained via pulse oximetry, reflecting pulmonary function; and $PtcO_2$ and $PtcCO_2$, reflecting tissue perfusion. The temporal patterns of these interacting noninvasive components were roughly comparable to the data obtained simultaneously with invasive monitoring.

4. The noninvasive systems may be used to characterize the physiology of surviving and nonsurviving patients beginning with ED admission. The data obtained with the three simultaneously monitored noninvasive systems (thoracic electric bioimpedance or other noninvasive measures of cardiac output, pulse oximetry, and transcutaneous O_2 tension) instituted shortly after ED admission were comparable with data from the invasive PA catheter when this became available. These three noninvasive systems provided evaluation of cardiac, pulmonary, and tissue perfusion.

5. When large volumes of fluid are required, central venous pressure or PA catheters may be used to monitor venous pressures to avoid fluid overload. The noninvasive systems are less hazardous than invasive catheters for the patient in terms of catheter complications and for the staff in terms of exposure to hepatitis, human immunodeficiency virus, and other infections.

6. Hardware and software innovations have provided much greater accuracy and reliability for the impedance method, when criteria are met.

7. Continuous online noninvasively monitored data provide a means to calculate the net cumulative deficits or excesses of each monitored variable. Discriminant analysis gives a more quantitative estimate of circulatory dysfunction and a powerful view of rapidly changing circulatory dynamics, transcending the boundaries of our old concepts of shock.

8. Because noninvasive monitoring can provide the essential circulatory information for patients in the hospital and prehospital locations, the data may be used to describe survivor and nonsurvivor patterns, to predict outcome, to define therapeutic goals, to titrate therapy to achieve these goals, and eventually to improve outcome. This may change the standard way we manage acutely ill patients.

References

1. Nyboer J: Impedance Plethysmography. Springfield, IL, Charles C Thomas, 1959.
2. Kubicek WG, Karnegis JN, Patterson RP, et al: Development and evaluation of an impedance cardiac output system. Aerospace Med 1966;37:1208–1219.
3. Bernstein DP: A new stroke volume equation for thoracic electrical bioimpedance: Theory and rationale. Crit Care Med 1986; 14:904–909.
4. Bernstein DP: Noninvasive cardiac output measurement. In Shoemaker WC, Ayres S, Grenvik A (eds): Textbook of Critical Care, 2nd ed. Philadelphia, WB Saunders, 1989, pp 159–185.
5. Sageman WS, Amundson DE: Thoracic electrical bioimpedance measurement of cardiac output in postaortocoronary bypass patients. Crit Care Med 1993;21:1139–1142.
6. Fuller HD: The validity of cardiac output measurement by thoracic impedance: A meta-analysis. Clin Invest Med 1992;15:103–112.
7. Raaijmakers E, Faes TJC, Scholten RJ, et al: A meta-analysis of three decades of validating thoracic impedance cardiography. Crit Care Med 1999;27:1203–1213.
8. Wang XA, Sun HH, Adamson D, Van de Water JM: An impedance cardiography system: A new design. Ann Biomed Eng 1989;17:535–556.
9. Wang XA, Van de Water JM, Sun HH, et al: Hemodynamic monitoring by impedance cardiography with an improved signal processing technique. IEEE Eng Med Biol 1993;15:699–700.
10. Wang XA, Sun HH, Van de Water JM: Time-frequency distribution technique in biological signal processing. Biomed Instrum Technol 1995;29:203–212.
11. Shoemaker WC, Wo CJ, Bishop MH, et al: Multicenter trial of a new thoracic electrical bioimpedance system for cardiac output estimation. Crit Care Med 1994;22:1907–1912.
12. Shoemaker WC, Belzberg H, Wo CC, et al: Multicenter study of noninvasive monitoring as alternative to invasive monitoring of acutely ill emergency patients. Chest 1998;114:1645–1652.
13. Wo CC, Shoemaker WC, Bishop MH, et al: Noninvasive estimations of cardiac output and circulatory dynamics in critically ill patients. Curr Opin Crit Care 1995;1:211–218.
14. Belzberg H, Shoemaker WC: Methods and concepts for noninvasive cardiac output measurements. Curr Opin Crit Care 1997; 3:238–242.
15. Shoemaker WC, Appel PL, Kram HB, et al: Multicomponent noninvasive physiologic monitoring of circulatory function. Crit Care Med 1988;16:482–490.
16. Shoemaker WC, Appel PL, Kram HB: Incidence, physiologic description, compensatory mechanisms, and therapeutic implications of monitored events. Crit Care Med 1989;17:1277–1285.
17. Bishop MH, Shoemaker WC, Shuleshko J, Wo CC: Noninvasive cardiac index monitoring in gunshot wound victims. Acad Emerg Med 1996;3:682–688.
18. Shoemaker WC: Invasive and noninvasive hemodynamic monitoring of high risk patients to improve outcome. Semin Anesth 1999;18:63–70.
19. Shoemaker WC, Wo CC, Bishop MH, et al: Noninvasive physiologic monitoring of high-risk surgical patients. Arch Surg 1996;131:732–737.
20. Shoemaker WC, Wo CC, Demetriades D, et al: Early physiologic patterns in acute illness and accidents: Toward a concept of

circulatory dysfunction and shock based on invasive and noninvasive hemodynamic monitoring. New Horiz 1996;4:395–412.

21. Shoemaker WC, Wo CC, Chan L, et al: Outcome predictors of severely injured patients by noninvasive hemodynamic monitoring beginning in the emergency department. Chest 2001; in press.

22. Shoemaker WC, Wo CC, Thangathurai D, et al: Outcome prediction of high risk surgical patients by noninvasive hemodynamic monitoring. Crit Care Med 2001; in press.

23. Shoemaker WC, Appel PL, Kram HB: Hemodynamic and oxygen transport responses in survivors and nonsurvivors of high-risk surgery. Crit Care Med 1993;21:977–990.

24. Gedeon A, Forslund L, Hedenstierna G, et al: A new method for noninvasive bedside determinations of pulmonary blood flow. Med Biol Eng Comput 1980;18:411–418.

25. Capek JM, Roy RJ: Noninvasive measurement of cardiac output using partial CO_2 rebreathing. IEEE Eng Med Biol 1998;35:653–661.

26. de Abreu M, Quntel M, Ragaller M, Albrecht M: Partial carbon dioxide rebreathing: A reliable technique for noninvasive measurement of nonshunted pulmonary capillary blood flow. Crit Care Med 1997;25:675–683.

27. Haryadi DG, Orr JA, Kuck K, et al: Evaluation of a partial CO_2 rebreathing Fick technique for measurement of cardiac output [abstract]. Anesthesiology 1998;89:A534.

28. Shoemaker WC, Sullivan MJ, Wo CCJ: Hemodynamic evolution and management of acute illness in the emergency department. In Shoemaker WC, Ayres SM, Grenvik A, Holbrook P (eds): Textbook of Critical Care, 4th ed. Philadelphia, WB Saunders, 2000, pp 258–272.

29. Shoemaker WC, Wo CC, Sullivan MJ, et al: Hemodynamic monitoring of septic shock patients in the emergency department. Eur J Emerg Med 2000; 7:169–175.

24 Transesophageal Doppler Monitoring

Mervyn Singer

History

In 1842, Doppler described what has come to be known as the Doppler effect: The shift in frequency emitted by, or reflected off, a moving object is proportional to the relative velocity between object and observer. A formula was derived relating frequency shift to velocity, encompassing other variables such as the angulation of the point of observation to the path of the moving object as well as the speed of sound. If these variables were kept constant, then the proportionality between changes in frequency shift and velocity would be maintained.

The first "industrial" application of Doppler ultrasound was an early sonar technique developed during World War I by Rutherford to detect German submarines. The Doppler effect has since been applied to many other areas, including radar speed traps, radioastronomy, and medicine. Its earliest medical application was in obstetric practice in the 1950s. In the following decade, the measurement of aortic blood flow was first reported by Light.[1] He directed a probe percutaneously at the aortic arch; this was initially placed over the second left intercostal space and, in subsequent studies, in the suprasternal notch, both being aimed toward the descending aorta. Huntsman and colleagues also used a suprasternal probe, albeit directed at the ascending aorta.[2] His group performed the first correlation with a comparative technique for measuring cardiac output (i.e., thermodilution), describing good agreement between the two.[3]

Disadvantages of the suprasternal Doppler technique include the need for adequate training to find and identify the optimal aortic flow signal; the loss of signal in patients with large air windows (e.g., emphysema), through which sound waves travel poorly; and the turbulent flow generated by aortic valve deformities, which invalidates flow measurement in the ascending or arch portions of the aorta. A further issue is the failure to fix the probe in the correct position to enable continuous monitoring. Alternative approaches being investigated concurrently included the transesophageal (Fig. 24–1) and the transtracheal routes. The latter technique, which employed an endotracheal tube, had a short commercial existence, owing in no small part to its lack of adequate validation before launch.[4] It is not discussed further in this chapter.

The transesophageal route has been incorporated into both standalone Doppler and combined echocardiographic-Doppler devices (transesophageal echocardiography). This chapter concentrates only on those techniques directed solely at measuring blood flow velocity in the descending thoracic aorta, from which a variety of parameters describing hemodynamic status can be obtained.

In 1971, Side and Gosling recorded velocity waveforms of blood flow in the aortic arch using a 1-cm esophageal probe emitting and receiving 5 MHz of continuous-wave Doppler ultrasound.[5] They did not publish further on the topic but, with prescient foresight, suggested possible applications in the detection of aortic valve disease and in perioperative hemodynamic management: "Beat-to-beat changes in the flow pattern and peak velocity and acceleration can be of considerable value to the surgeon by giving immediate warning of deteriorating cardiac efficiency."[5]

Three years later, Olson and Cooke reported their design for a combined esophageal Doppler and pulse-echo system whereby continuous measurement of flow could be combined with an aortic diameter value to provide volumetric measures.[6] Though the paper concentrated on canine studies, mention was made of five human subjects who underwent instrumentation with good results. They demonstrated in their animal work that aortic diameter only increased from 16.9 to 17.8 mm over the cardiac cycle, with most of this change occurring in early systole. Thus, most of the forward flow in systole passes through an aorta of constant diameter. In the same year, Duck and colleagues described a prototype esophageal Doppler flow probe, with the first detailed account of insertion, focusing, and difficulties encountered in human subjects.[7] Their transducer was 5.5 mm in diameter, emitting 8 MHz of continuous-wave Doppler ultrasound at an angle of 45 degrees, assuming parallel axes of descending aorta and esophagus. Fifteen anesthetized adults were investigated, with the transducer passed a distance of 30 to 40 cm beyond the lips. High-quality signals with a signal-to-noise ratio in excess of 20:1 developed within 10 minutes, the delay being ascribed to either the

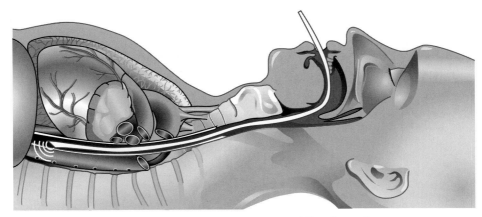

FIGURE 24–1. Positioning of esophageal Doppler probe.

initial presence of air or the buildup of a mucus coating over the probe head, which acted as a good coupling agent. Directional orientation was achieved by probe rotation using the maximal pitch of an audible signal. Incorrect probe positioning gave characteristically different Doppler signals from other flows (e.g., intracardiac or the hemiazygos vein).

In 1975, Daigle and colleagues described their esophageal probe, which incorporated 7.5-MHz pulsed-wave Doppler with an echo-ranging system to measure aortic diameter.[8] They validated flow measurements against electromagnetic flowmeters and pulsed-Doppler flow cuffs placed around the aortas of beagles at the level of the diaphragm. A blunt velocity profile was demonstrated during forward flow in the descending thoracic aorta. They too observed small fluctuations in aortic diameter over the cardiac cycle, mainly occurring in early systole, reaching 1.2 mm at the level of the aortic arch and 0.6 mm near the diaphragm. They concluded, "The simplicity of the oesophageal probe technique and its ability to obtain haemodynamic information non-traumatically are important assets which should lead to increasing use of such probes in numerous measurement applications."[8]

Another device, developed by Lavandier and associates, was 6.8 mm in diameter and combined a 5-MHz continuous-wave Doppler ultrasound system angled at 40 degrees with an A-scan echo transducer to measure aortic diameter.[9, 10] A latex balloon surrounded the distal end of the tube; it was claimed that when the balloon was inflated, it maintained probe position and provided good transducer coupling. A probe inserted to a depth of 35 cm from the lips would be at the level of the 5th or 6th thoracic vertebra, at which point the esophagus runs parallel to the descending aorta. Reproducibility between two observers was very close, with a maximum difference of 1.9% in 11 patients. Doppler cardiac output was compared with thermodilution in 21 patients. Although the coefficient of correlation was high (0.98 with a standard error of 0.54 L/minute), the Doppler values (6.67 ± 2.3 L/minute)

underestimated thermodilution values (7.88 ± 2.6 L/minute). They attributed this variation to numerous factors inherent in their device, yet did not consider the imperfect gold standard provided by thermodilution. This device is now commercially available as the Dynemo 3000 (Sometec, Stoneham, Mass). It measures descending aortic blood flow rather than total cardiac output. Though trend following is likely to be reasonable, it is still affected by inaccuracies generated through aortic diameter measurement; these differ by as much as 30% from echocardiographically derived data.[11]

In 1986, Mark and coworkers reported the first use of a commercial Doppler device, the Ultracom (Lawrence Medical Systems).[12] A later reincarnation, the Accucom, was developed by Lawrence and was subsequently taken over by Datascope (Montvale, NJ). The Ultracom had a 6-mm continuous-wave esophageal Doppler transducer with two additional inputs to provide a volumetric measure of total-body cardiac output: a suprasternal Doppler probe to calibrate descending aortic blood flow to total body blood flow, and provision for pulsed A-mode echocardiography to measure ascending aortic diameter. The result was optimized by means of an audio signal and a signal level seen on a digital LED display. This manipulation required 2 to 10 minutes, and the suprasternal calibration required a further 2 to 10 minutes. Doppler cardiac output was compared against simultaneous thermodilution in 16 patients undergoing surgery. Echocardiographic estimation of aortic diameter was compared with direct intraoperative measurement in 23 patients. For each patient, there was a fairly constant calibration error between Doppler and thermodilution cardiac output measurement, which accounted for much of the variability. In particular, aortic diameter measurements showed poor overall correlation. After excluding patients in whom it was difficult to obtain a clear echo image, only 71% were within 3 mm of one another (approximately 10% of aortic diameter dimensions). Nevertheless, trend following of cardiac output was

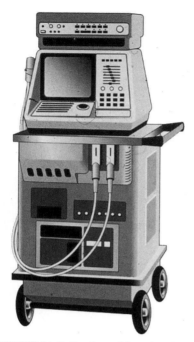

FIGURE 24–2. Esophageal Doppler device.

satisfactory. Mark concluded that significant errors were introduced by the calibration steps of measuring aortic diameter and ascending aortic flow. He suggested that further investigations should address the need for absolute cardiac output values and that trends alone may be sufficient to aid management in many instances.

The Accucom did away with the echocardiographic technique by utilizing a nomogram that calculated ascending aortic diameter. The calibration step, which employed a suprasternal Doppler probe, remained. A number of studies assessed the Accucom, demonstrating reasonable correlation with thermodilution results but rather variable absolute values for cardiac output.[13–15] Unfortunately, this device was not particularly user friendly and failed to achieve acceptance by the clinical community, resulting in its discontinuation.

Singer and colleagues described a new continuous-wave esophageal Doppler system, which in various stages of evolution has been called the ODM-1, the ODM-2, and the CardioQ (Deltex Medical, Chichester, UK) (Fig. 24–2).[16] This device incorporates only Doppler flow velocity measurement. Initially, the system was used to compare trends between descending aortic blood flow and total cardiac output measured by thermodilution, but Singer subsequently developed a nomogram (incorporating the patient's age, height, and weight) that translated the descending aortic Doppler values into an estimate of total left ventricular cardiac output without the need for other measurements. A number of studies in numerous countries employing a variety of comparative techniques (e.g., thermodilution, echocardiography, and dye dilution)

have generally shown high agreement.[17–20] The correlation in cardiac output measurements implies that blood flowing down the descending thoracic aorta remains in a fairly fixed proportion of total left ventricular cardiac output. This holds true despite changes in blood pressure, cardiac output, and body temperature, though changes in posture have not been formally examined. The great advantage of this finding is that the requirement to measure aortic diameter is obviated; this removes a further source of error, which is magnified twofold because the square of the radius is used in the calculation of aortic cross-sectional area. A 2-mm error in measuring a 25-mm aortic diameter would introduce a 16% error in aortic cross-sectional area.

Waveform Characteristics

Most esophageal Doppler devices display a velocity-time waveform in real time (Fig. 24–3). The area of the waveform (the velocity-time integral or the stroke distance) is proportional to blood flow traveling down the descending thoracic aorta, assuming, as stated previously, an aortic diameter that changes little during systole. This waveform area is also proportional to left ventricular stroke volume. The assumption that there is a fixed proportion of cardiac output traveling down the descending thoracic aorta appears to be borne out by numerous validation studies.

Apart from the waveform size, further information regarding hemodynamic status can be derived from the waveform shape (Fig. 24–4). The peak velocity declines by approximately 1% per annum of adult life, with normal values of 90 to 120 cm/second in a resting 20-year-old to 50 to 80 cm/second in a resting 70-year-old. Values falling outside the age-expected normal ranges are indicative of hypo- or hyperdynamic circulation. The former is clearly seen in left ventricular failure, whereas the latter is observed in conditions as diverse as sepsis and pregnancy. The peak velocity and the mean acceleration provide information on left ventricular contractility, such that a positive inotrope

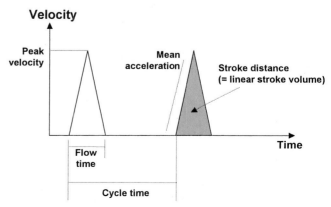

FIGURE 24–3. Doppler velocity-time waveform.

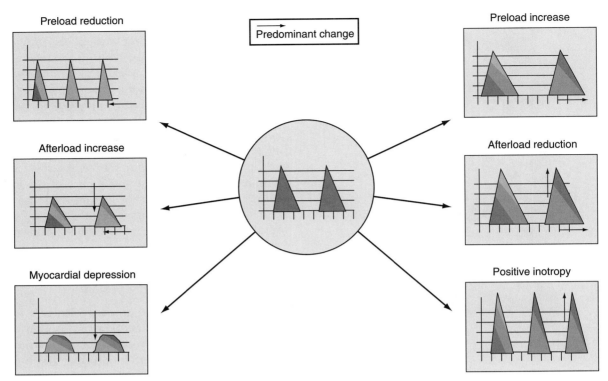

FIGURE 24–4. Changes in waveform shape with hemodynamic maneuvers.

will increase both variables, whereas myocardial depression resulting from drugs or ischemia will reduce values. These variables provide information similar to dP/dt data obtained from intraventricular pressure transducers; they reflect changes in left ventricular contractility though they are similarly affected by other factors, including changes in afterload and, to a lesser degree, preload.

The flow time—the base of the waveform—is obviously dependent on heart rate. Systolic and diastolic time intervals are reduced during tachycardia and are lengthened during bradycardia. By using a derivation of Bazett's equation to correct the QT interval to a heart rate of 60 beats per minute, the flow time can be corrected in a like manner by dividing it by the square root of the cycle time. Thus, for a heart rate of 60 beats per minute, the cycle time will be 1 second, and the systolic flow time will be approximately one third of this. The corrected flow time (FTc) has a range of 0.33 to 0.36 second in the normal individual. The FTc is inversely related to the systemic vascular resistance; thus, in vasoconstricted states (e.g., hypovolemia, excess vasopressor therapy, or hypothermia), the FTc narrows, whereas in low-resistance conditions (e.g., sepsis), the FTc widens.

The abovementioned characteristics of the waveform can be used both diagnostically and therapeutically. Diagnostic information is provided by the height of the waveform and the slope of the upstroke, which give an indication of contractile status, whereas the width (corrected for heart rate) describes the degree of constriction or dilatation within the circulation.[21] Moderate or severe aortic regurgitation is denoted by reverse blood flow occurring throughout diastole. The flow equivalent of pulsus paradoxus or respiratory swing is clearly seen in conditions such as severe asthma or pericardial tamponade. A narrow, reduced-size waveform in conjunction with increased central venous pressure suggests a major obstruction within the heart or the pulmonary tree (e.g., pulmonary embolus, tension pneumothorax, right ventricular infarction, or pericardial tamponade). The monitor also provides online support for clinical management, because the cardiovascular effects of a maneuver can be appreciated immediately. For example, a Starling-type ventricular function curve can be constructed by viewing the response to fluid challenges. Optimal filling is reached at the point where no further improvement occurs in stroke volume. If evidence of organ perfusion persists, alternative therapies should be sought (e.g., vasodilatation). Subsequent rechallenge with fluid may be necessary. Similarly, other challenges (e.g., inotrope administration) can be attempted and the benefit (or the harm) can be viewed, altering the level of positive end-expiratory pressure or other ventilator settings or pericardiocentesis.

Perioperative Outcome Studies

To my knowledge, the esophageal Doppler technique is unique among noninvasive monitoring technologies

TABLE 24–1. Results from a Cardiac Patient Study

	Protocol (*n* = 30)	Control (*n* = 30)	*P* Value
Intraoperative colloid (approx. mean)	900	1100	.05
Intraoperative crystalloid (approx. mean)	750	1400	.001
Mean intraoperative change in stroke volume	+29%	−9%	.001
Major complications	0	6	.01
Length of intensive care unit stay, mean (range)	1 (1–1)	1.7 (1–11)	.023
Length of hospital stay, mean (range)	6.4 (5–9)	10.1 (5–48)	.011

From Mythen MG, Webb AP: Perioperative plasma volume expansion reduces the incidence of gut mucosal hypoperfusion during cardiac surgery. Arch Surg 1995;130:423–429.

in that it has been successfully used in more than four prospective, randomized, controlled perioperative trials to guide management and improve outcome. All have used the Deltex ODM/CardioQ device. The first such trial was performed by Mythen and Webb in 60 cardiac surgical patients at the Middlesex Hospital in London.[22] An earlier interventional study by the same pair had demonstrated a significantly worse outcome with prolonged morbidity and hospital stay in those patients whose stroke volume had fallen over the perioperative period.[23] The trial used a simple protocol of fluid loading every 15 minutes during the intraoperative period to achieve optimal filling, with pre- and postoperative care being identical in both protocol and control groups. The control group received management that was standard for that institution, which did not include pulmonary artery catheterization. Results are shown in Table 24–1. Overall, a 37% reduction in hospital stay was noted. A similar protocol has been repeated recently in Dallas, although in that instance, pulmonary artery catheters were used in control patients who received the standard level of care. Although this study is yet to be published, a marked difference in outcome was also observed, with a significant reduction in intensive care unit stay (the primary study end point).

Sinclair and colleagues studied 40 patients undergoing repair of a fractured femoral neck, half of whom received intraoperative fluid loading at 15-minute intervals and half of whom were managed in standard fashion.[24] A 39% reduction in hospital stay was achieved in the protocol group, with similar results for time spent in an acute bed and time until being deemed medically fit for hospital discharge (Table 24–2). Venn and colleagues have recently repeated this study at St. George's Hospital in London with 29 control and 31 protocol patients. Again, similar results were obtained, with a reduction in total days spent in the hospital from 870 to 704 (D. Bennett, personal communication).

Another intraoperative study was recently reported in an abstract by Gan and associates from Duke University Medical Center.[25] One hundred patients undergoing general surgical procedures with an anticipated blood loss in excess of 500 mL were recruited; half received additional fluid loading at 15-minute intervals, as before. The protocol group had a shorter hospital stay (5 ± 3 days vs. 7 ± 5 days; *P* = .03) and tolerated a solid diet earlier (3 ± 2 days vs. 5 ± 4 days; *P* = .01).

Apart from the abovementioned interventional trials, a recent observational study by Poeze and associates in cardiac surgical patients revealed that a low stroke index immediately on admission to the intensive care unit was the best indicator of a poor outcome, and that specificity and sensitivity were even higher at 4 hours in those patients whose stroke index had decreased.[26] We have used this finding as the basis of an ongoing prospective study whereby patients are randomized shortly after admission to the intensive care unit to receive either standard postoperative care or aggressive fluid loading to the optimal point of a Starling curve. An inotrope is added if stroke index remains less than 35 mL/m². This protocol is nurse

TABLE 24–2. Results from a Cardiac Patient Study

	Protocol (*n* = 20)	Control (*n* = 20)	*P* Value
Intraoperative colloid	750 (550–950)	0 (0–450)	.001
Intraoperative crystalloid	725 (500–1000)	1000 (700–1250)	NS
Mean intraoperative change in stroke volume	+20%	−13%	.001
Length of hospital stay, median (95% CI)	12 (8–13)	20 (10–61)	.05

CI, confidence interval; NS, not significant.
From Sinclair J, James S, Singer M: Intraoperative intravascular volume optimisation and length of hospital stay after repair of proximal femoral fracture: Randomised controlled trial. BMJ 1997;315:909–912.

led and lasts 4 hours, management thereafter reverting to conventional methods. To date, 40 patients have been recruited, and a 19% reduction in hospital stay has been achieved in the protocol group. These preliminary data suggest that benefit can still be obtained in the immediate postoperative period through active management of the circulation.

Conclusion

Transesophageal Doppler monitoring of aortic blood flow is a quick, simple technique that with a relatively short period of training takes minutes to perform. Correct signal acquisition is easy to achieve and to recognize, and from both the size and the shape of the waveform, hemodynamic management is facilitated. Decisions regarding the use of fluid therapy, inotropes, pressors, and dilators are assisted by the additional information provided. Outcome benefit has been demonstrated in high-risk surgical patients through the use of this technique to optimize fluid loading.

References

1. Light LH: Non-injurious ultrasonic technique for observing flow in the human aorta. Nature 1969;224:1119–1121.
2. Huntsman LL, Gams E, Johnson CC, Fairbanks E: Transcutaneous determination of aortic blood flow velocities in man. Am Heart J 1975;89:605–612.
3. Huntsman LL, Stewart DK, Barnes SR, et al: Noninvasive Doppler determination of cardiac output in man. Circulation 1983;67:593–602.
4. Hausen B, Schafers HJ, Rohde R, Haverich A: Clinical evaluation of transtracheal Doppler for continuous cardiac output estimation. Anesth Analg 1992;74:800–804.
5. Side CD, Gosling RJ: Non-surgical assessment of cardiac function. Nature 1971;232:335–336.
6. Olson RM, Cooke JP: A nondestructive ultrasonic technique to measure diameter and blood flow in arteries. IEEE Trans Biomed Eng 1974;21:168–171.
7. Duck FA, Hodson CJ, Tomlin PJ: An esophageal Doppler probe for aortic flow velocity monitoring. Ultrasound Med Biol 1974;1:233–241.
8. Daigle RE, Miller CW, Histand MB, et al: Nontraumatic aortic blood flow sensing by use of an ultrasonic esophageal probe. J Appl Physiol 1975;38:1153–1160.
9. Lavandier B, Cathignol D, Muchada R, et al: Noninvasive aortic blood flow measurement using an intraesophageal probe. Ultrasound Med Biol 1985;11:451–460.
10. Cathignol D, Lavandier B, Muchada R: Debitmetrie aortique par effet Doppler transoesophagien. Ann Fr Anesth Reanim 1985;4:438–443.
11. Cariou A, Monchi M, Joly LM, et al: Noninvasive cardiac output monitoring by aortic blood flow determination: Evaluation of the Sometec Dynemo-3000 system. Crit Care Med 1998;26:2066–2072.
12. Mark NB, Steinbrook RA, Gugino LD, et al: Continuous noninvasive monitoring of cardiac output with esophageal Doppler ultrasound during cardiac surgery. Anesth Analg 1986;65:1013–1020.
13. Freund P: Transesophageal Doppler scanning versus thermodilution during general anesthesia. An initial comparison of cardiac output techniques. Am J Surg 1987;153:490–494.
14. Seyde WC, Stephan H, Rieke H: Non-invasive Doppler-ultrasound determination of cardiac output. Results and experiences with the ACCUCOM. Anaesthesist 1987;36:504–509.
15. Kumar A, Minagoe S, Thangathurai D, et al: Non-invasive measurement of cardiac output during general anesthesia by continuous wave Doppler esophageal probe: Comparison with simultaneous thermodilution cardiac output [abstract]. Anesthesiology 1987;67:A181.
16. Singer M, Clarke J, Bennett D: Continuous hemodynamic monitoring by esophageal Doppler. Crit Care Med 1989;17:447–452.
17. Valtier B, Cholley BP, Belot JP, et al: Noninvasive monitoring of cardiac output in critically ill patients using transesophageal Doppler. Am J Respir Crit Care Med 1998;158:77–83.
18. Lefrant JY, Bruelle P, Aya AG, et al: Training is required to improve the reliability of esophageal Doppler to measure cardiac output in critically ill patients. Intensive Care Med 1998;24:347–352.
19. Madan AK, UyBarreta VV, Aliabadi-Wahle S, et al: Esophageal Doppler ultrasound monitor versus pulmonary artery catheter in the hemodynamic management of critically ill surgical patients. J Trauma 1999;46:607–611.
20. Baillard C, Cohen Y, Fosse JP, et al: Haemodynamic measurements (continuous cardiac output and systemic vascular resistance) in critically ill patients: transoesophageal Doppler versus continuous thermodilution. Anaesth Intensive Care 1999;27:33–37.
21. Singer M, Allen MJ, Webb AR, Bennett ED: Effects of alterations in left ventricular filling, contractility and systemic vascular resistance on the ascending aortic blood velocity waveform of normal subjects. Crit Care Med 1991;19:1138–1145.
22. Mythen MG, Webb AR: Perioperative plasma volume expansion reduces the incidence of gut mucosal hypoperfusion during cardiac surgery. Arch Surg 1995;130:423–429.
23. Mythen MG, Webb AR: Intra-operative gut mucosal hypoperfusion is associated with increased post-operative complications and cost. Intensive Care Med 1994;20:99–104.
24. Sinclair S, James S, Singer M: Intraoperative intravascular volume optimisation and length of hospital stay after repair of proximal femoral fracture: Randomised controlled trial. BMJ 1997;315:909–912.
25. Gan TJ, Soppitt A, Maroof M, et al: Intraoperative volume expansion guided by esophageal Doppler improves postoperative outcome and shortens hospital stay [abstract]. Anesthesiology 1999;91(suppl 3):A537.
26. Poeze M, Ramsay G, Greve JW, Singer M: Prediction of postoperative cardiac surgical morbidity and organ failure within 4 hours of intensive care unit admission using esophageal Doppler ultrasonography. Crit Care Med 1999;27:1288–1294.

25 Gastric Tonometry

John M. Porter

An adequate method of assessing organ perfusion remains the "holy grail" in the monitoring of critically ill patients. The goal is to measure oxygenation at the cellular level. Shock—inadequate tissue perfusion—leads to impaired organ function because of either insufficient supply of oxygen (e.g., hemorrhage, trauma) or the inability of the cells to use the supplied oxygen (e.g., cytotoxic effect of sepsis). The optimal method of assessing cellular oxygenation would be to measure cellular oxygen tension or adenosine triphosphate levels; however, those techniques are not presently available. Currently, we can measure cellular oxygenation indirectly and globally. The two most common measurements are lactate levels and base deficit. Even when the sum for all tissue beds suggests adequate perfusion, however, there may be regional beds that are still underperfused. The optimal tissue bed has not been defined, but skin, muscle, and gut mucosa have been studied as sites of regional monitoring. This chapter focuses on gastric tonometry as a method of determining cellular oxygenation and the clinical relevance of this technique as a monitoring tool in the intensive care unit.

The basic principle of gastric tonometry is the equilibration of intramucosal and intraluminal partial carbon dioxide tensions. It is precisely this effect that makes tonometry useful as a monitoring tool in critically ill patients. In 1982, it was shown in canine experiments that both H^+ and CO_2 ions can diffuse from the lumen of the stomach. The concept of measuring the pH of the superficial layers of the gastric mucosa by determining mucosal carbon dioxide tension was thus born.

The Rationale for Gut Mucosal pH as a Measure of Regional Oxygenation

The health of any cell or tissue bed depends on the matching of the delivery of oxygen to the demand for oxygen at that particular time. Whenever the demand exceeds the supply, anaerobic metabolism occurs, leading to the development of acidosis. This is defined as dysoxia. Monitoring the tissue pH to assess the extent of acidosis will provide an indirect assessment of oxygen use at that time. As stated previously, global markers of perfusion assess the regional beds in aggregate. Thus, there may be beds with adequate perfusion and other beds that are inadequately perfused. The splanchnic bed, along with muscle and the subcutaneous tissues, is one of the first regional beds to be affected during shock and the last to be restored to normalcy after resuscitation. In fact, one of the most characteristic hemodynamic responses to hypovolemic or cardiogenic shock is profound splanchnic vasoconstriction, which is also disproportionate to that of the systemic circulation. Because of this physiology of the splanchnic vascular bed, intramucosal pH (pHi) can serve as both a marker for the presence of inadequate tissue oxygenation (shock) and an end point of resuscitation from that shock.

Gastric tonometry is the method whereby gastric pHi is estimated. The underlying principle is that CO_2, which is freely diffusible, equilibrates across a semipermeable membrane between two regions with different partial pressures of the gas. The partial carbon dioxide tension ($PiCO_2$) of the gastric mucosa, therefore, will be equal to that in a balloon with a Silastic membrane placed in contact with the gastric mucosa.

As defined previously, dysoxia occurs when cellular energy requirements exceed cellular oxygen delivery. The physiologic basis of gastric tonometry as a monitor of dysoxia is the increase in tissue CO_2 production that accompanies anaerobic metabolism. During aerobic metabolism, cellular production of CO_2 is a function of oxygen consumption. Anaerobic metabolism, however, results in the generation of hydrogen ions, which are buffered by tissue bicarbonate, resulting in increased CO_2 production. There is substantial evidence that increased mucosal $PiCO_2$ is a reliable signal of tissue hypoxia. Thus, if tonometry can accurately and consistently estimate intramucosal $PiCO_2$, it will be a reliable marker of tissue dysoxia, serving as a marker for shock and an end point of resuscitation.

Methodology

Gastric tonometry requires the use of a specialized nasogastric tube called a tonometer. The gastric tonometer (TRIP NACS catheter; Tonometrics Division, Datex-Ohmeda, Helsinki, Finland) consists of a gas-permeable silicone balloon attached to a gas-imperme-

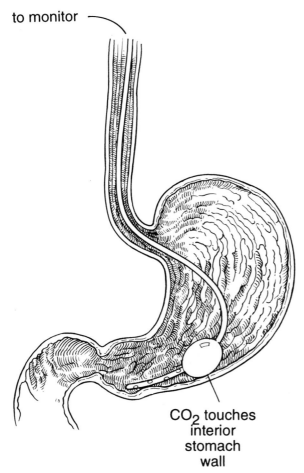

to monitor —

CO_2 touches
interior
stomach
wall

FIGURE 25–1. Tonometer with the semipermeable Silastic balloon in the lumen of the stomach. The holes distal to the balloon allow the tonometer to function as a nasogastric tube.

able sampling tube. This balloon is located at the tip of a conventional nasogastric sump tube. It can, therefore, function as a standard nasogastric tube and is inserted in a similar fashion (Fig. 25–1). There are two techniques for measuring $PiCO_2$. The first is fluid tonometry, in which the balloon is filled with saline

solution; the second is air tonometry, in which the balloon is filled with air. For the latter, a special monitor, the Tonocap (Tonometrics Division, Datex-Ohmeda, Helsinki, Finland), is required (shown in Figure 25–2).

In the saline technique, the silicone balloon is filled with saline solution. The balloon is gas permeable; therefore, CO_2 diffuses and equilibrates between the mucosa and the saline solution in the balloon to a steady state in about 30 to 90 minutes. Saline solution is then aspirated from the balloon in an anaerobic fashion. The initial 1.5 mL of saline solution is discarded, and the rest of the sample is sent for blood gas analysis to determine the $PiCO_2$ in the balloon, which at steady state is presumed to be equal to the luminal and the intramucosal CO_2. To obtain the pHi, arterial blood gas is measured simultaneously to obtain the arterial bicarbonate level. It is assumed that arterial bicarbonate equals intramucosal bicarbonate because bicarbonate is permeable and freely diffusible. This is a major assumption in determining the pHi. With intramucosal $PiCO_2$ and bicarbonate known, one calculates the pHi from the Henderson-Hasselbalch equation:

$$pHi = 6.1 + \log (HCO_3/PiCO_2 \times 0.03)$$

The slide calculator supplied by the manufacturer facilitates rapid calculation of pHi.

In air tonometry, a similar tonometer is used, but it is filled with air instead of saline solution. This technique involves the use of the Tonocap monitor, which is a multiparameter bedside monitor that provides an interface with the patient's gastric lumen $PiCO_2$ and the end-tidal CO_2 if the patient is intubated. The same equilibration assumptions hold with this technique, although the equilibration time is shorter (usually only 15 minutes versus 30 to 90 minutes with saline tonometry). At specified intervals, as short as every 5 minutes, air is aspirated automatically by the Tonocap. The

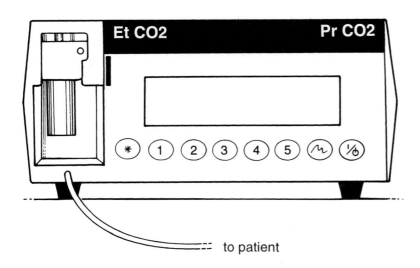

to patient

FIGURE 25–2. Tonocap machine, which can "continuously" measure both the end-tidal CO_2, if the patient is intubated, and the $PiCO_2$ in the tonometric balloon. This eliminates the sampling of the balloon by the nurses as well as the frequent drawing of arterial blood gases.

$PiCO_2$ of the air is measured using the same infrared technology as for capnography to measure end-tidal CO_2. The pHi can then be calculated by the Tonocap if arterial blood gas is measured simultaneously to obtain the bicarbonate level. This critical assumption can be avoided by determining the mucosal-to-arterial $PiCO_2$ gap, the so-called Pi-aCO_2 gap. This gap is independent of systemic acid-base balance and is not affected by changes in ventilation unless those changes affect cardiac output. Moreover, because $PiCO_2$ and pHi are inversely proportional, one could follow just the $PiCO_2$ measured semicontinuously by the Tonocap.

When gastric tonometry is being used, the patient should be administered H_2 blockers, and the tonometer should be placed on low intermittent suction. Air tonometry is used more frequently than saline tonometry.

Normal Values

Studies have determined that the normal value for pHi in children and adults varies from 7.33 to 7.41. A normal Pi-aCO_2 gap is less than 10 mm Hg. Some investigations have shown that a gap of more than 18 mm Hg correlates with death after severe trauma. As a predictor of mortality, an indicator of shock, or an end point for resuscitation, pHi levels as low as 7.25 have been used. I use a pH of 7.30 and a gap of 18 mm Hg as cutoffs. Of note, the values for $PiCO_2$ obtained via air tonometry are consistently higher than those obtained via saline tonometry, but the correlation is good.

Pitfalls in the Measurement of pHi

Assumption That Intramucosal Bicarbonate Level Equals Arterial Bicarbonate Level. As discussed previously, one of the primary assumptions in the calculation of pHi is that arterial bicarbonate level equals mucosal bicarbonate level. In certain systemic acid-base disturbances, especially when there are changes in ventilation (specifically hyperventilation) and low systemic pH, the actual mucosal bicarbonate level is lower than the measured arterial bicarbonate level. This causes the calculated pHi to be falsely elevated. Despite the problem with this assumption, most of the current literature supporting the clinical use of tonometry has employed pHi and not the PCO_2 gap. One of the major reasons for this is that there is still a downward trend for pHi when the bicarbonate levels are dissimilar, so that the clinician has information suggesting regional hypoperfusion and can treat the patient accordingly. Currently, there is a trend to use the direct number (i.e., Pi-aCO_2) rather than the derived number (i.e., pHi). A gap of more than 10 to 15 mm Hg is considered abnormal.

Gastric Acid Secretion. The presence of H^+ in the gastric lumen, a normal occurrence, can falsely increase the measured $PiCO_2$ and thus falsely lower the pHi, independent of mucosal perfusion. The main reason for this is that the presence of H^+ in the gastric lumen, when combined with bicarbonate, leads to increased intraluminal $PiCO_2$. This CO_2 equilibrates with the CO_2 in the balloon, falsely increasing the $PiCO_2$ in the absence of inadequate perfusion. Because of this, the use of H_2 blockers is highly recommended.

Blood Gas Analyzers. The use of blood gas analyzers calibrated for routine blood gas analysis has been reported to underestimate the value of $PiCO_2$ in the saline solution. It is a small error and can be minimized by using the same machine for all measurements to reduce intermachine bias. It is also recommended to run a saline solution quality control test. This small error can be eliminated by using the Tonocap, which is specifically designed to measure the $PiCO_2$ in the air in the balloon.

Anaerobic Sampling of Balloon Saline Solution. To avoid false elevation of atmospheric CO_2 due to CO_2 in the balloon, the tube needs to be carefully primed, and the sample must be obtained so as not to allow air to come into contact with it. For the same reason, the nasogastric tube must not be on continuous sump suction, which could cause air to be sucked into the stomach, again falsely elevating intraluminal $PiCO_2$. Intermittent suction at low levels is appropriate.

Enteral Feeding. Enteral feeding into the stomach can stimulate acid secretion, which can falsely increase the measured $PiCO_2$. This effect can be eliminated by either feeding postpylorically, keeping the patient on nothing-by-mouth status, or emptying the stomach before measuring pHi. Of note, some authors recommend not starting any enteral feedings until gut perfusion has been restored to normal (i.e., normal pHi), because there have been case reports of small bowel necrosis from enteral feeding in the face of inadequate gut perfusion. My practice has been to delay feeding until the pHi has been normalized.

Clinical Applications of Gastric Tonometry

The goals of monitoring in the intensive care unit include early detection of abnormalities, guidance of therapy toward correction of the abnormality, improvement of outcome, and provision of prognostic information early in the stay.

Early Detection of Inadequate Perfusion

Theoretically, as discussed, pHi should be a marker of regional hypoperfusion. In healthy volunteers in whom

25% of blood volume was depleted, it was found that pHi was the best predictor of hypovolemia, compared with standard vital signs, stroke volume, base deficit, and lactate. In fact, after the first depletion of 12.5% of the blood volume, only the pHi had changed. The information obtained with the tonometer was compared with the judgments made by experienced intensivists concerning the adequacy of splanchnic perfusion. It was concluded that experienced intensive care physicians tended to overestimate visceral perfusion, which suggests that gastric tonometry adds useful information to routine hemodynamic indices.

Prediction of Intensive Care Unit Morbidity and Mortality

Monitoring of pHi has been shown to predict the subsequent course of the intensive care unit stay as early as the initial 24 hours after admission. When pHi was measured by means of gastric aspiration on admission in 59 postoperative patients, the 72-hour mortality rate was significantly greater in patients with a pHi of less than 7.32 than in those with a higher pHi (37% vs. 0%). A prospective study compared pHi with standard oxygen transport variables and found a low pHi to be the best predictor of mortality.[4] When 83 intensive care unit patients were studied, it was found that compared with oxygen transport variables, lactate, and base excess, pHi at 24 hours had the highest sensitivity (88%) in predicting death. Among 17 consecutive patients with pancreatitis, the lowest pHi recorded during the first 48 hours was the best predictor of intensive care unit admission and death. Among 19 consecutive critically ill trauma patients, those patients in whom resuscitative efforts could not raise the pHi to greater than 7.32 in 24 hours had a significantly increased likelihood of developing multiple system organ failure. The findings in these studies support the use of pHi as a prognostic variable in intensive care unit patients.

pHi as a Goal-directed End Point in Therapy

Predicting morbidity and mortality is indeed important; however, two prospective trials have been performed showing that pHi has value as a goal-directed end point to improve survival.[1, 5] In a randomized study, 260 patients were grouped based on admission pHi (>7.35 or <7.35) and were then randomized to therapeutic interventions to (1) keep the pHi at 7.35 or raise it to greater than 7.35 or (2) maximize standard oxygen transport variables.[5] In patients admitted with low pHi, survival was similar between the protocol and the control groups (37% vs. 36%). This lack of

improvement was thought to be related to the duration of inadequate perfusion before entering the study. In patients admitted with a normal pHi, survival was significantly greater in the protocol group (58% vs. 42%, $P < .01$).

Another study included 20 critically injured trauma patients who had mucosal ischemia based on a pHi of less than 7.25.[1] Seven patients received standard therapy, whereas 13 received a "cocktail," which included folate, mannitol, and low-dose isoproterenol, to increase splanchnic perfusion. The protocol group had fewer organ system failures and a decrease in both intensive care unit and hospital length of stay. These studies show that pHi-directed therapy is a promising technique, although further studies need to be performed.

pHi as an End Point for Resuscitation in Trauma Patients

The search for an optimal end point in the resuscitation of trauma patients continues. In a study of 15 multiple trauma patients with monitoring of pHi, base deficit, and lactate, there was poor correlation between the regional marker, pHi, and the global markers, lactate and base deficit.[12] In the seven patients in whom the pHi remained normal (>7.32), there were no deaths or complications. Of the eight patients in whom one or more determinations of pHi were less than 7.32 in the first 48 hours, three developed major complications, and two subsequently died. In a similar prospective study of 20 critically injured trauma patients who had global evidence of inadequate perfusion—base deficit worse than −5 or lactate greater than 5—there was a poor correlation between global and regional markers.[3] Patients who had a low pHi (<7.32) on admission and who continued to have a low pHi at 24 hours had a higher mortality rate than those who had a normal pHi at 24 hours (50% vs. 0%, $P < .03$).

Ivatury and associates randomized 57 severely injured trauma patients into two groups.[8] The end points for resuscitation in the control group were the standard oxygen transport variables. Normalization of the pHi (>7.30) was the end point for resuscitation in the protocol group. pHi was measured in all patients but was used to guide therapy only in the protocol group. Of the 44 patients with pHi greater than 7.30 at 24 hours, three (6.8%) died of multiple organ dysfunction, as compared with seven of the 13 (53.9%) in whom pHi was not optimized ($P = .006$). Optimization times for oxygen transport variables, lactate, and base excess were similar in survivors and nonsurvivors. The time to pHi optimization was significantly longer in nonsurvivors. Of note, Ivatury's group also found that a persistently low pHi was frequently associated with systemic or intra-abdominal complications.

These studies point not only to the effectiveness of pHi as an end point for resuscitation but also to the 24-hour time period in which this normalization should occur. Resuscitation of the gut mucosa to a normal pHi should be one of the important goals of resuscitation.

Conclusion

There are good data to suggest that incomplete splanchnic cellular resuscitation is associated with the development of multiple organ failure and death in critically ill patients. Gastric tonometry is a promising technique that assesses the adequacy of splanchnic perfusion. It appears to be superior to global indicators in assessing the adequacy of perfusion. Given the prime role of the gut in the development of multiple organ failure and death, it appears that the ability to recognize gut ischemia early and to correct it promptly is important to the physician managing critically ill patients. Gastric tonometry is the only current noninvasive technology that allows the clinician to do that. It would seem that pHi should be monitored in all patients at risk of developing overt or covert shock, not only to assess the adequacy of tissue oxygenation but also because it may reduce the mortality rate.

References

1. Barquist E, Kirton O, Windsor J, et al: The impact of antioxidant and splanchnic-directed therapy on persistent uncorrected gastric mucosal pH in the critically injured trauma patient. J Trauma 1998;44:355–360.
2. Bonham MJ, Abu-Zidan FM, Simovic MO, Windsor JA: Gastric intramucosal pH predicts death in severe acute pancreatitis. Br J Surg 1997;84:1670–1674.
3. Chang MC, Cheatham ML, Nelson LD, et al: Gastric tonometry supplements information provided by systemic indicators of oxygen transport. J Trauma 1994;34:488–494.
4. Gutierrez G, Bismar H, Dantzker D, Silva N: Comparison of gastric intramucosal pH with measures of oxygen transport and consumption in critically ill patients. Crit Care Med 1992;20:451–457.
5. Gutierrez G, Palizas F, Doglio G, et al: Gastric intramucosal pH as a therapeutic index of tissue oxygenation in critically ill patients. Lancet 1992;339:195–199.
6. Gys T, Hubens A, Neels H, et al: Prognostic values of gastric intramural pH in surgical intensive care patients. Crit Care Med 1988;16:1222–1224.
7. Hamilton-Davies C, Mythen MG, Salmon JB, et al: Comparison of commonly used clinical indicators of hypovolaemia with gastrointestinal tonometry. Intensive Care Med 1997;23:276–281.
8. Ivatury R, Simon R, Islam S, et al: A prospective randomized study of end points of resuscitation after major trauma: Global oxygen transport indices versus organ-specific gastric mucosal pH. J Am Coll Surg 1996;183:145–154.
9. Kirton OC, Windsor J, Wedderburn R, et al: Failure of splanchnic resuscitation in the acutely injured trauma patient correlates with multiple organ system failure and length of stay in the ICU. Chest 1998;113:1064–1069.
10. Maynard N, Bihari D, Beale R, et al: Assessment of splanchnic oxygenation by gastric tonometry in patients with acute circulatory failure. JAMA 1993;270:1203–1210.
11. Porter JM, Ivatury RR: In search of the optimal endpoints of resuscitation. J Trauma 1998;44:908–914.
12. Roumen RMH, Vreugde JPC, Goris RJA: Gastric tonometry in multiple trauma patients. J Trauma 1994;36:313–316.
13. Salzman AL, Strong KE, Wang H, et al: Air tonometry: A new method for determination of gastrointestinal mucosal PCO2 [abstract]. Crit Care Med 1993;21:S202.
14. Santoso JT, Wisner DH, Battistella FD, Owings JT: Comparison of gastric mucosal pH and clinical judgement in critically ill patients. Eur J Surg 1998;164:521–526.

Renal Function and Support

Howard Belzberg and James Murray

Renal failure in the critically ill or injured patient is crucial from a variety of perspectives. Renal failure remains one of the complications associated with the highest mortality rate in the intensive care unit. In addition, the cost of dialysis is a major factor, and the ability to provide fluid and nutrition is limited by renal failure. Despite advances in renal replacement therapy, the mortality rate associated with acute renal failure exceeds 50%, especially in the setting of acute surgical disease.

This observation is particularly disappointing in light of the improved ability to provide renal support and advanced methods of hemodynamic monitoring. It is most likely that the inability to improve the outcome in patients with renal failure has been due to a variety of factors over the past few years, including higher acuity and severity of illness in patients surviving critical medical or surgical illnesses and the increase in toxicity and volume of diagnostic and therapeutic interventions.

The causes of renal dysfunction are numerous, and their effect is often compound. It is usually impossible to identify a single causal factor for renal failure. Some of the common factors that may induce acute renal dysfunction in critically ill patients include hypotension, blood transfusion, contrast media, rhabdomyolysis, aminoglycoside therapy, sepsis, vasopressor therapy, and autoimmune disease.

Monitoring

Close monitoring of both glomerular and tubular function is of utmost importance in the assessment of renal function in the critical care unit. Focusing only on urinary output may seriously underestimate the degree of renal failure. Many extrarenal factors may contribute to increased or decreased urine flow. For example, hyperglycemia may induce diuresis despite a decrease in glomerular function. Agents such as mannitol or contrast media may induce osmotic diuresis, which does not reflect the volume status or the renal function. Factors that may decrease urinary flow include abdominal compartment syndrome and hepatic failure, both of which are characterized by oliguria caused by insufficient flow to the kidneys, which reverts to normal renal function once the flow is re-established.

It is important to recognize that the renal system has a tremendous reserve. The serum creatinine level will not begin to increase until more than 50% of glomerular function is lost, and urinary flow may continue to appear normal even after 90% of glomerular units have been lost.

In addition to the glomerular (filtering) component of the renal system, the tubular (concentrating) component is subject to many of the insults associated with critical illness. In terms of volume status, the tubular component is most responsible for controlling intravascular volume and most sensitive to injury from severe hypovolemic insults.

Approach to Acute Renal Failure

The traditional classification of acute renal failure (prerenal, renal, obstructive) remains useful for categorizing the area to be evaluated as the focus for further evaluation and therapy. In particular, the use of urinary electrolytes to separate prerenal (usually associated with a low urinary sodium level and low [< 1] fractional excretion of sodium) from renal failure can be rapid and helpful (Table 26–1).

The glomerular function is best assessed by analysis of the creatinine clearance. Although there are many formulas that attempt to estimate the creatinine clearance, they are subject to significant error in the critically ill patient. The 2-hour creatinine clearance is a rapid and reliable method of measuring the creatinine clearance on a daily basis. The intrinsic accuracy of the 2-hour creatinine clearance is similar to that of the 24-hour test; however, because of the smaller volumes and times, it is essential that both time and volume be recorded accurately.

TABLE 26–1. Important Renal Equations

Creatinine Clearance

$$CrCl = \frac{\text{urine creatinine}}{\text{serum creatinine}} \times \text{urine volume} \times \frac{1.73}{\text{BSA}}$$

Fractional Excretion of Filtered Sodium

$$FeNa = \frac{\text{urine Na/plasma Na}}{\text{urine Cr/plasma Cr}} \times 100$$

BSA, body surface area; Cr, creatinine; CrCl, creatinine clearance; FeNa, fractional excretion of filtered sodium.

Fluid and electrolyte control is largely dependent on renal function. These functions can be divided into two categories: (1) acid/base balance, predominantly dictated by bicarbonate metabolism and organic acid clearance, and (2) sodium/potassium/chloride balance, predominantly dictated by tubular function.

Metabolic acidosis is a common complication of renal dysfunction. The acidosis may be anion gap acidosis, which is most commonly due to increased organic acid production and catabolic states in which there is increased production of phosphoric and sulfuric acids. In the setting of nonanion gap acidosis, there is typically an elevated chloride concentration. When the kidney is unable to generate bicarbonate, a progressive deficit develops, amplified by the addition of alkali-free fluid, inducing further dilution of bicarbonate and consequent acidosis.

Therapeutic Approach

As for most problems in medicine, prevention is the most effective method of reducing the morbidity and the mortality of renal dysfunction. Of primary importance is the maintenance of intravascular volume and perfusion of the kidneys. The use of dopamine in doses targeted at increasing blood flow in the renal and splenic circulation is widely believed to reduce the risk of acute renal failure. Although large-scale prospective randomized clinical trials are lacking, there are several studies supporting the theory that low-dose dopamine (<5 μg/kg/hour) improves flow to the kidneys and urine output.

Adequate volume loading has been shown to reduce significantly the risk associated with contrast media administration. The avoidance of nephrotoxic agents may reduce the incidence of renal failure; however, it should be noted that many of the risks of these agents could be reduced by adequate volume loading with normal saline solution before exposure.

Early intervention may be beneficial in the setting of rhabdomyolysis. The diagnosis of rhabdomyolysis should be considered in any patient with muscle injury. In the presence of a positive urine dipstick test for hemoglobin without a commensurate number of red blood cells on microscopic examination, the diagnosis of myoglobinuria secondary to rhabdomyolysis should be made presumptively. In this setting, treatment with a mixture of 150 mEq of sodium bicarbonate (3 ampules) in 1 L of 5% dextrose in water with 25 g of mannitol—initially administered at a rate of 250 mL/hour for 4 hours, then titrated to maintain a urine output of greater than 100 mL/hour—may be used. This therapy will provide alkalinization of the urine and osmotic flow to reduce the risk of tubular dysfunction. The therapy should be continued until there is no evidence of myoglobinuria.

If renal failure occurs, the most common major problem in the critical patient is acute tubular necrosis. This form of renal failure typically presents with oliguria followed by polyuria, which usually leads to return of significant but incomplete renal function in 6 to 8 weeks. Although the conversion of oliguric renal failure to polyuric renal failure is not of major prognostic significance, the management of polyuria is much simpler than that of oliguria. For this reason, an attempt to induce urine flow with loop diuretics during the oliguric phase is reasonable. A trial of progressive doses of furosemide with or without ethacrynic acid is worthwhile as an effort to induce polyuria and to allow for simpler fluid and electrolyte management.

Renal Replacement Therapy

In critically ill trauma patients who are hemodynamically stable and are not suffering from major pulmonary or bleeding complications, intermittent hemodialysis is an acceptable method of renal replacement therapy. Intermittent hemodialysis is widely available and does not require 24-hour monitoring. Large volumes of fluid and electrolytes can be removed rapidly, and nitrogenous waste can be cleared very effectively. Unfortunately, hemodialysis usually requires some degree of anticoagulation; is associated with sudden fluid shifts, often causing hypotension; and may be associated with transient pulmonary deterioration. Owing to the presence of surgical wounds and logistic complications, peritoneal dialysis is rarely practical in patients with acute trauma.

Continuous renal replacement therapy (CRRT) is performed by placing a filter, usually a hollow-fiber microfilter, in line with the patient's circulation. This is accomplished either via arterial and venous access, which uses the patient's blood pressure to drive the system, or via venovenous access, which uses a roller pump to drive the system. If dialysis is desired in addition to filtration, a solution may be instilled into a space surrounding the hollow fibers, creating an osmotic gradient. Fluid and electrolytes are removed continuously, and replacement of essential components and excess removed volume is performed via intravenous infusion.

In most cases, this technique can be performed with little or no anticoagulation. Owing to the slow and continuous nature of the system, there is no hemodynamic instability, and pulmonary deterioration is uncommon. The system does remove nitrogenous waste at a slower rate than hemodialysis, however; thus, it should be started at the earliest opportunity once the diagnosis of renal failure is confirmed. Although solute removal is slow with continuous therapy, the ability to remove large volumes of fluid gently offers the opportunity to control volume status very effectively.

Continuous renal replacement therapy is within the capabilities of most surgical intensive care unit nurses with appropriate training and the supervision of knowledgeable physicians. CRRT includes continuous venovenous hemofiltration (CVVH) or continuous venovenous hemodialysis (CVVHD) and continuous arteriovenous hemofiltration (CAVH) or continuous arteriovenous hemodialysis (CAVHD).

The basic elements of the procedure include blood supply (access), filter, filtrate collector, and blood return (access). A pressure gradient between the supply blood access and the return blood access across the filter is required. This is provided either by the gradient between the mean arterial pressure and the mean venous pressure (CAVH, CAVHD) or by a peristaltic pump (CVVH, CVVHD). In the most basic configuration, CRRT is provided as CAVH. In this system, the gradient between the mean arterial blood pressure and the mean central venous pressure provides the pressure to drive the system. No pump is required, and two catheters provide the required access: an arterial catheter from the supply side and a venous catheter from the return side. In patients who do not have the necessary gradient between arterial and venous pressure, do not have adequate arterial access, or require high filtration rates, a peristaltic pump can be used, and venovenous access can be employed.

The indications for CRRT include fluid overload, hyperkalemia, metabolic acidosis, uremic encephalopathy, coagulopathy, and acute poisoning. Renal replacement should be started early in the course of acute renal failure.

Technical Application of Continuous Renal Replacement Therapy

Continuous hemofiltration consists of extracorporeal ultrafiltration designed to remove water and uremic toxins while conserving the cellular and the protein content of plasma. The hemofilter is composed of several thousand hollow-fiber capillaries and is connected between supply (arterial) and return (venous) access sites. Water and solutes of less than 50,000 daltons in size filter across a synthetic membrane, propelled by the hydrostatic pressure gradient into the extracapillary space as an ultrafiltrate. This allows for continuous therapy that can be employed as long as renal replacement is necessary.

Percutaneous femoral cannulation provides the best access for CRRT (Fig. 26–1). Wide-bore, relatively short catheters are preferred to allow maximum blood flow with minimal vessel trauma. The technique of vascular access is described elsewhere in this text.

Continuous arteriovenous hemofiltration removes an ultrafiltrate at a rate of approximately 500 to 1000 mL/hour in most settings. A CAVH system is shown in Figure 26–2. The supply to the filter is from an artery, and the return is into a vein. The pressure gradient across the filter is dependent on the difference between the mean arterial pressure and the mean central venous pressure. A replacement fluid is infused either through a separate venous line or via the venous line of the filter. A negative net balance is maintained by replacing only a portion of the ultrafiltrate each hour.

Continuous arteriovenous hemodialysis combines CAVH with concurrent dialysis. An isotonic solution is infused through an extracapillary port into the extracapillary space. This provides an osmotic concentration gradient for the selective removal of solutes.

Continuous venovenous hemofiltration is performed with a blood pump. This allows hemofiltration to occur without arterial access. The peristaltic pump generates the pressure gradient, and access is achieved through a double-lumen venous catheter. A CVVH system is shown in Figure 26–3.

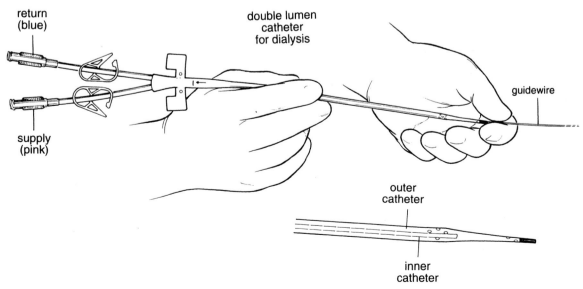

FIGURE 26–1. Introduction of special double-lumen catheter for renal replacement therapy.

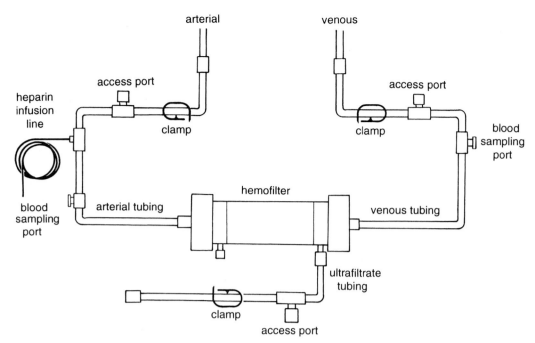

FIGURE 26–2. Continuous arteriovenous hemofiltration.

Strict aseptic technique must be observed for each procedure. The following steps should be performed.

Blood Circuit Setup

- A hemofilter kit containing arterial, venous, and ultrafiltrate tubing must be obtained.
- All devices and accessories for the construction of CAVH are opened and are unpacked onto a sterile field.
- The arterial (red) and the venous (blue) lines should be securely attached to the corresponding ends of the hemofilter.
- The ultrafiltrate tubing should be attached to the ultrafiltrate port.
- For CAVH, the ultrafiltrate port is located at the venous end of the hemofilter. The second extracapillary port should be capped.
- For CAVHD, the ultrafiltrate tubing is connected to the port at the arterial end of the hemofilter. The port at the venous end is used for the infusion of dialysate. This port should be capped with a Luer–Lok during the setup procedure.
- For CVVH, the ultrafiltrate port is located at the venous end.
- For CVVHD, the ultrafiltrate port is located at the arterial end.

Gravity Rinsing and Priming Procedure

Before use, the filter must be flushed, and air must be removed from the hemofilter circuit.

1. Add 5000 U of heparin to each liter of normal saline solution.

2. Close all clamps on the filter lines (arterial, venous, ultrafiltrate, and heparin infusion lines).
3. Place a clamp on the arterial tubing between the filter and the heparin infusion line. Make sure the cap on the ultrafiltrate ports is securely closed.
4. Place the first liter into a flush bag, and reconnect the arterial line.
5. Secure the end of the venous line to a collection basin on the floor.
6. Open and flush the heparin infusion line, first by removing the proximal clamp from the arterial line. Open the stopcock on the end of the heparin infusion line. Once the heparin line has been completely flushed, replace the stopcock.
7. Position the hemofilter vertically, and remove the clamps from the arterial and the venous lines. Continue to infuse the remainder of the first liter of saline solution. Gentle tapping of the filter will assist in removing air bubbles. Do not completely empty the entire liter, so as not to allow air to reenter the filter and the tubing. Once it has been adequately flushed, clamp the venous line.
8. Replace the saline flush bag with the second liter of saline (with 5000 U of added heparin).
9. Connect this line to the arterial line. With the venous line clamped, open the ultrafiltrate tubing. Infuse the liter to prime the extracapillary space. Position the hemofilter to remove the air from the extracapillary chamber. Once the liter is almost completely infused, clamp the ultrafiltrate line.
10. Once complete, clamp all lines, and replace the caps on the arterial and the venous tubing.

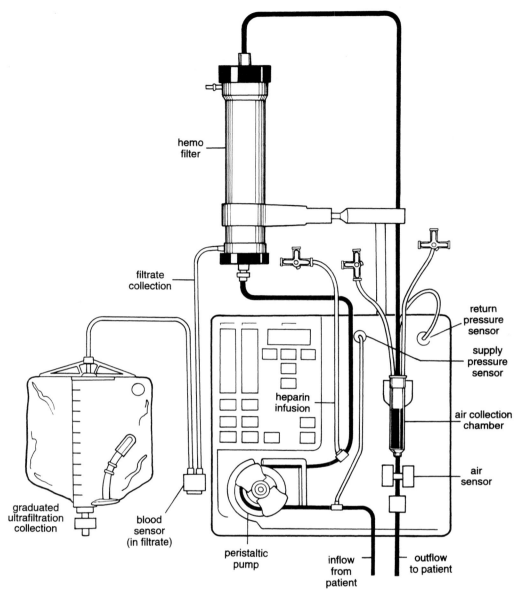

FIGURE 26–3. Setup for continuous venovenous hemofiltration and dialysis.

Attachment of Hemofilter Circuit

1. Prepare a sterile field around the arterial and the venous access sites. Clean all surfaces of the cannulas with Betadine (povidone-iodine).
2. Clamp the arterial and the venous access lines on the soft silicone portions of the catheter, and remove the Luer caps from each catheter. Connect the arterial hemofilter tubing to the catheter securely, then the venous line to the venous access port.
3. The heparin line can be connected to intravenous tubing attached to a heparin solution.
4. Remove the clamps from the access cannulas. Pulsation should be noted in the arterial line at this time. If this is not present, disconnect the hemofilter, and ensure the patency of the arterial tubing.
5. Unclamp the lines of the hemofilter. Unclamp the

ultrafiltrate line. Place a collection chamber below the level of the filter.
6. For CAVHD, connect 1 L of isotonic solution to the extracapillary port on the venous end of the hemofilter.

Management and Maintenance
Replacement Fluids
QUANTITY

The volume of replacement fluid depends on the desired fluid balance. Replacement of the ultrafiltrate should be done on an hourly basis, according to the following formula:

$$RF = UF - D - X$$

where RF equals replacement fluid, UF equals ultrafiltrate fluid, D equals dialysate, and X equals desired negative fluid balance per hour. Example: UF = 1800, D = 1000, and X = 200. Therefore, RF = 1800 − 1000 − 200 = 600. RF for the subsequent hour will be 600 mL. Instruct the nurses what hourly negative fluid balance is desired. If CAVHD is not being employed, then D equals zero.

The dialysate fluid is not reflected in the input/output section of the patient's chart. In the previous example, because 1800 mL of fluid was collected in 1 hour, the chart will reflect an ultrafiltrate of 800 mL, with a 600-mL input of replacement fluid in the following hour.

The ultrafiltrate will contain uremic solutes and electrolytes. The patient's fluid status and electrolyte balance need to be monitored regularly when CRRT is employed.

FLUIDS
1. Normal saline solution (dialysate).
2. Normal saline solution with 1 to 2 ampules of calcium chloride (replacement fluid).
3. One-half normal saline solution with 1 to 2 ampules of sodium bicarbonate (replacement fluid).

The type and the amount of replacement fluid will need to be modified regularly according to the patient's needs and electrolyte balance.

To begin, alternate normal saline solution with 1 ampule of calcium chloride and one-half normal saline solution with 2 ampules of sodium bicarbonate. Alternate the two solutions every hour. The amount of calcium chloride or sodium bicarbonate can be decreased. The frequency of alternation may also vary (i.e., 1:1 to 1:2, 1:3, 2:1, 3:1, and so forth).

Dialysate Fluid

The dialysate fluid should be isotonic. Hypotonic solutions will cause a net flux of fluid from the extracapillary space into the filter.

FLUIDS
1. Normal saline solution.
2. One-half normal saline solution with 2 ampules of sodium bicarbonate. This is used to correct additional acidosis, which may be difficult to control with the replacement fluid alone.

These may also be alternated as needed.

Heparin

Heparin may be added to the arterial line of the filter to prevent clotting in the filter. It will not resolve established clot or prevent clotting when the flow through the filter is insufficient.

A total of 500 to 1000 U/hour of heparin can be infused through the side port on the arterial side. The filter will remove approximately 75% of the administered heparin. This should not cause additional bleeding problems in a uremic patient.

Perfusion of the Filter

Perfusion of the filter is determined by the difference between the mean arterial pressure and the central venous pressure or, in the case of CVVH, by the pressure difference between the inflow site of the filter and the venous return site. Adequate perfusion requires a difference of at least 50 to 60 mm Hg. Adequate flow through the filter requires that there be no obstruction of the catheters or the lines. Clotting or kinking of the arterial line will decrease the inflow rate. Likewise, obstruction of the venous line or thrombus in the veins will reduce outflow from the filter.

The longevity and the efficiency of the filter are dependent on unobstructed inflow and outflow. Mechanical obstruction of the lines and the catheters must be excluded when filters fail. In fact, the most common cause of filter failure is a mechanical problem with the vascular access devices.

Filter performance routinely decreases over time, requiring replacement approximately every 2 to 5 days. Normally, a well-functioning filter will provide an ultrafiltrate of at least 500 to 1000 mL/hour (excluding dialysate). When the amount of ultrafiltrate falls below this level, the filter will soon become clotted. A new filter should be primed at this time and should be used to replace the old one before it becomes clotted. This will prevent thrombosis of the access catheters. An additional filter can be primed and kept ready, wrapped in a sterile towel, for up to 24 hours. If a filter is not ready when another becomes clotted, place clamps on the silicone portions of the catheters, remove the filter and the tubing, and connect the catheters to heparinized saline solution in flush bags. The lines should be flushed continuously to prevent thrombus formation in the catheters until the new filter can be applied.

Discontinuation of Hemofiltration

Improvement of the creatinine clearance to a minimum of 20 mg/minute is usually required before hemofiltration can be discontinued. The patient's serum creatinine and blood urea nitrogen levels cannot continue to rise, and adequate fluid balance must be maintained by the patient's urine output.

The filter can be removed, connecting the catheters to the heparin flush bags. The patient can be observed over the next 24 hours without hemofiltration to determine if intrinsic renal function is adequate before removing the vascular access catheters.

Complications

- Bleeding from the catheter sites.
- Infection of the catheter sites.
- Arterial pseudoaneurysms.

- Arteriovenous fistula (when both catheters are placed in the same leg).
- Arterial thrombosis and extremity ischemia. Pulses distal to the arterial catheter should be checked before placement of the filter and frequently after the catheter is placed.
- Air embolus. Extreme caution should be taken during connection of the lines.
- Venous thrombosis at the access sites.
- Rupture of the capillaries, noted by a change in the ultrafiltrate color to pink or red. This mandates that the filter be removed immediately and replaced.

References

1. Belzberg H, Cornwell EE III, Berne TV: Critical care of the surgical patient-II. Pulmonary and renal support. Surg Clin North Am 1996;76:971–983.
2. Frost L, Pedersen RS, Bentzen S, et al: Short and long term outcome in a consecutive series of 419 patients with acute dialysis-requiring renal failure. Scand J Urol Nephrol 1993;27:453–462.
3. Kellen M, Aronson S, Roizen MF, et al: Predictive and diagnostic tests of renal failure: A review. Anesth Analg 1994;78:134–142.
4. Koch SM (ed): Problems in Critical Care: Critical Care Catalog: 1992. Philadelphia, JB Lippincott, 1992, p 571.
5. McCarthy JT: Prognosis of patients with acute renal failure in the intensive-care unit: A tale of two eras. Mayo Clin Proc 1996;71:117–126.
6. Morris JA Jr, Mucha P Jr, Ross SE, et al: Acute posttraumatic renal failure: A multicenter perspective. J Trauma 1991;31:1584–1590.
7. Nichols L: Can 12-hour creatinine clearances be substituted for 24-hour creatinine clearances in monitoring for nephrotoxicity from cancer chemotherapy? A pilot study and preliminary data. Am J Clin Pathol 1988;90:373–374.
8. Reynolds HN, Borg U, Belzberg H, Wiles CE III: Efficacy of continuous arteriovenous hemofiltration with dialysis in patients with renal failure. Crit Care Med 1991;19:1387–1394.
9. Ronco C, Barbacini S, Digito A, Zoccali G: Achievements and new directions in continuous renal replacement therapies. New Horiz 1995;3:708–716.
10. Rudnick MR, Berns JS, Cohen RM, Goldfarb S: Nephrotoxic risks of renal angiography: Contrast media-associated nephrotoxicity and atheroembolism—A critical review. Am J Kidney Dis 1994;24:713–727.
11. Venegas JG, Fredberg JJ: Understanding the pressure cost of ventilation: Why does high-frequency ventilation work? Crit Care Med 1994;22:S49–S57.

27 Noninvasive Autonomic Nervous System Monitoring in Critical Care

J. Colombo and William C. Shoemaker

Living things, including people, go to a considerable amount of trouble to stay alive. Some of the work and effort involved in staying alive is expended at the level of consciousness but fortunately much of it is carried out automatically under the direction of a great communication system of the body—the autonomic nervous system.

JAY TUPPERMAN, *Metabolic Physiology*

The autonomic nervous system (ANS), through its two branches—the parasympathetic nervous system (PSNS) and the sympathetic nervous system (SNS)—is continually cycling. It has long been a desire of clinicians to be able to monitor the ANS simply and noninvasively and to understand how its cycles correlate with health. ANS monitoring with analysis based on heart rate variability (HRV) is a noninvasive technologic innovation that is simple to apply in a clinical or a hospital setting. It has been demonstrated to be of significant help in identifying and managing patients in a variety of clinical states.

Heart rate variability is defined as recurrent changes in beat-to-beat (or RR) intervals characteristic of balanced cardiac control. Research suggests that decreased variability with normal RR intervals can be a prognostic indicator of a number of disease states. The ANS has considerable effect on the integrity of cardiovascular and, indeed, overall homeostasis. The antagonistic components of the ANS compose the core of HRV-based ANS monitoring.

Added to the HRV component of ANS monitoring is an analysis of the cyclic nature of respiratory activity (RA). In free-breathing individuals, subtle changes in the respiratory cycle are indicative of autonomic outflow and the influence of the ANS on the integrity of pulmonary homeostasis. Even during regulated breathing or in mechanically ventilated patients, RA analysis provides information regarding how the ANS is responding to and compensating for the RA that is present. Together, HRV and RA provide two noninvasive measurements of ANS activity, allowing for assessment of the underlying component branches of the ANS and their relative energy levels. Thus, it is now possible to quantify the independent power in the SNS and the PSNS as well as the power in the total ANS (Fig. 27–1).

Monitoring of the ANS that is HRV based is a simple, noninvasive clinical method of assessing the integrity of autonomic input to cardiovascular, pulmonary, and other visceral and neural systems. Numerous research studies have analyzed sequential RR intervals in stunningly diverse clinical populations. Some of these conditions include sudden cardiac death (SCD) associated with myocardial infarction (MI), diabetic neuropathy, congestive heart failure, sleep apnea, hypertension, alcohol abuse, hypovolemia, Chagas' disease, neonatal disorders, and syncope. As a measure of the body's autonomic response, ANS monitoring is a versatile test, providing a window to a previously difficult-to-obtain measurement. The test seems to be exquisitely sensitive, and the proof of specificity is rapidly emerging.

Recommendations of the American College of Cardiology

Heart rate variability exists in a variety of forms: time-domain, frequency-domain, linear, and nonlinear. All these can provide clinical insight into the state of the ANS, but only a few can actually provide reliable and repeatable clinical information about the two individual component branches of the ANS. The more acceptable form of ANS monitoring uses power spectral, or frequency-domain, analysis of HRV.[1] Results of HRV spectral analysis combined with the results of RA spectral analysis represent the tone of, or the power in, the total ANS as well as in the PSNS and the SNS. The clinical usefulness of these values is based on the concept that in the normal state of ANS, the PSNS and the SNS work harmoniously to maintain homeostasis. This results in a stable power spectral content, with a balance of power contained in the high-frequency (HF) components and the low-frequency (LF) components. Should homeostasis be upset owing to damage, disease, or dysfunction, this harmony is broken, and the balance is lost, providing another, sometimes earlier, indication of pathologic conditions.

Only recently has it been appreciated that disturbances in HRV are of clinical significance. Specifically, it has been found that the HF components are highly correlated with PSNS tone.[2, 3] As an example, in respi-

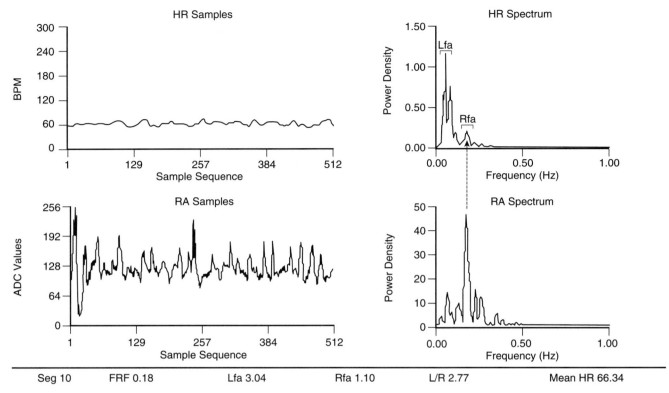

| Seg 10 | FRF 0.18 | Lfa 3.04 | Rfa 1.10 | L/R 2.77 | Mean HR 66.34 |

FIGURE 27–1. Method of computing autonomic nervous system monitoring parameters: low frequency (LF), high frequency (HF), and ratio. The *left* panels show the 512 samples of the instantaneous heart rate *(top)* and the respiratory activity *(bottom)* time-varying waveforms. The *right* panels show the spectra for the two time-domain signals: heart rate (HR; *top*) and respiratory activity *(bottom)*. The peak mode of the respiratory activity (RA) spectrum, the fundamental respiratory frequency, provides the center frequency for the HF area (HFa, sometimes referred to as the respiratory frequency area [RFa]) analysis window. The HF analysis window is 0.12 Hz, wide. The LF analysis window, spanning frequencies from 0.04 to 0.10 Hz, is placed based on "classic" heart rate variability methods. The area under the HR spectral curve within these two windows is computed to provide the HF and LF monitoring components, respectively. The ratio is computed by dividing LF by HF. The low frequency area (Lfa) is indicative of total autonomic tone. The HFa is indicative of parasympathetic nervous system tone. The ratio (L/R) is indicative of sympathetic nervous system tone. Every 32 seconds, a new segment (seg) of data is analyzed, thereby updating the autonomic nervous system monitoring parameters. ADC, analog-to-digital converter; BPM, beats per minute; FRF, fundamental respiratory frequency; L/R, low-frequency area to high-frequency area ratio.

ratory sinus arrhythmia in a young healthy subject, HRV is synchronized to a cycle with a period that corresponds to the respiratory pattern. (The beat-to-beat intervals are in phase with the respiratory cycle.) This is a sign of good parasympathetic tone and cardiovascular health.

History

Akselrod and colleagues stated, "As a response to the long-standing recognition of beat-to-beat variation and its clinical relevance, researchers have explored the physiologic mechanisms that generate these fluctuations. Spectral analysis characterizes mathematically the physiologic mechanisms that generate variation in RR intervals. Spectral analysis calculates the frequency content of time-varying signals, offering a breakdown of the successive RR intervals to their frequency components."[2] In experiments dating back 100 years, chemical and, later, electrical stimulation of brain centers of anesthetized animals showed a link between

changes in neural activity and cardiac arrhythmias, including ventricular ectopic beats, ventricular tachycardia, and ventricular fibrillation. The observation that heart rate and blood pressure vary from beat to beat was first made by Hales, who, in the 18th century, performed the first quantitative measurements of arterial blood pressure. He observed a correlation between respiratory cycle, beat-to-beat systolic pressure, and interbeat interval.

During the ensuing century, it was shown that sympathetic stimulation has a provocative or a facilitative effect with respect to ventricular arrhythmias and that this effect may be favorably modulated by parasympathetic activity, which seems to be protective. Subjects who are young, healthy, and physically fit have high parasympathetic tone and are extremely unlikely to experience fatal ventricular arrhythmias, even if cardiac ischemia occurs. On the other hand, patients with impaired left ventricular function, heart failure, or recent MI have high sympathetic tone and are at high risk of sudden death.

The interrelationships between sympathovagal balance, hemodynamic changes, and cardiac arrhythmias are complex. Whether the autonomic effects are primarily responsible for the occurrence of arrhythmias (which is a necessary but an insufficient condition) or are merely epiphenomena is debatable. The clinical studies performed suggest, however, that measurement of HRV does provide information independent from what is perceived to be the clinical severity of infarction and ejection fraction. This imparts clinical value to HRV measurement as a basis for testing the state of the ANS and its constituent branches.

Heart Rate Variability

Time-Domain Measures

Until the latter 1970s, only the beat-to-beat information from the electrocardiogram (ECG) was considered, and many time-domain measures were developed (discussed later in this chapter). Few of the time-domain measures are predictive, however; they are mostly historical, requiring long periods of stable data. Only the standard deviation of normal-to-normal heartbeat interval has been associated with any significant prognostic indices (e.g., a risk of sudden death in patients who have experienced an MI).[4] A comparison of the time-domain measures is presented in Table 27-1.[5-12] Note the wide ranges and standard deviations, leading to overlapping, the primary reason for the lack of sensitivity and specificity of time-domain data.

Frequency-Domain Measures

Even after visual analysis of the waveform generated by plotting the beat-to-beat interval with respect to time, it is obvious that HRV is composed of more than one frequency component. Hence, spectral analysis of HRV was introduced; it has shown greater correlation with pathologic states and has gained greater acceptance as a prognostic indicator.[1]

For the most part, classic HRV—whether time-domain or frequency-domain measures were employed—was based solely on the analysis of the ECG, and strict global correlation with the individual underlying components of the ANS was weak.[13] This was due in large part to the attempts to describe a two-component system with a single parameter. An example is the standard deviation of normal-to-normal heartbeat interval, which is based on 15 minutes of ECG data. It has been accepted as an indicator of total autonomic tone but does not correlate well with the SNS or the PSNS information. More recently, a number of nonlinear analysis methods (e.g., chaos theory, approximate entropy, and detrended fluctuation analysis) have been applied to the HRV signal, mostly with disappointing results.

The breakthrough came when a group of researchers from the Massachusetts Institute of Technology–Harvard biomedical engineering program added spectral analysis of the RA to the spectral analysis of the HRV. Now two variables (HRV measured in the classic way and variations in the RA) were being used to

TABLE 27-1. Comparison of Time-Domain Measures for Normal (or Control) and Abnormal Ranges

Measure	Normal Value	Abnormal Value	Study Group	Researcher
mNN	907 ± 26 ms	907 ± 35 ms	Patients 2 weeks after MI	Lombardi[5]
		862 ± 28 ms	Patients 12 months after MI	
	830 ± 100 ms	770 ± 180 ms	SCD patients (all causes)	Martin[6]
	833 ± 52 ms	857 ± 198 ms	Noninducible cardiac patients	Myers[7]
		732 ± 162 ms	Inducible cardiac patients	
	770 ± 62 ms	702 ± 112 ms	CHF patients from 15 minutes	Saul[8]
SDNN		<50 ms	34.4% all-cause mortality after MI	Kleiger[4]
		50 to 100 ms	13.8% all-cause mortality after MI	
		>100 ms	9.0% all-cause mortality after MI	
	195 ± 31 ms	102 ± 94 ms	Noninducible cardiac patients	Myers[7]
		49 ± 32 ms	Inducible cardiac patients	
SDANN	154 ± 40 ms	56 ± 23 ms	SCD patients (all causes)	Martin[6]
		71 ± 33 ms	Noninducible cardiac patients	Magdid[9]
		55 ± 24 ms	SCD patients	
	170 ± 23 ms	89 ± 69 ms	Noninducible cardiac patients	Myers[7]
		34 ± 17 ms	Inducible cardiac patients	
		87 ± 11 ms	Non–SCD VT patients	Van Hoogenhuyze[10]
		54 ± 7 ms	SCD patients	
pNN50		16.5 ± 15.9%	Patients from the >100 ms group[4]	Bigger[11]
	18 ± 7%	3.3 ± 4.3%	Patients from the <50 ms group[4]	
		22 ± 2%	Noninducible cardiac patients	Myers[7]
		2 ± 1%	Inducible cardiac patients	
rMSSD	25 ± 8 ms			Bruggemann[12]

CHF, congestive heart failure; MI, myocardial infarction; mNN, mean of all beat-to-beat intervals between normal beats; pNN50, percentage of successive RR intervals that differ by >50 ms; rMSSD, root-mean-square difference between immediately successive normal-to-normal RR intervals; SCD, sudden cardiac death; SDANN, standard deviation of 5-minute averages of normal-to-normal RR intervals; SDNN, standard deviation of the mean of the normal-to-normal RR intervals; VT, ventricular tachycardia.

characterize the two underlying parameters of the ANS (i.e., the SNS and the PSNS). With this method, the LF information, the HF information, and the ratio (the division of the power in the LF component by the power in the HF component) were developed and became the basis for ANS monitoring.

Real-Time Autonomic Nervous System Monitoring

The spectrogram of HRV displays the power that exists in the various components of the ANS and in the ANS as a whole. The more power and the greater the balance among its components, the better health the ANS can maintain. Conversely, the less power or the greater the imbalance, the greater the state of disease or dysfunction, either within the ANS itself or in one of its effector organs or processes.

The medical community now has at its discretion an industry-accepted, reimbursable means of independently monitoring the SNS and the PSNS simultaneously, along with the ANS. Canine research has demonstrated three components (HF, midfrequency, LF) from the frequency-domain analyses and has attributed physiologic origins to each (Fig. 27–2).

Humans on average have a lower respiratory rate than dogs, and the midfrequency and the LF are not easily separated; thus, the LF and the MF components from canine studies (see Fig. 27–2) are combined in the LF parameter referred to in Figure 27–1. This research has shown that higher frequencies are mediated by the PSNS alone, because the frequency response of the sympathetic system is too slow to reflect changes at this frequency. In fact, the PSNS can respond over a wide range of frequencies, whereas the SNS can respond only in a narrow band at relatively low frequencies (less than approximately 0.15 Hz). Therefore, only the PSNS can mediate heart rate fluctuations of greater than 0.15 Hz, whereas both systems mediate functions of less than 0.15 Hz.

Clinical Significance

Autonomic nervous system monitoring through spectral analysis of HRV and RA indicates the proportional amount of variation at each component frequency. The comparative height of a point on the spectrum demonstrates its relative contribution to overall HRV. The digitization of these frequency areas (LF and HF) provides numerical data (low-frequency area [LFa],

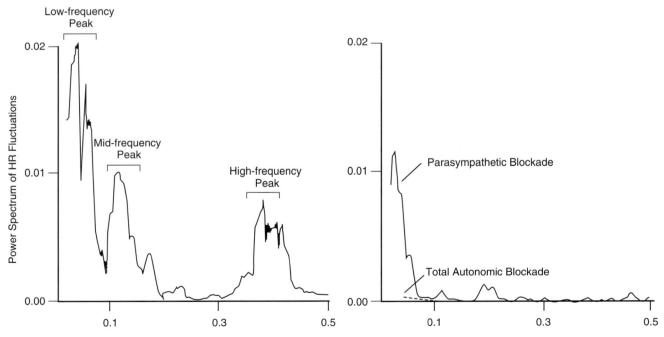

FIGURE 27–2. Spectral components of autonomic nervous system monitoring in the dog and the response to autonomic blockade. Three components are identified: a high-frequency (HF) peak at 0.4 Hz (Hz region from 0.15 to 1.0), corresponding to the respiratory rate (faster in dogs than in humans); a midfrequency (MF) peak at 0.12 Hz (MF region from 0.09 to 0.15 Hz), corresponding to the baroreceptor reflex frequency response; and a low-frequency (LF) peak (LF region from 0.02 to 0.09 Hz), corresponding to various slow changes in vasomotor tone, such as those of thermoregulation. Parasympathetic blockade (using glycopyrrolate, a muscarinic blocker analogous to atropine) removes HF and sinus arrhythmia peaks and reduces MF and LF peaks considerably (*solid line in right panel*). Sympathetic blockade (with propranolol) reduced only the LF peak, whereas a converting enzyme inhibitor (which blocks the effect of angiotensin) increased the variability in the LF and the MF band, suggesting a damping effect. Total autonomic blockade eliminates the residual heart rate (HR) variability entirely (*broken line in right panel*; virtually not seen). (Adapted from Akselrod S, Gordon D, Ubel FA, et al: Power spectrum analysis of heart fluctuations: A quantitative probe of beat-to-beat cardiovascular control. Science 1981;213:220–222. Copyright 1981 American Association for the Advancement of Science.)

high-frequency area [HFa], and ratio) that can be compared and easily used by the physician. In this way, HRV together with RA spectral calculations provides a "quantification" of the state and well-being of the ANS.

An example is illustrated in Figure 27–3. Pomeranz and coworkers studied the effect of postural change and respiration on HRV.[14] They found that the LF band increases 10-fold from a supine position to a standing position in healthy individuals. Their data suggest that LF frequency fluctuations (less than 0.12 Hz, in this case) in the supine position are mediated entirely by the PSNS. On standing, the LF fluctuations increase and are jointly mediated by the SNS and the PSNS. HF fluctuations are decreased by standing and are mediated solely by the PSNS. This is supported by data from the hourly spectral plots over a 24-hour period, which allow the respiratory influence on HRV to be visualized. During sleeping hours, the respiratory peak is more prominent as a result of supine positioning and increased parasympathetic tone (see Fig. 27–3).

The absolute values of the ANS parameters (LFa, HFa, and ratio) change from individual to individual; thus, it is the trends that are of greatest importance. Should the absolute values of any of these parameters be dangerously low (<0.1) in the unanesthetized state or extremely high (>40), they indicate signs of disease. In the emergency room or other short-term intensive care situation, trends can be developed in less than 15 minutes and provide immediate feedback whether the therapy or the intervention is sufficient, too little, or too much. Medical interventions, whether pharmaceu-

tical or not, can be titrated, and the patient's response can be monitored to determine in real time (the physiologic response can actually be seen as it happens) if the intervention was appropriate for the level of response desired by the physician.

Whether the patient is monitored continuously or intermittently is ultimately based on the physician's assessment of the patient. In general, until the patient is stable, continuous monitoring is recommended. Once the patient has stabilized, intermittent monitoring (similar to blood pressure measurement) is suggested to monitor the patient's progress.

In its current form, HRV-based ANS monitoring is still a general monitoring technique. Its sensitivity, its reliability, and its repeatability have been accepted. Its specificity, however, is still an issue. Similar to blood pressure measurement or ECG testing, ANS monitoring is currently an indicator of health, illness, or dysfunction. The standards by which specific diseases or dysfunctions can be measured are still being developed. Thus, it is another perspective to be correlated with other available information. The general feeling is that regardless of what monitoring results indicate specifically, when there is an indication for ANS monitoring, it is usually sensitive enough to provide information earlier than any other currently available monitor or diagnostic test. This relates to the underlying theory, in that the power in and the tone of the control system itself are being monitored in real time. Therefore, before an end-organ begins to fail or work too hard, the control system can be seen struggling to prevent the unhealthy state. This struggle is what is

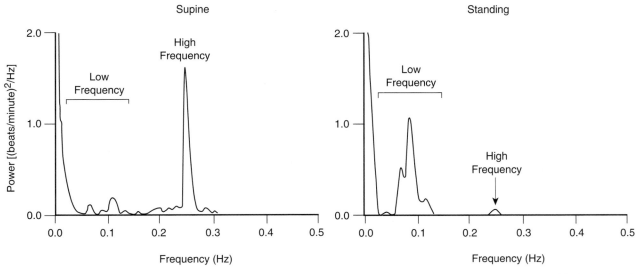

FIGURE 27–3. Heart rate variability response to changes in posture. The *left panel* depicts the power spectrum of a healthy individual in a supine position (the high-frequency [HF] or the respiratory frequency peak is at a lower frequency owing to the slower respiratory rate in humans). Note that a small low-frequency (LF) peak is an indication of reduced sympathetic activity and a prominent HF peak corresponds to the normal respiratory sinus arrhythmia and increased parasympathetic activity. The *right panel* depicts the power spectrum of the same individual in a standing position. Note the prominent LF peak as a result of a sympathetic surge corresponding to the gravitational challenge and the small HF peak owing to decreased parasympathetic activity. (Adapted from Pomeranz B, Macaulay RJ, Caudill MA, et al: Assessment of autonomic function in humans by heart rate spectral analysis. Am J Physiol 1985;248:H151–H153.)

being quantified and digitized by the ANS monitoring system. The latter technology supports and enhances the art of medicine.

Clinical Applications

Clinical usefulness is based on the hypothesis that ANS monitoring can determine when a particular level of treatment is too little, sufficient, or too much. ANS monitoring provides this information noninvasively as numerical trends in real time. The goal is to titrate interventions to the particular level that is most effective at that given time. For comparison, Table 27–2 contains data from researchers at the Cleveland Clinic, who have suggested the ranges of ANS monitoring values in normal healthy adults.[15] ANS monitoring has been useful in critical care situations in the emergency department or the trauma unit, the operating room, and the intensive care unit and on the hospital floors. It provides an early indication of improving health or increasing severity of acute illness in patients of all ages and may lead to a better understanding of the developing patterns in nonsurvivors. This chapter summarizes a few reported clinical applications in critical care situations.

Trauma and Shock

Autonomic nervous system monitoring is a noninvasive means of evaluating internal bleeding and hypovolemia in general. When the level of hypovolemia increases, the level of sympathetic excitation also increases as the ANS attempts to maintain proper central nervous system perfusion. In the late hypovolemic state, the two components of the ANS become uncoordinated and begin to "flail" (see Fig. 27–5).

Preliminary results from a study of 160 consecutively monitored patients with major traumatic injuries were studied at the Los Angeles County, University of Southern California Trauma Center beginning shortly after their admission to the emergency department. The patients were followed to the radiology suite when

TABLE 27–2. Sample Ranges of Normal (Stable) for the Three Parameters Subserving ANS Monitoring*

	LF	RF	L/R
Stable (supine)	5.2 ± 1.0	2.17 ± 0.5	2.4 ± 0.5
Stable (60-degree tilt)	15.7 ± 2.5	1.33 ± 0.92	11.8 ± 2.3

Data from 1991 Cleveland Clinic Study of 27 normal healthy adult volunteers (age, 30 ± 2.0 years) followed for 4 months. All subjects with abnormal histories during that time were rejected. Subjects' results at 30-degree tilt were statistically the same as supine ($P < .01$). All values carry units of power (msec²/Hz).

ANS, autonomic nervous system; LF, low frequency; L/R, low-frequency to high-frequency ratio; RF, respiratory (high) frequency.

TABLE 27–3. ANS Monitoring Parameters and HRV During and After the Septic Period

Variable	Septic Period	Recovery Period	P Value
HR (beats/min)	105 ± 20	106 ± 17	
HRV (beats/min² Hz)	0.51 ± 0.42	1.64 ± 1.11	$P < .0001$
LFa (beats/min² Hz)	0.43 ± 0.25	0.68 ± 0.17	$P < .0012$
L/R ratio	1.34 ± 1.61	4.27 ± 7.06	$P < .001$

ANS, autonomic nervous system; HR, heart rate; HRV, heart rate variability; LFa, low-frequency area; L/R ratio, low-frequency to high-frequency ratio.

studies were required, to the operating room, through the postanesthesia recovery area, and to the intensive care unit. The results have shown that HF values greater than 40 bpm²/Hz during the first 72 hours after admission correlate highly with nonsurvival. The converse also holds: Patients with nonzero HF values of less than 40 bpm²/Hz during the first 72 hours after admission survive (Unpublished data).

Sepsis

During sepsis, analysis of variance (ANOVA) showed that total HRV ($P < .0001$) and the LF value ($P < 0.01$) were significantly lower than in the subsequent recovery phase. Both Acute Physiology and Chronic Health Evaluation (APACHE II) and Therapeutic Intervention Scoring System (TISS) scores were inversely correlated with the total HRV, the logarithm of LF, the LF value, and the ratio ($P < .002$ to $P < .0001$). The LF value was significantly lower during the sepsis syndrome and was inversely proportional to disease severity. The LF component (<0.1 Hz) was often undetectable during sepsis syndrome but returned to normal during the recovery period. Average heart rate was not significantly different during sepsis and recovery. HRV and the sympathetically mediated ratio were reduced during sepsis (Table 27–3).

These patients were maintained with combinations of morphine, alfentanil, midazolam, or propofol. These data are confounded owing to the large standard deviations; however, they show reduced activity in the overall ANS (HRV) and the sympathetically mediated parameters with increasing severity of illness. The disturbance in autonomic control could result from alterations in central nervous system vasomotor activity resulting from impaired neural transmission to the heart or from changes in end-organ responsiveness. Respiratory rates were ventilator dependent during the period of sepsis and were significantly higher during recovery, when the patients were breathing freely. The LF value was also reduced in hypotensive sepsis (not shown in Table 27–3) but was increased in non–sepsis-related hypotension, consistent with the expected homeostatic responses.[16]

Depth of Anesthesia

Autonomic nervous system monitoring provides a window into the depth of anesthesia as it relates to SNS and PSNS responses to the depressant effect of anesthetic agents. Also, during the perioperative period, ANS monitoring can provide real-time feedback on the adequacy of treatment and is a potentially early indicator of sudden death. The amount of power in the SNS and the PSNS before anesthesia induction is recorded as the baseline for that patient at that specific time regardless of previous medicated or mental state. After anesthesia induction, the objective is to maintain enough power in the ANS to support life by titrating sufficient quantities of anesthetic agent for that patient at that time. In the operating room, prolonged (more than 30 minutes) LF and HF values of less than 0.1 indicate an extremely unstable physiologic condition and may warn of possible cardiac arrest. During reversal, the doses may be titrated more appropriately for the specific patient, which aids the physician in determining his or her stability and readiness for ICU discharge.

Autonomic nervous system monitoring detects and records in real time subtle brainstem responses to all stimuli (e.g., responses to slight table tilts are recorded as sympathetic surges, and responses to peritoneal manipulations are recorded as parasympathetic surges). The observed anesthetized states are suggested in Table 27–4 for adults after skin incision. The overanesthetized state is characterized by LF and HF values of less than 0.1 and a ratio of less than 1.0. Table 27–5 suggests data for children in the stable and the overanesthetized states.

In reported depth-of-anesthesia studies, there were no significant changes in heart rate during anesthesia.[17, 18] The data show that induction of anesthesia

TABLE 27–4. ANS Monitoring Parameters During the Period of Anesthesia*

Anesthesia Period	LF (bpm²)	HF (bpm²)	Ratio
Before induction	2.54 ± 0.95	1.88 ± 0.25	2.06 ± 0.57
3 minutes after induction	0.09 ± 0.02	0.58 ± 0.16	8.88 ± 2.32
After tracheal intubation	1.13 ± 0.84	1.43 ± 0.55	3.45 ± 1.08
Immediately before skin incision	0.95 ± 0.75	0.47 ± 0.31	1.73 ± 0.60
Immediately after skin incision	0.17 ± 0.10	0.25 ± 0.11	2.87 ± 0.86
During maximal surgical stimulation	0.20 ± 0.08	0.29 ± 0.10	2.14 ± 0.43
During skin closure	0.26 ± 0.11	0.44 ± 0.28	2.23 ± 0.62

*Recent unpublished data suggest refinements to these ranges: LF and HF values of 0.5 ± 0.4 when the patient is quiet (i.e., not including any sympathetic or parasympathetic surges) and ratio values of approximately 2.5.

ANS, autonomic nervous system; HF, high frequency; LF, low frequency.

Adapted from Brum JM: Power spectrum of heart rate variability: Synopsis of research activities. Division of Anesthesia and Department of Brain and Vascular Research, Cleveland Clinic Foundation, May 1991.

TABLE 27–5. Summary Data from Children During and Following Cardiac Surgery*

	LF	RF	L/R
Stable	0.1 < 10.0	<5.0	1.0 < 40.0
Cardiovascular unstable	<0.05	<3.0	<1.0
Cardiovascular stress	>10.0	<3.0	>50.0
Anesthetized	0.1 < 5.0	<5.0	0.6 < 3.0
Overanesthetized	<0.1	10 to 30 × > LF	<0.01

*A blinded University of Illinois study performed at Children's Hospital of Philadelphia involving 158 children studied for a 24-hour period (1989).

LF, low frequency; L/R, low-frequency to high-frequency ratio; RF, respiratory (high) frequency.

significantly decreases both ANS components (see Table 27–4); however, the effect on HF values predominated. Tracheal intubation temporarily restored HRV to its preinduction levels, possibly owing to the sympathetic surges, which are brainstem rather than cortical responses. With continued anesthesia and controlled ventilation, both ANS components (LF and HF) remained in a low state.

Heart rhythm changes during induction of anesthesia can cause myocardial ischemia in patients with coronary artery disease. The ANS, which may be involved in this phenomenon, can supply information on its control of cardiac chronotropic activity. ANS monitoring showed significant differences ($P < .05$) between bradycardic and nonbradycardic patients before and after induction (sufentanil, 5 to 8 µg/kg, and vecuronium, 0.12 to 0.15 mg/kg), whereas there was no significant difference in heart rate, mean arterial pressure, cardiac output, or cardiac index between the two groups (Table 27–6).[15]

In mechanical ventilation, the accuracy of ANS readings when free breathing is not occurring is questioned. There is anecdotal evidence that in the anesthetized state, there is still measurable activity. During the typical anesthetized state, the time-varying instantaneous heart rate and the RA show sympathetic and parasympathetic surges (brainstem responses) owing to the surgeon's and the anesthesiologist's interventions. The spectral measures of LF, HF, and ratio over time reflect ANS compensations for ventilation, even though the ANS is not mediating ventilation. With regard to cardiac pacing, so long as there are regular beats—especially with mechanical ventilation—there is no HRV, and monitored ANS activity can be misleading.

TABLE 27–6. Differences Between Bradycardic and Nonbradycardic Patients Before and After Induction of Anesthesia

	LF (bpm²)	HF (bpm²)	Ratio
Bradycardic	1.36 ± 0.30	0.34 ± 0.08	7.30 ± 1.31
Nonbradycardic	1.91 ± 0.32	1.04 ± 0.22	4.38 ± 0.63

HF, high frequency; LF, low frequency.

Adapted from Brum JM: Power spectrum of heart rate variability: Synopsis of research activities. Division of Anesthesia and Department of Brain and Vascular Research, Cleveland Clinic Foundation, May 1991.

Sudden Cardiac Death

Spectral techniques provide more specific information about the physiologic systems that control heart rhythm; thus, use of these techniques allows for better separation of patients according to risk.[7] Studies have shown that decreased HRV is an independent long-term statistical predictor of overall and sudden arrhythmic death after MI. The prevailing hypothesis is that HRV is dependent on intact neurocardiac autonomic regulation and that decreased HRV reflects autonomic dysfunction associated with cardiac electrical instability. Adrenergic hyperactivity or lack of presumably protective parasympathetic autonomic tone is the purported pathophysiologic mechanism of such arrhythmogenesis.[19]

Post–Myocardial Infarction Risk Stratification. Cardiac electrical instability (LF < 0.05, HF < 3.0, and L/R ratio < 1.0) is a sign of ill health and has been identified as one of the primary factors responsible for SCD. Electrical stability of the heart has been found to be reduced by elevation of sympathetic efferent activity and to be increased by a major increase in vagal efferent activity. Studies suggest that patients with decreased HRV have decreased parasympathetic tone with or without increased sympathetic tone and may have more than a fivefold higher risk of developing ventricular fibrillation; thus, decreased HRV carries an adverse prognosis.[4, 8, 20] In conjunction with this, diminished HRV has been reported to occur in patients at risk of sudden death as opposed to those not at risk.[6] The American College of Cardiology has recommended power spectral analysis of HRV to stratify the risk of developing SCD following acute MI.[1]

Identifying this high-risk group allows the initiation of aggressive treatment to improve survival.[1, 21] Impaired HRV is independently associated with an increased mortality rate and is superior to other factors (late potentials, ventricular ectopic beats per hour, couplets, and ejection fraction) in predicting death in postinfarction patients.[11, 12, 20–22] Kleiger and colleagues found that decreased HRV was associated with markedly increased mortality rates at ejection fractions of less than 30%.[4] Low HRV and, therefore, low ANS parameters (especially HF values) more than double the risk. ANS monitoring parameters were lower in patients at high risk of SCD than in patients with asymptomatic ventricular ectopy. Other investigations suggest that an altered balance between the beta-sympathetic and the parasympathetic systems in patients with low ANS parameters predisposes them to ventricular fibrillation and sudden death.[9] The use of reduced values for ANS monitoring parameters in the stratification of postinfarction risk is attractive because this type of monitoring is sensitive and noninvasive. It is speculated that decreased HF, LF, and L/R ratio values

(indicating high risk) might be prevented by prophylactic drug therapy.[23]

Chest Pain: Cardiac Dysfunction and Cardiopulmonary Disease

Many patients with possible MI present with chest pain, which may or may not be of cardiac origin. ANS monitoring is a quick, simple, nonstressful, and noninvasive test that may be helpful in determining if the chest pain is life threatening. If the chest pain is a result of cardiac arrhythmias, the ANS power may indicate cardiac instability (all spectral components are very low) or cardiovascular stress (the LF value and the L/R ratio are extremely high). Throughout most of a 10- to 15-minute test in nonarrhythmic patients, the LF and the ratio values will be elevated but otherwise within the normal range.

Myocardial Dysfunction Monitoring. Reduced ANS parameters in children recovering from cardiac surgery have been shown to predict a fatal outcome (see Table 27–5). In general, reduced HRV has been observed consistently in patients with acute cardiac dysfunction characterized by signs of sympathetic activation (e.g., faster heart rate and high levels of circulating catecholamines); a relationship between changes in HRV and the extent of left ventricular dysfunction was reported.[24] In most patients with advanced ventricular dysfunction and drastically reduced ANS parameters, an LF component could not be detected despite clinical signs of sympathetic activation. In conditions characterized by markedly persistent and unopposed sympathetic excitation, the responsiveness of the sinus node to neural input may drastically diminish. As a result, it becomes independent of the ANS and therefore regular in its activity (i.e., HRV is greatly reduced or nonexistent).

Congestive Heart Failure Monitoring. The net cardiovascular response in patients with congestive heart failure is less HRV, as manifested by lower LF, HF, and L/R ratio values. Declines in these values may be detected in some cases before weight gain. ANS-monitored parameters in patients with congestive heart failure are reduced by a factor of 10 as compared with normal, with the power in the HF values virtually absent.[25] In addition to showing reduced ANS parameters in all frequencies, the spectra display a shift to the low frequencies, which are disproportionately higher than in normals. Casolo and associates showed that although the spectral composition of HRV varies both quantitatively and qualitatively during the day in normal subjects, it does not vary appreciably in patients with congestive heart failure (Fig. 27–4; Table 27–7).[24]

Monitoring of ANS based on HRV identifies various severities of congestive heart failure and has prognostic value. In one study, patients with different New York

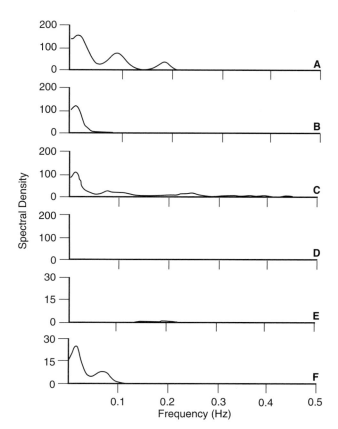

FIGURE 27–4. Examples of stereotypical spectra from 4-minute segments of heart rate from a normal subject (A), a patient with congestive heart failure (B), a patient with diabetes and mild neuropathy (C), a patient with diabetes and severe neuropathy (D), a patient shortly after heart transplantation (E), and a patient 7 months after heart transplantation (F). Note that the spectral density scale in plots A through D is the same (0 to 200 bpm²/Hz) and that of the plots for E and F is significantly reduced (0 to 30 bpm²/Hz) to illustrate the frequency-specific differences between the two transplant patients. (Adapted from Saul JP: Beat-to-beat variations of heart rate reflect modulation of cardiac outflow. News Physiol Sci 1990;3:32–37.)

terventions changed the spectra. For example, physical therapy significantly increased HF power with concurrent decreases in LF power. Prolonged use of angiotensin-converting enzyme inhibitors significantly increased total and HF power with no significant change in LF power.[25] Binkley and colleagues found significant decreases in HF power with increases in ratios in patients with congestive heart failure, which indicates withdrawal of parasympathetic tone with an imbalance in autonomic tone, predominantly sympathetic.[26a] This was in addition to an overall decrease in spectral power at all frequencies compared with normal individuals. The reduced parasympathetic tone was partially reversed after 12 weeks of treatment with angiotensin-converting enzyme inhibitors.

Cardiac Transplant Monitoring. When the patient is in the resting supine position after heart transplantation, the beating heart is essentially metronomic, with a fixed stable heart rate and essentially no HRV. Under conditions of increased cardiovascular demand, heart rate changes, presumably in response to circulating catecholamine levels, but this change is slower than normal. The return to rest is also slower than normal because of the need to metabolize the circulating catecholamines. In addition, the resting heart rate and the circadian modulation of heart rate in transplanted hearts are less than normal. Clinical findings show that ANS monitoring parameters are reduced in denervated transplanted hearts (see Fig. 27–4, A and E). Power in all frequencies from 0.02 to 1.0 Hz is reduced by 90% in heart transplant patients. After some time, circadian modulations along with variations in LF values return, suggesting some reinnervation; however, the amplitude of the LF values is significantly lower than normal (see Fig. 27–4, E and F).

The spectra from transplanted hearts during rejection have elevated power levels (with respect to normal transplants) in all frequencies from 0.1 to 1.2 Hz. Overall power levels are decreased compared with normal, however. ANS parameters derived from these spectra are similar to those seen in cardiovascular instability (see Table 27–5), with slightly higher LF values (e.g., LF < 2.0, HF < 3.0, and ratios < 1.0).

Heart Association functional classes of disease had different ANS values: the higher the functional class, the lower the values.[26] Also, clinical deterioration was associated with further decreases in ANS values, whereas patients who improved showed no significant change in values. On the other hand, therapeutic in-

TABLE 27–7. Comparison of HRV in Control Subjects and Patients with Congestive Heart Failure

Time	LF Normal	LF CHF	HF Normal	HF CHF	Ratio Normal	Ratio CHF
7 to 12 AM	245 ± 205	21 ± 23	49 ± 46	4 ± 6	8 ± 11	20 ± 26
1 to 6 PM	196 ± 143	19 ± 22	29 ± 34	3 ± 4	19 ± 18	15 ± 20
7 to 12 PM	236 ± 195	20 ± 17	49 ± 58	3 ± 4	13 ± 17	15 ± 19
1 to 6 AM	243 ± 204	17 ± 16	106 ± 75	5 ± 6	4 ± 4	11 ± 19

All values carry a significance of $P < .001$ except the AM ratios for CHF patients, which carry a significance of $P < .005$, and PM ratios for those patients, which carry no significance.

CHF, congestive heart failure; HF, high frequency; HRV, heart rate variability; LF, low frequency.

Adapted from Casolo GC: Heart rate variability in patients with heart failure. In Malik M, Camm AJ (eds): Heart Rate Variability. Armonk, NY, Futura, 1995, pp 449–465.

Hypertension

The baroreceptor reflex in hypertensive patients appears to be operating near its saturation level (toward the higher blood pressure values), limiting heart rate control.[27] Others have found that hypertension is characterized by increased LF power and decreased HF power compared with normals as well as blunting of circadian rhythmicity of the LF values. The difference between the results of ANS monitoring in patients with congestive heart failure and the results in patients with hypertension is that in congestive heart failure, the overall power levels are severely depressed (by up to 10 times) compared with normals. In patients with hypertension, however, the overall power levels are near normal.

Administration of 300 mg of clonidine to patients in the supine position induced increases in HF values in both hypertensive and healthy subjects; LF and L/R ratio values decreased in healthy subjects but not in patients with hypertension. Overall, patients with mild hypertension had lower HF values than healthy subjects. On assuming the sitting position, both groups showed reduced HF values and increased LF and L/R ratio values. In healthy subjects, the response to postural change was unaffected by clonidine. In contrast, patients with hypertension who took clonidine showed no changes in LF and L/R ratio values and a significantly lower decrease in HF values. Results suggest that patients with hypertension have altered sympathovagal balance, which can be unmasked by clonidine. This phenomenon should be considered when attempting to achieve better control of cardiovascular risk in patients with hypertension.[28]

Ventricular Tachycardia

In patients with ventricular tachycardia, all power spectra of HRV were significantly decreased before the onset of sustained tachycardia but not before the onset of unsustained tachycardia.[1] This indicates a temporal relationship between changes in the ANS-monitored parameters and the onset of sustained ventricular tachycardia. In supraventricular arrhythmias, there were significant increases in heart rate with overall decreases in ANS parameters.[1]

Tilt Table Testing. Increased heart rate and increased blood pressure during passive head-up tilting are normal hemodynamic responses. These responses are complex and may be attributed to either augmented sympathetic or reduced parasympathetic activity. In normal adults, there were no significant changes in heart rate in response to the change from a supine position to a 30-degree head-up tilt.[15] The 60-degree head-up tilt caused an increase ($P < .01$) in LF value (15.7 ± 2.5) and L/R ratio (11.8 ± 2.3) compared

with the values in the supine position (LF value, 5.2 ± 1.0; L/R ratio, 2.4 ± 0.5) (see Table 27–2). The HF value was slightly altered with tilting. In normal teenagers, the ANS parameters were similar to those in adults except for the LF value, which also increased in the 30-degree head-up tilt position. Significant deviations from these ranges and responses are an indication of an abnormally functioning ANS, and this technique can be used in place of other more strenuous or invasive tests to indicate dysfunction.[15]

In patients susceptible to syncope of unknown origin, head-up tilting can initiate inadequate autonomic responses, resulting in bradycardia or tachycardia. No differences were observed between this group and normal individuals in heart rate, HF value, and ratio.[15] The LF measure was significantly lower ($P < .05$) in the syncopal group, however—who had syncope during tilting (1.7 ± 1.4)—than in the normal group (3.8 ± 3.2). Thus, patients developing syncope during head-up tilting have lower sympathetic activity at rest than do healthy subjects.[15]

Measuring extrinsic ANS modulation of intrinsic sinus node activity can be more revealing in patients suspected of sick sinus syndrome. ANS monitoring during head-up tilting can elevate the SNS and the PSNS controls of the sinus node. Because sinus node disorders account for 50% of new pacemaker implants, better assessments of the disease can aid in more appropriate use of pacemakers. ANS monitoring is noninvasive and nonpharmaceutical, is simpler to administer, and is without pharmaceutical side effects.[15]

Diabetic Autonomic Dysfunction

Autonomic nervous system monitoring based on HRV has been found to be a suitable noninvasive clinical test of diabetic autonomic dysfunction. It can provide another early diagnostic parameter for coronary artery disease. In neuropathy associated with diabetes mellitus characterized by alteration of small nerve fibers, reduction in ANS parameters carries a negative prognostic value and precedes the clinical expression of autonomic neuropathy.[9] Furthermore, in patients with diabetes without evidence of autonomic neuropathy, reduction of the absolute power of LF and HF values was also reported.[29] The origins of this abnormal response have been traced to the parasympathetic portion of the ANS in the early stages of the disease. As the disease begins, the power in all components decreases, with a greater drop in HF components relative to LF components (see Fig. 27–4, A and C). As the disease progresses, eventually all HRV disappears, and all the ANS-monitored parameters decrease to near zero (see Fig. 27–4, A and D).

Coronary heart disease is twice as likely to develop as a result of autonomic neuropathy in diabetes mellitus.

Indeed, 75% of excess deaths in men with diabetes in the first National Health and Nutrition Survey were due to coronary artery disease.[17] It has been shown that ANS monitoring predicts the progression of neuropathy in patients with diabetes and the risk of SCD and secondary MIs in patients after MI. A study of asymptomatic myocardial ischemia in patients with diabetes with and without autonomic dysfunction showed that painless ischemia was significantly more frequent in patients with dysfunction than in those without dysfunction (38% vs. 5%).[30] Thus, ANS monitoring may help improve the detection of silent events, including ischemia, and may help stratify the risk of sudden death in the patient with diabetes.

Cardiovascular autonomic neuropathy has been linked to the following clinical manifestations: postural hypotension, exercise intolerance, enhanced intraoperative cardiovascular liability, increased incidence of asymptomatic ischemia and MI, and decreased rate of survival after MI. The earliest subclinical indicator of this complication is reduced HRV. Although clinical symptoms of autonomic neuropathy generally do not occur until after a long duration of diabetes, the presence of subclinical autonomic dysfunction has been demonstrated within 12 months of diagnosis in patients with type 2 diabetes and within 24 months in patients with type 1 diabetes.[31]

As the duration of diabetes lengthens, increased HR occurs first (owing to decreased PSNS tone), and then decreased HR occurs (owing to continuing loss of SNS tone). Finally, when the heart is denervated, a fixed heart rate is present.[6] As autonomic dysfunction progresses, the HR response to posture or the Valsalva maneuver is diminished. Symptomatic autonomic neuropathy identifies individuals at increased risk of sudden death. Whether cardiac autonomic neuropathy contributes to silent ischemia is unclear, but the pain response to ischemia is often blunted in patients with diabetes, complicating detection of coronary artery disease. As a result, patients with diabetes may be asymptomatic or may present with symptoms of easy fatigability, exertional dyspnea, or indigestion.[32] These are potential causes of inconclusive or negative stress tests. ANS monitoring is a simple, noninvasive, less stressful test that provides meaningful clinical information using tilt table, postural, or Valsalva challenges.

The 5-year survival rate in patients with diabetes who are free of neurologic complications is greater than 99%, whereas patients with clinically overt autonomic neuropathy have a 25% to 40% chance of dying within 5 years. Subtle tests of autonomic function reveal minor abnormalities in almost 100% of patients with even newly diagnosed diabetes. These asymptomatic findings do not constitute a risk of progression of diabetes; however, those individuals with symptoms are at risk of sudden death, MI, or renal failure. Thus, the potential benefits of diagnosing asymptomatic coronary artery disease in patients with diabetes include (1) the implementation of preventative programs aimed at reducing the risk of future coronary morbidity and mortality, (2) the initiation of treatment with anti-ischemic medications, and (3) the early identification of the patient for whom revascularization is appropriate.[33]

Pain Management

An increase in the level of pain is typically accompanied by concurrent elevations in SNS activity, primarily mediated by adrenal outflow. Significant increases in LF and ratio values resulting from ANS monitoring can aid in evaluation of actual versus perceived pain. Furthermore, the reduction in the ratio component in response to the administration of pain-masking pharmaceuticals (e.g., morphine) can permit the titration of these potentially addictive agents and can reduce the likelihood of overprescribing, while maintaining patient comfort.

Neonatal Development and Infant Monitoring

Although physicians have been long aware of the beat-to-beat variation in heart rate, or so-called normal sinus arrhythmia, as a salutary cardiovascular sign, its direct clinical importance was perhaps first demonstrated in the area of fetal monitoring. Beat-to-beat variations in fetal heart rate during labor signify fetal distress and the need for rapid delivery.[22] Furthermore, given that the use of HRV as the basis for ANS monitoring is indicative of a healthy ANS, it seems reasonable that a set of normal ANS parameters could serve as the basis for determining the maturity and the health of developing fetal autonomic innervation. On the other hand, a decrease in, or an absence of, HRV may appear as the result of a variety of pathologic states (e.g., fetal metabolic acidosis or hypoxia, neurologic abnormality, cardiac arrhythmia, marked prematurity, or chemical substance dependency). Diminished ANS parameters, as measured before intrauterine fetal death, were found to be a better indicator of impending death than late or variable decelerations.[21] A reduction in ANS parameters can also accompany fetal sleep and fetal inactivity, however, which signal a healthy fetus.[21] Therefore, as with children and adults, ANS monitoring is not the ultimate measure. It is merely another sensitive parameter of health and a potential earlier indicator of disease. Additional evaluations must be considered to ensure fetal well-being.

In the premature neonate, a stay of 10 days or more in the neonatal intensive care unit is often required before the child is mature enough to be released.

Early evidence from studies of ANS monitoring during feeding show that immature infants manifest frequent and life-threatening bradycardia while attempting to coordinate sucking, breathing, and swallowing. Preliminary data suggest that ANS monitoring can be an early indicator of the onset of bradycardia and can also help determine the neonate's level of maturity and potential for earlier discharge from the neonatal intensive care unit.

Pharmaceutical Interactions

Pharmaceuticals may enhance the protective nature of the PSNS in guarding against SCD.

Beta-Adrenergic Blockers. Beta-adrenergic blockade significantly raises the HF variable in ANS monitoring, which may be indicative of increased parasympathetic tone. Although this increase is significant and can place a patient at lower risk of SCD, it is not very large in absolute amplitude. In addition, beta-adrenergic blockade prevents the increase in the LF component observed in the morning.[1]

Antiarrhythmic Drugs. Antiarrhythmic drugs (e.g., flecainide, propafenone, encainide, and moricizine) decrease HRV in patients with chronic ventricular arrhythmia and post-MI conditions. Specifically, they reduce the LF value much more than the HF value, resulting in a smaller ratio, which indicates reduced HRV. There is no correlation between the effects of these drugs and death during follow-up, however. In fact, given that reduced HRV can be an indicator of an increased risk of death in post-MI patients, it may be that some antiarrhythmic drugs are associated with an increased rate of mortality.

Muscarinic Receptor Blockers. Low-dose muscarinic receptor blockers (e.g., atropine and scopolamine) produce paradoxical increases in cardioparasympathetic activity. Muscarinic blockers significantly increase HRV, specifically the HF component. Thus, they enhance the protective nature of a high level of parasympathetic tone.

Brain Death

In the brain-dead patient, the time-varying instantaneous heart rate is absolutely flat (no variation), and the LF and the HF values are both less than 0.08 ± 0.02 (unpublished data). Unlike the anesthetized patient—in whom brainstem responses can still be elicited through pharmacologic, surgical, or clinical interventions—the brain-dead patient shows none of these responses. ANS and HRV data, even when the patient is in the anesthetized state, have been shown to be sensitive to a nurse's touch or to movement (tilting or raising) of the bed, in addition to other more invasive manipulations. None of these responses is present in a brain-dead patient. With no activity in either branch of the ANS, the patient is unable to maintain homeostasis.

The Terminal State

Autonomic nervous system data from records of LF, HF, and ratio values (unpublished data) suggest that just before death, the parasympathetic and the sympathetic branches lose coordination and begin to flail (similar to the late hypovolemic state). It has been

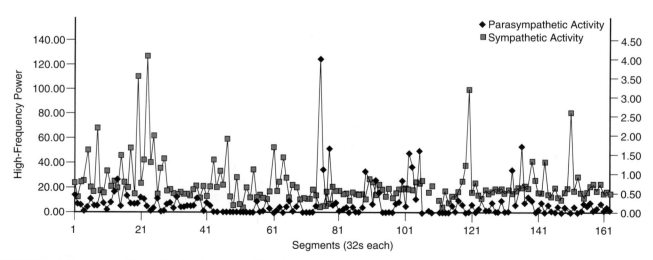

FIGURE 27–5. Power recordings of high frequency and low frequency–to–high frequency ratio. This is an example of the loss of autonomic nervous system coordination (e.g., parasympathetic and sympathetic "flailing" typical of autonomic activity) toward the end of a patient's life. This patient was eventually resuscitated and survived. Notice how the sympathetic activity spends a significant amount of time at or below 0.05 (a sign of disease), with excursions into the healthy range. Similarly, the parasympathetic activity is abnormally low for a significant period of time, with excursions into the healthy range and beyond. Also, the excursions of the two systems are mostly out of phase with each other. This is thought to be indicative of the two components working independently in an attempt to find a strategy that will work to return homeostasis. 32s, 32 seconds.

suggested that this behavior is a last attempt of the ANS to reestablish homeostasis. As in Figure 27–5, the parasympathetic (represented by the power in the HF component of the data) and the sympathetic (represented by the Ratio component) systems surge apparently at random, seeking to resolve the homeostatic instability. Note that medical intervention revived this patient.

References

1. Heart rate variability: Standards of measurement, physiological interpretation and clinical use. Task Force of the European Society of Cardiology and the North American Society of Pacing and Electrophysiology. Circulation 1996;93:1043–1065.
2. Akselrod S, Gordon D, Ubel FA, et al: Power spectrum analysis of heart fluctuations: A quantitative probe of beat-to-beat cardiovascular control. Science 1981;213:220–222.
3. Akselrod S, Gordon D, Madwed JB, et al: Hemodynamic regulation: Investigation by spectral analysis. Am J Physiol 1985;249:H867-H875.
4. Kleiger RE, Miller JP, Bigger JT, et al: Decreased heart rate variability and its association with increased mortality after acute myocardial infarction. Am J Cardiol 1987;59:256–262.
5. Lombardi F, Sandrone G, Pernpruner S, et al: Heart rate variability as an index of sympathovagal interaction after acute myocardial infarction. Am J Cardiol 1987;60:1239–1245.
6. Martin GJ, Magid NM, Myers G, et al: Heart rate variability and sudden death secondary to coronary artery disease during ambulatory electrocardiographic monitoring. Am J Cardiol 1987;60:86–89.
7. Myers GA, Martin GJ, Magid NM, et al: Power spectral analysis of heart rate variability in sudden cardiac death: Comparison to other methods. IEEE Trans Biomed Eng 1986;33:1149–1156.
8. Saul JP, Arai Y, Berger RD, et al: Assessment of autonomic regulation in chronic congestive heart failure by heart rate spectral analysis. Am J Cardiol 1988;61:1292–1299.
9. Magdid NM, Martin GJ, Kehoe RF, et al: Diminished heart rate variability in patients with sudden cardiac death. Circulation 1985;72(suppl III):241.
10. Van Hoogenhuyze D, Weinstein N, Martin GJ, et al: Reproducibility and relation to mean heart rate of heart rate variability in normal subjects and in patients with congestive heart failure secondary to coronary artery disease. Am J Cardiol 1991;68:1668–1676.
11. Bigger JT Jr, Kleiger RE, Fleiss JL, et al: Components of heart rate variability measured during healing of acute myocardial infarction. Am J Cardiol 1988;61:208–215.
12. Bruggemann T, Andresen D, Voller H, et al: Heart rate variability from Holter monitoring in a normal population. Am J Cardiol 1993;72:8–13.
13. Houle MS, Billman GE: Low-frequency component of the heart rate variability spectrum: A poor marker of sympathetic activity. Am J Physiol 1999;276:H215–H223.
14. Pomeranz B, Macaulay RJ, Caudill MA, et al: Assessment of autonomic function in humans by heart rate spectral analysis. Am J Physiol 1985;248:H151–H153.
15. Brum JM, Ribeiro MP, Estafanous FG, et al: Power spectrum of heart rate variability: Synopsis of research activities. Division of Anesthesia and Department of Brain and Vascular Research, Cleveland Clinic Foundation, May 1991, pp 1–15.
16. Garrard CS, Kontoyannis DA, Piepoli M: Spectral analysis of heart rate variability in the sepsis syndrome. Clin Auton Res 1993;3:5–13.
17. Butler R, MacDonald TM, Struthers AD, Morris AD: The clinical implications of diabetic heart disease. Eur Heart J 1998;19:1617–1627.
18. Genovely H, Pfeifer MA: RR-variation: The autonomic test of choice in diabetes. Diabetes Metabol Rev 1988;4:255–271.
19. Vybiral T, Glaeser DH: Changes in heart rate variability preceding ventricular arrhythmias. In Malik M, Camm AJ (eds): Heart Rate Variability. Armonk, NY, Futura, 1995, pp 421–428.
20. Saul JP: Beat-to-beat variations of heart rate reflect modulation of cardiac outflow. News Physiol Sci 1990;5:32–37.
21. Hirsch M: Heart rate variability in the fetus. In Malik M, Camm AJ (eds): Heart Rate Variability. Armonk, NY, Futura, 1995, pp 517–531.
22. Hon EH, Lee ST: Electronic evaluation of the fetal heart rate patterns preceding fetal death. Am J Obstet Gynecol 1965;87:814–826.
23. Bosner MS, Kleiger RE, Rottman JN: Heart rate variability and risk stratification after myocardial infarction. Cardiol Clin 1992;10:487–498.
24. Casolo G, Balli E, Taddei T, et al: Decreased spontaneous heart rate variability in congestive heart failure. Am J Cardiol 1989;64:1162–1167.
25. Casolo GC: Heart rate variability in patients with heart failure. In Malik M, Camm AJ (eds): Heart Rate Variability. Armonk, NY, Futura, 1995, pp 449–465.
26. Stenfenelli T, Bergler-Klein J, Globits S, et al: Heart rate behaviour at different stages of congestive heart failure. Eur Heart J 1992;13:902–907.
26a. Binkley PF, Nunziata E, Haas GJ, et al: Parasympathetic withdrawal is an integral component of autonomic imbalance in congestive heart failure: Demonstration in human subjects and verification in a paced canine model of ventricular failure. J Am Coll Cardiol 1991;18:464–472.
27. Parati G: Heart rate and blood pressure variability and their interaction in hypertension. In Malik M, Camm AJ (eds): Heart Rate Variability. Armonk, NY, Futura, 1995, pp 467–478.
28. Lazzeri C, La Villa G, Mannelli M, et al: Effects of clonidine on power spectral analysis of heart rate variability in mild essential hypertension. J Auton Nerv Syst 1998;74:152–159.
29. Pagani M, Malfatto G, Pierini S, et al: Spectral analysis of heart rate variability in the assessment of autonomic diabetic neuropathy. J Auton Nerv Syst 1988;23:143–153.
30. Langer A, Freeman MR, Josse RG, et al: Detection of myocardial ischemia in diabetes mellitus. Am J Cardiol 1991;67:1073–1078.
31. Schumer MP, Joyner SA, Pfeifer MA: Cardiovascular autonomic neuropathy testing in patients with diabetes. Diabetes Spectrum 1998;11:227–231.
32. Consensus development conference on the diagnosis of coronary heart disease in people with diabetes: 10-11 February 1998, Miami, Florida. American Diabetes Association. Diabetes Care 1998;21:1551–1559.
33. Singer DH, Martin GJ, Magid N, et al: Low heart rate variability and sudden cardiac death. J Electrocardiol 1998;21(suppl):S46–S55.

28 Physiology of Shock and Acute Circulatory Failure

William C. Shoemaker and Charles C. J. Wo

To . . . end . . . the thousand natural shocks that flesh is heir to.

'Tis a consummation devoutly to be wish'd.

WILLIAM SHAKESPEARE, *Hamlet*

More than 2.1 million people in the United States die per year; half die acutely with or of shock. Shock plays a role in all fatal illnesses, however, because circulatory failure is a part of the final common pathway. Moreover, circulatory dysfunction or shock is a common complication of many acute life-threatening illnesses and is central to most nonfatal circulatory disorders. The shock syndrome is a symptom complex easily diagnosed from the presence of hypotension in the late stage, but it is initially recognized by nonspecific signs and subjective symptoms that are secondary effects of acute circulatory failure unrelated to the primary physiologic problem. The lack of objective physiologic criteria to replace these imprecise signs and symptoms has been a major deterrent to development of optimal therapeutic goals. For maximal therapeutic effectiveness, it is necessary to understand the underlying physiology.

Monitoring, which is a major reason for admission to the intensive care unit, is frequently used to measure mean arterial pressure, heart rate, central venous pressure (CVP), hematocrit, urine output, and arterial oxygen tension (PaO_2). These traditionally monitored variables characterize circulatory failure in advanced stages of shock. They are not measures of the adequacy of circulatory function or of tissue perfusion in the early stages. Moreover, the appearance of hypotension or other signs and symptoms of shock does not mark the beginning of circulatory failure, but rather it represents decompensation or the failure of compensatory mechanisms that maintain blood pressure in the face of falling blood flow. Clearly, hemodynamic and oxygen transport variables, not the secondary manifestations of the syndrome, should be used to evaluate circulatory function and shock. Measurements begun after the appearance of hypotension usually reflect late mechanisms.

Evolution of Shock Syndromes

The normal function of the circulation is to supply oxygen and oxidative substrates (glucose, amino acids, and fatty acids) and to remove CO_2, hydrogen ion, organic acids, lactate, pyruvate, and other partially metabolized compounds. As with many other diseases, circulatory disorders are evaluated on the basis of the normal range of hemodynamic variables; values outside the normal range establish criteria for diagnosis and therapy. This approach is inappropriate for circulatory disorders, however, because the body normally responds to diurnal bodily activity, exercise, and other common stresses with increased hemodynamic function. Similar compensatory responses occur with fever, surgery, trauma, and infection to maintain the normal intracellular milieu.

Shock, although recognized by secondary signs and symptoms, begins as inadequate tissue perfusion and oxygenation, measured by cardiac output or index (CI), oxygen delivery (DO_2), and oxygen consumption (VO_2) patterns.[1] Most circulatory disorders involve changes in the three major physiologic components of the circulation: cardiac, respiratory, and tissue perfusion functions.[2–6] Therefore, monitoring of all three circulatory components is needed to describe survivor and nonsurvivor patterns and to predict and improve outcome. The common initial problem in most acute critical illnesses is circulatory failure from inadequate tissue perfusion and tissue hypoxia, which leads to organ failure and death.

Conventional Etiologic Approach to Physiology and Therapy of Shock

Most textbooks of medicine, surgery, pediatrics, and emergency medicine classify shock by cause: hemorrhagic, traumatic, septic, or cardiogenic. These etiologic categories are then described according to clinical signs and symptoms, laboratory findings, their presumed pathophysiology, and recommended therapy. This approach is widely accepted, simple, clear, and understandable. It suggests that traumatic and hemorrhagic shock should be treated with fluids; cardiogenic shock should be treated with inotropic agents and fluid restriction; and septic shock should be treated with antibiotics, drainage, and débridement. This widely held therapeutic paradigm is sufficient to normalize the vital signs, arterial blood gases, hematocrit, urine output, and other symptoms of shock.

Monitored variables are evaluated independently, and each abnormality is corrected when discovered. When they are first recognized, hypotension and oliguria are usually normalized by use of vasopressors, crystalloids, and diuretics. The assumption is that normal values for these parameters are criteria of circulatory normalcy and that their attainment ensures adequate resuscitation. Shock is not that simple, however; complex etiologic events rarely begin and end with a single alteration that can be corrected by a single therapy. Moreover, when superficial manifestations of the shock syndrome are corrected by crystalloids, diuretics, and vasopressors, the underlying low or uneven flow, inadequate tissue perfusion, and tissue hypoxia may remain unnoticed and untreated until organ failure appears. Unfortunately, blood pressure early in the course of high-risk surgery, injury, and other types of shock does not correlate well with blood flow.[1]

This overly simplistic description of complex pathophysiology is seriously misleading. A major limitation is that this one-dimensional approach ignores the interactions of the various components of the circulation (e.g., the capacity of the heart to compensate for inadequacies of pulmonary function or tissue perfusion). Therapy based on a one-dimensional etiologic approach is unlikely to be optimal. Moreover, the lack of objective physiologic criteria has been a major deterrent to early effective therapy.[1-7]

Myocardial Performance in Shock Physiology

The conventional approach to assessment of myocardial performance is to measure cardiac output by means of thermodilution together with venous inflow pressure (the Starling curve). Since the development of the pulmonary artery (PA) balloon-tipped flow-directed (Swan-Ganz) catheter, the myocardial performance curve has been used routinely by cardiologists to evaluate circulatory function.[8, 9] The CI (or some function of the heart, such as cardiac output, stroke volume, stroke work, or cardiac work) is plotted against the corresponding inflow pressure (PA occlusion or wedge pressure). This is usually plotted as one line representing the lower limit of normal CI (2.5 L/min/m²) and a second line representing the upper limit of normal for PA wedge pressure (20 mm Hg). These two lines divide the field into four quadrants, which define four clinical subgroups according to flow and inflow

pressures. Hemodynamics and therapy are suggested by these criteria; low flow, low wedge pressure suggests hypovolemia; low flow, high wedge pressure suggests cardiogenic shock; high flow, low pressure suggests compensation for sepsis and stress; and high flow, high pressure suggests blood volume overload or possible cardiac problems.

This approach was thought to provide sufficient information to adjust fluids, inotropes, and diuretics in shock, but it is primarily relevant to cardiac patients and the cardiac component of noncardiac patients in the intensive care unit. In essence, this diagnostic and therapeutic paradigm relates only to cardiac function; it does not evaluate pulmonary function, tissue perfusion, or tissue oxygenation. It was developed for cardiac patients and has limited usefulness in patients with traumatic, septic, or postoperative shock, because death in these patients is usually due to tissue hypoxia resulting from inadequate tissue perfusion, capillary leak, and multiple organ failure.

An Alternative Approach to Physiology and Therapy of Shock

Hemodynamic monitoring displays frequent, repetitive, or continuous measurement of circulatory function at the bedside to describe patterns of shock, organ failure, and death in patients who undergo high-risk surgery or who have severe trauma, hemorrhage, sepsis, or other acute illnesses. Clinical judgment, on the other hand, may be difficult to define precisely in terms of therapeutic goals. Monitoring, like laboratory values and radiographic studies, supplements rather than supplants clinical opinions, which are often subjective and difficult to quantify for titration of therapy. Monitoring provides objective criteria for the evaluation of physiologic deficiencies separate from diagnostic anatomic pathology; this distinction is particularly important, because most people die not from their diagnosis but from physiologic deficiencies. The purpose of early invasive or noninvasive monitoring of hemodynamics, oxygen transport, and tissue perfusion is to correct the major primary circulatory problems before they become lethal.[1-6]

An alternative therapeutic paradigm is to use survivors' hemodynamic values as a first empiric approximation of therapeutic goals.[2-6, 10-28] The assumption here is that normal hemodynamic and oxygen transport values are appropriate for normal healthy volunteers, but supranormal values observed in survivors represent compensatory hemodynamic responses needed to meet increased metabolic needs. These responses have survival value. Specific circulatory problems associated with the patient in early shock include inadequate tissue perfusion from uneven microcirculatory blood flow, changes due to the effects of anesthetics, and oxygen debt from delays in keeping up with blood losses. Moreover, the increased metabolic need due to tissue repair, fever, immunochemical responses, sepsis, and organ failure requires increased tissue metabolism and perfusion.

The survivors' patterns are assumed to represent the effects of the initiating stress or illnesses and the body's successful compensatory responses. The nonsurvivors' patterns are assumed to reflect the effects of severe illnesses and the body's inadequate compensatory responses with subsequent decompensations.

Normal Circulatory Response to Exercise

The circulatory response to injury and disease is similar to the normal compensatory response to exercise. In Olympic-class athletes, increased body metabolism, which may exceed VO_2 values of 5000 mL/minute as a result of exercise sprinting, is compensated for by increased cardiac output values of 50 L/minute. Increased circulatory function is a normal regulatory response to exercise. Similarly, in injury and acute illness, the basic assumption is that the major circulatory function is to provide for body metabolism, which if suddenly increased requires commensurate circulatory increases. On a moment-to-moment basis, the circulation responds to changes in bodily activity to maintain the "milieu interior" for normal cellular metabolism.

Early Hemodynamic and Oxygen Transport Patterns in Postoperative Shock

Although instances of relatively "pure" types of shock are seen, most clinical conditions are accompanied by combinations of several types of shock, which are affected by age, prior illnesses, comorbid conditions, and cardiac reserve capacities. Shock in high-risk surgical patients may be used as a model for other etiologic types of shock because time relationships are documented precisely in the chart after elective surgery.[3] In contrast, temporal patterns are not clearly apparent in sepsis, occult hemorrhage, and incipient medical shock.

The temporal patterns of mean arterial pressure, CI, PA wedge pressure, systemic vascular resistance, DO_2, and VO_2 in a series of 708 high-risk postoperative survivors and nonsurvivors are shown in Figure 22–2.[20] The survivors, compared with the nonsurvivors, had (1) greater increases in CI and flow-related variables, with lower CVP and wedge pressure; (2) less pulmonary vasoconstriction (lower PVR and mean pulmonary arterial pressure [MPAP]); (3) greater increases in DO_2 and VO_2, with lower oxygen extraction rates and normal blood gases; (4) greater hematocrit, blood volume, and red cell mass; and (5) less pulmonary shunt (Qsp/Qt).[1–4, 20] The assumption was that early changes statistically related to survival represent the effects of surgery plus adequate physiologic compensation; therefore, these values could be used as therapeutic goals. Early changes related to death, however, reflect the overwhelming effects of surgery plus inadequate compensation. On the other hand, these values may be used as early warning criteria for impending disaster and death.

Preoperative patients with sepsis, severe stress, accidental injury, or advanced cirrhosis often had hyperdynamic preoperative baseline CI values.[20] Preoperative patients with heart failure or hypovolemic shock had hypotension, high PA occlusion pressure, and reduced values for CI, DO_2, and VO_2; in the early postoperative period, however, CI, DO_2, and VO_2 in the average survivor were appreciably higher than in comparable groups of nonsurvivors, who had minimal increases in CI, DO_2, and VO_2 despite higher CVP and PA occlusion pressure. Thus, patients may start with higher or lower baseline values for preoperative cardiac output, but the differences in postoperative patterns between survivors and nonsurvivors should be related to their own preoperative baseline (control) values.[20] Similar differences in the survivor/nonsurvivor patterns were observed in many other conditions, including severe trauma, hemorrhage, medical and surgical sepsis, cardiogenic shock, acute myocardial infarction, congestive heart failure, acute respiratory failure, late-stage cirrhosis, and head injury.[10–27]

Pathophysiology of Shock and Acute Circulatory Failure in Trauma, Sepsis, and Stress

The body's initial neuroadrenal stress response increases heart rate and cardiac output, which compensate for tissue oxygen debt from low or maldistributed microcirculatory flow. The earliest changes observed in trauma, elective surgery, sepsis, and other types of stress were increases in heart rate, CI, and DO_2, unless hypovolemia or impaired cardiac function was present.[2–6, 10–26]

Use of Oxygen Transport Variables to Measure Tissue Perfusion

The bulk movement of oxygen is a useful measure of both tissue perfusion and overall circulatory function. The rate of oxygen consumption (VO_2) represents all oxidative metabolic reactions; as such, it reflects the status of body metabolism. It represents the actual amount of oxygen consumed, not necessarily how much is needed, which may be more than is burned. VO_2 is supply dependent: The rate of oxygen consumed is limited by the CI and the DO_2.[29] The body compensates for inadequate VO_2 by increasing DO_2, which is the amount of oxygen delivered to the tissues. As such, DO_2 reflects perfusion to peripheral tissues; its increase compensates for earlier inadequate tissue oxygenation. The temporal patterns of changes in DO_2 and VO_2 are more informative than a single set of measurements because the sequential patterns of change provide a history of physiologic events that lead to shock and subsequent organ failure.

Oxygen Debt, Organ Failure, and Mortality

Organ Failure as a Sequela of Inadequately Treated Shock

With increasing degrees of illness, circulatory compensations may not be adequate to supply increasing metabolic requirements for oxygen and oxidative substrates. When the stress or the illness is excessive and there is inadequate blood flow and oxygen supply, tissue hypoxia may occur. Decreased DO_2 occurs in cardiac failure, hypoxemia, respiratory failure, trauma, hemorrhage, dehydration, cardiopulmonary arrest, and other acute circulatory catastrophes. Thus, the extensive metabolic demands of acute illness may overwhelm the capacity of the circulation to respond effectively. Failure of the circulation to meet the added needs of acute illness leads to decompensation, shock, organ failure, and death. Shock, therefore, may be due to inadequate hemodynamic responsiveness to acute illnesses.

Inadequate tissue oxygenation due to inadequate perfusion is the common pathophysiologic defect underlying shock syndromes. Low flow or uneven (i.e., maldistributed) flow successively leads to tissue hypoxia, organ dysfunction, organ failure, and death.[2–6, 10–26, 30, 31] In acute illness, oxygen debt may occur as a result of increased metabolic demand or reduced oxygen supply. Decreased DO_2 occurs in cardiac insufficiency, hypovolemia, hypoxemia, respiratory failure, trauma, hemorrhage, dehydration, cardiopulmonary arrest, and other acute circulatory catastrophes. In trauma, postoperative states, and other acute illnesses, the most common life-threatening hypodynamic state is hypovolemia due to inadequate volume resuscitation. In the terminal state of many chronic disorders, hypovolemia, low CI, and low DO_2 may develop insidiously.

Oxygen Debt in Experimental Hemorrhagic Shock and in High-Risk Patients

The degree and the duration of tissue hypoxia may be estimated under experimental conditions as the net cumulative deficit of VO_2. Guyton and colleagues measured VO_2 in dogs subjected to hemorrhage; when the net accumulated O_2 debt was less than 100 m/kg, all dogs survived, and when the O_2 debt was greater than 140 mL/kg, all died. Fifty percent mortality occurred at 120 mL/kg.[32, 33]

A semiquantitative method of estimating oxygen debt was developed for high-risk patients monitored before, during, and immediately after surgery. The preoperative VO_2 was measured, this value was corrected for the effects of anesthesia, and the changes in temperature were used to calculate the oxygen need.[30] The patient's own oxygen need was extrapolated to the first 48 hours postoperatively. The rate of oxygen debt was calculated by subtracting the patient's measured VO_2 from the estimated oxygen need. The net cumulative oxygen debt could then be calculated from the area defined by time and the rate of oxygen debt; the integrated area under this time-rate curve gives the cumulative amount of oxygen debt at any given time (Fig. 28–1).[30]

Oxygen debt was measured in a series of 253 consecutively monitored high-risk surgical patients. The sequential patterns of CI, DO_2, and VO_2 and the net cumulative oxygen debt are shown for the preoperative, the intraoperative, and the 48-hour postoperative periods (see Fig. 28–1); this demonstrates the interrelationship between DO_2 and VO_2 for the survivors with and without organ failure as compared with nonsurvivors, all of whom had organ failure.[30] Although the groups started with similar baseline values, the nonsurvivors had significantly lower DO_2 and VO_2 values in the intraoperative period and throughout their subsequent course. The DO_2 and the VO_2 values of survivors without organ failure were higher throughout their perioperative courses; values for survivors with organ failure were intermediate. The oxygen debt began during the operation and reached a maximum 4.1 ± 0.6 hours postoperatively in survivors without organ failure, compared with 10.1 ± 2.7 hours in survivors with organ failure and 17.8 ± 2.2 hours in nonsurvivors, all of whom died with organ failure ($P < .05$).[30]

There was a higher incidence of organ failure, sepsis, and disseminated intravascular coagulation in high-risk postoperative patients with large oxygen debts when normal values were used as therapeutic goals. When oxygen debt was prevented or rapidly repaired by increasing CI and DO_2 to optimal values (determined empirically from survivors' patterns), the incidence of organ failure and death decreased significantly.[30] The time of appearance of organ failure was

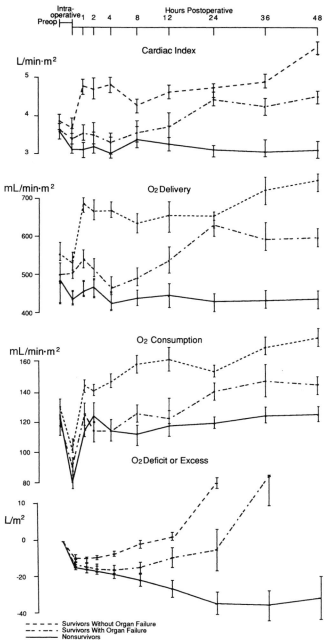

FIGURE 28–1. Temporal patterns for cardiac index, oxygen delivery, oxygen consumption, and calculated oxygen debt indicated by the net cumulative oxygen consumption deficit in a series of high-risk patients studied intraoperatively and at successive periods postoperatively. Nonsurvivors *(solid lines)* had essentially normal values; survivors without organ failure *(dashed lines)* had optimal values; survivors with organ failure *(dashed/dotted lines)* had intermediate values. (From Shoemaker WC, Appel PL, Bishop MH: Temporal patterns of blood volume, hemodynamics, and oxygen transport in pathogenesis and therapy of postoperative adult respiratory distress syndrome. New Horiz 1993;1:522–536.)

3.6 ± 3.1 (standard deviation) days in acute respiratory distress syndrome, 4.2 ± 4.8 days in cardiogenic problem, 5.9 ± 4.1 days in renal failure, 6.2 ± 5.6 days in disseminated intravascular coagulation, and 7.4 ± 4.9 days in sepsis. Although there were wide ranges

in temporal patterns, organ failure followed the time of appearance as well as the maximal oxygen debt.

In a prospective, preoperatively randomized trial in which supranormal "optimal" oxygen transport values were used as the goals of therapy, the protocol patients who had optimal values as therapeutic goals developed a maximum oxygen debt of 7.6 ± 3.4 L/min/m², which peaked at an average of 3 hours postoperatively and lasted an average of 13 hours.[30] In contrast, the control patients who had normal values as therapeutic goals developed a maximum oxygen debt of 17.3 ± 6.3 L/m², which peaked at 31 hours postoperatively (*P* < .05) and lasted approximately 48 hours.[30] This suggests that tissue oxygen debt from reduced tissue perfusion is the primary underlying mechanism that leads to organ failure and death.

Mathematical Coupling of DO_2 and VO_2 Values

There is a potential problem in the mathematical coupling of DO_2 values with VO_2 values because CI is a common term in the calculation of both DO_2 and VO_2. Obviously, if there is a spuriously high CI, then the calculated DO_2 and VO_2 will also be incorrectly high. Although this is theoretically possible, it is unlikely to be a frequent or consistent error when careful troubleshooting and quality controls are routinely performed. Moreover, there are a number of clinical conditions in which changes in DO_2 are not associated with similar changes in VO_2:

1. In late stages of sepsis, postoperative states, and severe cardiac conditions, small changes in DO_2 were sometimes associated with a large VO_2 response, indicating a large oxygen debt.
2. Early postoperative patients may have major increases in DO_2 with minimal changes in VO_2, suggestive of a small oxygen debt.
3. The use of packed red cells in septic patients often stimulates major changes in VO_2 with minimal or insignificant changes in CI and DO_2.
4. Normal unstressed or preoperative patients may have large increases in DO_2 with little or no VO_2 response because there was no oxygen debt.

In essence, when DO_2 and VO_2 increase together, there may be supply-dependent VO_2 or an error due to coupling. Coupling cannot explain the supply-independent VO_2, however, for which increased DO_2 values are not accompanied by increased VO_2 values; this relationship results in a nearly horizontal line when DO_2 values are plotted against their corresponding VO_2 values. Moreover, in the early postoperative period, the differences in the patterns of DO_2 values in survivors and nonsurvivors plotted against their corresponding VO_2 values (Fig. 28–2) were similar to CI data

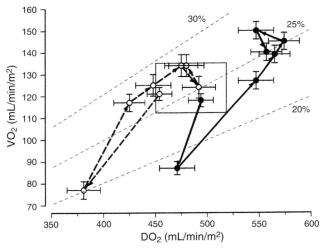

FIGURE 28–2. Oxygen consumption (VO₂) values plotted against their corresponding oxygen delivery (DO₂) values at preoperative baseline, intraoperatively, and during succeeding time periods. *Solid lines* represent survivors, *dashed lines* represent nonsurvivors. Note the higher values for survivors. The *boxed area* is the normal range. (From Shoemaker WC: Oxygen transport and oxygen metabolism in shock and critical illness. Crit Care Clin 1996;12:939–969.)

from the same series plotted against the corresponding oxygen extraction ratio (Fig. 28–3). The CI versus O₂ extraction relationship eliminates the problem of mathematical coupling.

Capillary Leak, Fluid Overload, and Water Distribution

In the early stage of shock, restoration of intravascular volume and the subsequent maintenance of blood volume depend on plasma oncotic pressure and the amount of intravenously administered fluids. Inadequacies of either may lead to progressive hypovolemic shock, organ failure, and death. Capillary leak occurs in the late stage of septic shock and, less commonly, in traumatic and hemorrhagic shock. It is characterized clinically by excessive peripheral edema and persistent hypovolemia despite adequate fluid administration. The leak of capillary membranes, augmented by immunochemical mediators, results in escape of plasma proteins and plasma water into the interstitium. In late stages, edema may worsen with belated efforts to keep up with plasma volume losses by administering fluids, including colloids, crystalloids, or even transfusions.

Local tissue hypoxia in association with a host of biochemical mediators is thought to initiate the capillary leak; however, the precise physiologic and biochemical mechanisms and the temporal order of their interactions are incompletely understood. Capillary leak occurs in septic postoperative patients during the late stage of shock. This is a clinical diagnosis, however, because quantitative measurements of capillary leak are not available at the bedside. Because of this, the

presence of a capillary leak is inferred clinically from failure of fluids, colloids, and blood transfusions to maintain blood volume while interstitial fluids continue to expand (as indicated by the continued progression of peripheral and pulmonary edema).

Capillary leak must be differentiated from both blood volume overload and excessive expansion of the interstitium with large volumes of crystalloids, which may greatly expand the interstitial space without adequately restoring plasma volume. As much as 30 to 50 L of Ringer's lactate solution have been advocated for severe trauma by several surgical groups. This may be tolerated in the early resuscitation of young, previously healthy patients; however, elderly patients with a history of cardiac disease, particularly those on salt-restricted diets, may not tolerate even a few liters of crystalloids. During their resuscitation, the latter may develop peripheral and pulmonary edema before restoration of PA wedge pressure and blood volume.

The distribution of administered fluids between plasma water and interstitial water during initial crystalloid resuscitation must be considered separately from the phenomenon of capillary leak. Capillary leak, plasma volume overload, and massive crystalloid infusions that expand the interstitial space may give rise to pulmonary and peripheral edema, but by different mechanisms. Capillary leak occurs when increased capillary permeability allows plasma proteins to escape from the intravascular space in amounts that compromise the maintenance of plasma volume. The pulmonary edema produced by blood volume overload or cardiac failure is characterized by high wedge pressures (>20 mm Hg) that drive plasma water into the

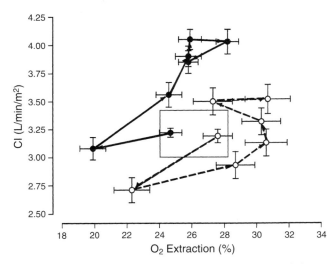

FIGURE 28–3. Cardiac index (CI) values plotted against their corresponding oxygen extraction values at preoperative baseline, intraoperatively, and during succeeding time periods. *Solid lines* represent survivors, *dashed lines* represent nonsurvivors. Note the marked differences in patterns between survivors and nonsurvivors. The *boxed area* is the normal range. (From Shoemaker WC: Oxygen transport and oxygen metabolism in shock and critical illness. Crit Care Clin 1996;12:939–969.)

interstitium by hydrostatic force. In contrast, increased interstitial lung water may be produced occasionally after massive crystalloid infusion while wedge pressures remain relatively normal, because 80% of administered crystalloids leave the intravascular space by the end of the infusion. In addition, by 40 minutes later, most of the rest has left the plasma volume to expand the interstitial space.[34, 35] Pulmonary and peripheral edema may also be produced by cardiac failure, low protein values due to malnutrition, renal failure, hepatic failure, hypermetabolic states, head injuries, high-altitude sickness, anaphylactic reactions, hyperthermia, and carcinomatosis and other terminal states.

Time Relationships of Capillary Leak and Oxygen Transport Responses

In the late stage of capillary leak, there were minimal increases in DO_2 and no significant improvement in VO_2 with maximal fluid volume loading and inotropic stimulation. In contrast, in the early (first 48 hours) postoperative period, there were significant improvements in both variables with volume and inotropic stimulation. Capillary leak, as observed clinically, began to appear in the middle period (3 to 5 days postoperatively) of the illness in some severely ill patients who were predominantly septic; it reached its zenith in the late or the terminal stage.[36] Capillary leak is not an all-or-none phenomenon; it develops gradually over several days. It is obviously best to give therapy early, before capillary leak appears, to achieve maximal effectiveness. Finally, capillary leak follows the occurrence of tissue hypoxia and oxygen debt and is likely to be the effect rather than the cause of tissue hypoxia.[36–39]

Falloff of Radiolabeled Albumin as a Measure of Capillary Leak

Measurement of plasma volume has been performed with ^{131}I- and ^{125}I-labeled human serum albumin. Shippy and colleagues reported results of a series of more than 1700 plasma volume measurements.[27] After two or more baseline control values were secured, radiolabeled iodinated human serum albumin was injected intravenously, and four to six timed blood samples were obtained over the subsequent 60-minute period. The radioactivity of plasma samples decreased about 1% to 2% per hour in normal preoperative conditions and 2% to 3% per hour 3 to 6 days after major life-threatening surgery. The falloff was 3% to 6% per hour in septic patients 3 to 7 days postoperatively but 5% to 9% per hour in late-stage or terminal septic patients.

Relation of Tissue Hypoxia to Mediators of Organ Failure

Tissue hypoxia and acidosis precipitate or trigger several cascades, including the arachidonic acid cascades to thromboxane, prostaglandins, and leukotrienes; histamine and other amines; serotonin; complement system; tumor necrosis factor; cytokines; and the continued elaboration of bacterial antigens, messengers, and oxygen free radicals by activated macrophages. These mediators are thought to initiate or intensify capillary leak and organ failure.

Fluid Challenge as a Measure of Circulatory Adequacy and Reserve Capacity

The increase in CI and DO_2 in response to standard fluid volume loading may also be a measure of circulatory reserve capacity and the ability to compensate. In practical terms, supply-dependent VO_2 is indicated by increased VO_2 of more than 15 mL/min/m^2 when DO_2 increases to more than 80 mL/min/m^2 after rapid administration of a standard volume of fluids (e.g., 1000 mL of crystalloids, 100 or 500 mL of 5% albumin, or 6% hydroxyethyl starch).[7, 27]

Prospective Clinical Trials of Supranormal CI and DO$_2$

The hypothesis was tested that increased CI and DO_2 represent compensations that have survival value when DO_2 increases and there is concomitant improvement in VO_2 indicative of improved tissue oxygenation.[2–6, 10–27] An early prospective clinical trial evaluated the effectiveness of supranormal values as therapeutic goals to improve outcomes over a 7½-year period. The initial clinical trial evaluated 252 high-risk surgical patients allocated to one of three clinical services; normal values were used as therapeutic goals for the control service and the supranormal values as goals for the protocol service. There were marked significant reductions in mortality rate in the patients in the protocol group (19% vs. 44%).[2] Subsequently, a randomized controlled trial was performed that preoperatively allocated patients to one of three groups: (1) CVP catheter group with normal values as goals; (2) PA catheter control group with normal values as goals; and (3) PA protocol group with supranormal values as goals. The result showed no significant differences in outcome between the CVP group and the PA control group; both used normal values as goals. Thus, if the intent is only to maintain normal values, the PA catheter has no real advantage over the CVP catheter. In contrast, the PA protocol group had significantly reduced mortality compared with the PA control group (4% vs. 33%, $P < .02$) as well as fewer days on mechanical ventilation, fewer hospital days, fewer days in the intensive care unit, and less cost.[2, 3]

Some recent reports have failed to confirm these observations. In an insightful meta-analysis, Boyd and Bennett showed no outcome improvement in seven randomized studies done several days postoperatively after organ failure had developed.[12] There was reduced mortality in six prospective randomized studies done early, however (i.e., 8 to 12 hours postoperatively).[2–5, 10–14, 22] Moreover, these trials showed improved survival, reduced organ failure, and lower costs when optimal values of CI, DO_2, and VO_2 were used as early goals. The concept of using supranormal values in survivors as optimal goals has been supported by a considerable number of studies. Hankeln and associates, Edwards and coworkers, Yu and colleagues, and Boyd and Bennett reported improved outcome with optimal values in postoperative patients[5, 7, 10, 12, 17, 19]; Scalea and associates, Bishop and coworkers, Pasquale and colleagues, and Moore and associates have reported improved outcome with supranormal values in trauma patients.[14–16, 29] Boyd and coworkers reported improved outcome in randomized trials by optimizing high-risk surgical patients preoperatively and then maintaining optimal values intraoperatively and postoperatively.[5, 12] Edwards and colleagues, Hankeln and coworkers, and Tuchschmidt and colleagues reported improved outcome in medical septic shock; the latter study was randomized.[5, 7, 19, 22, 26, 27] Creamer and associates demonstrated survival in 14 of 17 patients with cardiogenic shock after acute myocardial infarction when they were able to increase CI from 1.3 ± 0.5 to 2.6 ± 0.4 L/min/m². [24] Hankeln and coworkers and Edwards and associates also showed improved outcome in cardiac patients.[7, 17, 19] All these had some variations in their protocols, but each used supranormal values as early goals.

Moore and colleagues observed good outcome when optimal VO_2 was produced by increasing the DO_2 values.[16] When increasing DO_2 values failed to produced commensurate VO_2 values, however, there were higher incidences of organ failure and death. Similarly, Bishop and associates showed that severely traumatized patients resuscitated to optimal values less than 24 hours after injury had an 18% mortality rate, whereas those who reached optimal goals more than 24 hours later or who failed to reach them had a 38% mortality rate.[14] Other investigators have confirmed increased CI, DO_2, and VO_2 in survivors of septic shock.[21–23]

Early Therapeutic Goals for High-Risk Patients

Empirically determined supranormal values for CI, DO_2, and VO_2 observed in survivors of high-risk surgi-

cal operations, trauma, or sepsis were used as objective physiologic criteria or as "first approximations" of optimal physiologic goals for therapy. The relatively normal or low values in nonsurvivors serve as early warning of potentially lethal patterns of organ failure and death for which circulatory function cannot compensate.

Table 28–1 lists the mean CI, DO_2, and VO_2 values in survivors of high-risk surgical operations without associated preoperative sepsis or cardiovascular problems, in survivors of severe trauma, and in survivors of septic shock. These empirically determined supranormal values may be used as a first approximation of physiologic goals for therapy but must be adjusted for age, the presence of comorbid conditions, the patient's own baseline values, and the reserve capacity to compensate hemodynamically.[20] In patients older than 50 years of age, the CI and the DO_2 patterns started from the lower range of baseline values and reached lower peak values with each successive decade. Patients with sepsis, trauma, or cirrhosis had higher baseline values and reached higher peak values. The therapeutic goals may also be modified by various diagnostic and high-risk categories: the presence of previous preoperative hyperdynamic states (e.g., trauma, stress, sepsis, recent surgery, late-stage cirrhosis); the presence of previous hypodynamic states (e.g., hemorrhage, hypovolemia, cardiogenic problems); the time elapsed after onset of trauma or surgery; the presence of terminal and preterminal states; the presence of specific postoperative organ failure (e.g., respiratory, renal, hepatic, cardiac, central nervous system); and the presence of postoperative complications (e.g., sepsis, septic shock, disseminated intravascular coagulation, and nutritional failure).[20]

Time Relationships in Shock

Abnormal values for each variable are most often presented in terms of the mean plus or minus the standard error of the mean for various etiologic types of shock, especially septic shock (in which onset and progression to various stages are subtle). These values are usually presented without reference to time; that

TABLE 28–1. Goals of Therapy in Various High-Risk Conditions

Condition	Cardiac Index, mL/min/m²	DO_2 mL/min/m²	VO_2, mL/min/m²
Normal values	$3.2 \pm .2$	520 ± 57	130 ± 17
High-risk surgery	>4.5	>600	>167 ± 18
Severe trauma	5	>800	>180
Septic shock	>5.5	>900	>190
Cardiogenic shock	>2.6	>500	>120

DO_2, oxygen delivery; VO_2, volume of oxygen consumption.
Data from references 3, 4, and 31.

is, each piece of data is presented as though that same value occurred throughout the entire course of shock. Hemodynamic patterns have wide variations throughout the time course of shock syndromes, however, and are affected by associated comorbid conditions, delays in management, degrees of illness, and therapy.

The time of onset of circulatory problems is often obscure, and the time lines that identify major changes in the evolution of circulatory failure are rarely used to define the evolving stages of the various etiologic categories of shock. When temporal patterns are described, low or inadequate flow is frequently observed to be an antecedent event of subsequent hyperdynamic states, vital organ failure, and death.[7, 20] Moreover, low flow may also be the precipitating clinical event causing shock in critically ill postoperative, hemorrhagic, traumatic, or septic patients. Furthermore, low flow in the intraoperative or the immediate postoperative period has been identified as the cause of oxygen debt and subsequent multiple organ failure and death.[30] To understand time relationships of acute circulatory dysfunction or shock properly, it is necessary to describe the sequential patterns of circulatory variables in survivors and nonsurvivors, beginning with the normal baseline control period before the precipitating etiologic event. It is misleading to begin describing monitored events after hypotension has already appeared and shock is already established. When monitoring was started early (i.e., at or shortly after the precipitating event), we found that survivors started with low flow but promptly developed compensatory hyperdynamic states, whereas low or relatively normal flow and poor tissue perfusion and oxygenation continued in nonsurvivors. These led to organ failure, capillary leak, and, finally, death.[30]

Time Needed to Reach Goals

Time is the single most important outcome-related issue. When the aim in high-risk surgery was to achieve the optimal supranormal goals in the first 8 to 12 hours postoperatively, there was marked reduction in the number of organ failures and in mortality.[3, 4, 11, 12] Optimization of DO_2 and VO_2 occurred in the late stage after organ failure but did not improve the mortality rate.[12] In Bishop's study of patients with trauma, the mortality rate was 18% when optimal goals were achieved less than 24 hours after hospital admission; when optimal goals were not achieved until 24 hours or more after admission, however, the mortality rate increased to 39%.[14] In patients with severe trauma, low incommensurate VO_2 responses to increased DO_2 in the first day after injury were associated with an increase in organ failure and death. In contrast, increased DO_2 associated with increased VO_2 favorably

affected outcome. There was a 92% survival rate when the optimal goals were achieved within 24 hours of intensive care unit admission, but there was a 93% mortality rate when achievement of the goals was delayed or was not reached at all and when lactate levels did not return to satisfactory levels.[2–6, 14–20]

Summary

The major causes of inadequate tissue perfusion in the acutely ill patient are hypovolemia, low flow, maldistributed flow due to uneven vasoconstriction, and capillary leak. These common circulatory deficiencies underlie inadequate tissue perfusion; they are made worse by the increased metabolism produced by stress, trauma, surgery, and sepsis. Inadequate tissue perfusion leads to tissue hypoxia, organ dysfunction, and organ failure. In essence, the basic problem in acute circulatory failure is tissue hypoxia due to the failure of the circulation to provide oxygen and oxidative substrates for the body's metabolic needs. Appropriate monitoring should address the early recognition of these subtle problems. This approach has been shown to improve outcome in high-risk surgery, accidental trauma, septic shock, and cardiogenic shock.

The overall function of the circulation is to support body metabolism in both normal conditions and the rapidly changing metabolic activities of exercise, stress, and acute illness. Increased circulatory function is the tool that maintains the milieu interior of intracellular metabolism in conditions that suddenly require increased metabolism. The important circulatory functions are total body blood flow, reflecting cardiac function; arterial oxygenation, reflecting pulmonary function; and transcutaneous oxygen tension ($PtcO_2$) and transcutaneous partial pressure of carbon dioxide ($PtcCO_2$), reflecting tissue perfusion. Recognition and treatment of shock are traditionally guided by imprecise signs and subjective symptoms, but a more physiologic alternative is to evaluate and treat the major primary circulatory problems of hypovolemia, low or uneven distribution of microcirculatory flow, and increased metabolic demands. Increased metabolism may be augmented by proinflammatory responses, wound healing, and fever. The temporal patterns of these interacting components characterize the physiology of surviving and nonsurviving patients. Unless hypovolemia or impaired cardiac function is present, increased CI and DO_2 are the earliest changes in trauma, elective surgery, sepsis, and other types of stress. In survivors, increased CI and DO_2 occurred earlier and were greater in degree and duration than in comparable patients who subsequently died. Increased DO_2, as part of the body's stress response, is the principal physiologic response to acute circulatory deficits that limit body metabolism; this compensates for tissue oxygen debt due to inadequate tissue perfusion and oxygenation.

Tissue hypoxia also occurs with accidental trauma, hypovolemia, anesthesia, sepsis, and cardiac problems. These problems can be documented by early monitoring, which will enable evaluation of appropriate therapy to allow rapid achievement of physiologic goals and to prevent lethal organ failure. The alternative is to allow progressively increasing tissue hypoxia to lead to capillary leak and organ failure, which are widely regarded as major proximate causes of death.

Conclusions

1. The aim of physiologic monitoring is (1) to diagnose the etiologic and the functional basis of acute circulatory problems; (2) to evaluate cardiac function in terms of inflow pressure; (3) to evaluate pulmonary function in terms of arterial blood gases or pulse oximetry; (4) to evaluate tissue perfusion in terms of DO_2 and VO_2 or in terms of $PtcO_2$ and the $PtcO_2/FIO_2$ index; (5) to evaluate the relative effectiveness of alternative therapies on these interacting circulatory functions; and (6) to titrate therapy to achieve the optimal physiologic goals that effect the best outcome.

2. These aims are based on the assumption that acute circulatory dysfunction is easier to analyze and more effective to treat at its first appearance; the earlier it is treated, the more responsive it is to therapy.

3. The interactions of heart, lung, and tissue perfusion functions, as well as compensations for these, are more clearly evident in the early periods.

4. **Hypotension represents the beginning of decompensation, not the onset of shock.**

5. Circulatory dysfunction starts with the precipitating event (hemorrhage, trauma, surgery, sepsis), not with the onset of hypotension. When monitoring is not started until after hypotension appears, the first half of the circulatory dysfunction has been missed.

6. Increased CI and DO_2, which may precede the hypotensive episode, are early protective physiologic mechanisms stimulated by increased metabolic need and the adrenomedullary stress response.

7. The temporal patterns of high CI, DO_2, and VO_2 before the onset of hypotension in survivors of hemorrhagic, postoperative, traumatic, or septic shock indicate that increased CI and DO_2 are survival compensations that maintain the body's metabolic needs.

8. Increased CI and DO_2 values or their equivalent noninvasive monitored values may be used as therapeutic goals.

9. In nonsurvivors, the temporal pattern of lower CI, DO_2, and VO_2 before the onset of hypotension indicates overwhelming etiologic events, inadequate physiologic reserve capacity, or decompensation.

10. Increased CI and DO_2 often precede the hypotensive episode and are early protective physiologic mechanisms stimulated by increased metabolic need and the adrenomedullary stress response.

11. Inadequate tissue oxygenation due to inadequate perfusion is the basic pathophysiologic defect underlying most shock syndromes; low or uneven (i.e., maldistributed) flow is the direct cause of tissue hypoxia, organ dysfunction, organ failure, and death.

12. Oxygen debt may occur as a result of increased metabolic demand or reduced oxygen supply.

13. Decreased DO_2 occurs in cardiac failure, hypoxemia, respiratory failure, trauma, hemorrhage, dehydration, cardiopulmonary arrest, and other acute hypovolemic conditions.

14. Many chronic disorders may develop hypovolemia insidiously as well as low CI, which may be tolerated if there are no added stresses or infections.

15. The common life-threatening hypodynamic state is often associated with postoperative patients and patients with trauma who received inadequate volume resuscitation.

References

1. Wo CJ, Shoemaker WC, Appel PL, et al: Unreliability of blood pressure and heart rate to evaluate cardiac output in emergency resuscitation and critical illness. Crit Care Med 1993;21:218–223.
2. Bland R, Shoemaker WC, Shabot MM: Physiologic monitoring goals for the critically ill patient. Surg Gynecol Obstet 1978;147:833–841.
3. Shoemaker WC, Appel PL, Kram HB, et al: Prospective trial of supranormal values of survivors as therapeutic goals in high risk surgical patients. Chest 1988;94:1176–1186.
4. Shoemaker WC, Kram HB, Appel PL, et al: The efficacy of central venous and pulmonary artery catheters and therapy based upon them in reducing mortality and morbidity. Arch Surg 1990;125:1332–1338.
5. Boyd O, Grounds M, Bennett D: Preoperative increase of oxygen delivery reduces mortality in high risk surgical patients. JAMA 1993;270:2699–2704.
6. Berlauk JF, Abrams JH, Gilmour IJ, et al: Preoperative optimization of cardiovascular hemodynamics improves outcome in peripheral vascular surgery. Ann Surg 1991;214:289–297.
7. Hankeln KB, Sanker R, Schwarten JW, et al: Evaluation of prognostic indices based on hemodynamic and oxygen transport variables in shock patients with adult respiratory distress syndrome. Crit Care Med 1987;15:1–7.
8. Swan HJC, Ganz W, Forrester JS, et al: Catheterization of the heart in man with use of a flow-directed balloon-tipped catheter. N Engl J Med 1970;283:447–451.
9. Forrester JS, Diamond GA, Chatterjee K, et al: Medical therapy of acute myocardial information by application of hemodynamic subsets. N Engl J Med 1976;295:1356–1362.
10. Yu M, Levy MM, Smith P, et al: Effect of maximizing oxygen

delivery on mortality and mortality rates in critically ill patients: a prospective randomized controlled study. Crit Care Med 1993;21:830–838.

11. Wilson J, Woods I, Fawcett J, et al: Reducing the risk of major elective surgery: Randomized controlled trial of preoperative optimisation of oxygen delivery. BMJ 1999;318:1099–1103.

12. Boyd O, Bennett D: Enhancement of perioperative tissue perfusion as a therapeutic strategy for major surgery. New Horiz 1996;4:453–465.

13. Schulz RJ, Whitfield GF, La Mura JJ, et al: The role of physiologic monitoring in patients with fractures of hip. J Trauma 1985;25:309–316.

14. Bishop MW, Shoemaker WC, Kram HB, et al: Prospective randomized trial of survivor values of cardiac output, oxygen delivery, and oxygen consumption as resuscitation endpoints in severe trauma. J Trauma 1995;38:780–787.

15. Scalea TM, Simon HM, Duncan AO, et al: Geriatric blunt multiple trauma: Improved survival with early invasive monitoring. J Trauma 1990;30:129–136.

16. Moore FA, Haemel JB, Moore EE, et al: Incommensurate oxygen consumption in response to maximal oxygen availability predicts postinjury oxygen failure. J Trauma 1992;33:58–62.

17. Edwards JD, Redmond AD, Nightingale P, et al: Oxygen consumption following trauma. Br J Surg 1988;75:690–692.

18. Siegel JH, Rivkind AI, Dolal S, et al: Early physiologic predictors of injury and severity and death in blunt multiple trauma. Arch Surg 1990;125:498–508.

19. Edwards JD, Brown GCS, Nightingale P, et al: Use of survivors' cardiorespiratory values as therapeutic goals in septic shock. Crit Care Med 1989;17:1098–1103.

20. Shoemaker WC, Appel PL, Kram HB: Hemodynamic and oxygen transport responses in survivors and nonsurvivors of high risk surgery. Crit Care Med 1993;21:977–990.

21. Abraham E, Bland RD, Cobo JC, et al: Sequential cardiorespiratory patterns associated with outcome in septic shock. Chest 1984;85:75–80.

22. Tuchschmidt J, Fried J, Astiz M, Rackow E: Evaluation of cardiac output and oxygen delivery improves outcome in septic shock. Chest 1992;102:216–220.

23. Rackow EC, Kaufman BS, Falk JL, et al: Hemodynamic response to fluid repletion in patients with septic shock: Evidence for early depression of cardiac performance. Circ Shock 1987;22:11–22.

24. Creamer JE, Edwards JD, Nightingale P: Hemodynamic and oxygen transport variables in cardiogenic shock secondary to acute myocardial infarction. Am J Cardiol 1990;65:1297–1300.

25. Rady MY, Edwards JD, Rivers EP, et al: Measurement of oxygen consumption after uncomplicated acute myocardial infarction. Chest 1993;103:886–895.

26. Bishop MH, Shoemaker WC, Shuleshko J, Wo CCJ: Noninvasive cardiac index monitoring in gunshot wound victims. Acad Emerg Med 1996;3:682–688.

27. Shippy CR, Appel PL, Shoemaker WC: Reliability of clinical monitoring to assess blood volume in critically ill patients. Crit Care Med 1984;12:107–112.

28. Shoemaker WC, Belzberg H, Wo CCJ, et al: Multicenter study of noninvasive monitoring systems as alternatives to invasive monitoring of acutely ill emergency patients. Chest 1998;114:1643–1652.

29. Pasquale MD, Cipolle MD, Lundgren P, et al: Effect of oxygen delivery on outcome in trauma patients. Clin Intensive Care 1994;4:21–24.

30. Shoemaker WC, Appel PL, Kram HB: Role of oxygen debt in the development of organ failure, sepsis, and death in high-risk surgical patients. Chest 1992;102:208–215.

31. Dunham CM, Siegel JH, Weireter L, et al: Oxygen debt and metabolic acidemia as quantitative predictors of mortality and the severity of the ischemic insult in hemorrhagic shock. Crit Care Med 1991;19:231–243.

32. Crowell JW, Smith EE: Oxygen deficit and irreversible hemorrhagic shock. Am J Physiol 1964;106:313–319.

33. Guyton AC, Crowell JW: Dynamics of the heart in shock. Fed Proc 1961;10:51–54.

34. Hauser CJ, Shoemaker WC, Turpin I, et al: Hemodynamic and oxygen transport responses to body water shifts produced by colloids and crystalloids in critically ill patients. Surg Gynecol Obstet 1980;150: 811–818.

35. Lazrove S, Wawman K, Shoemaker WC: Hemodynamic, blood volume, and oxygen transport responses to albumin and hydroxyethyl starch infusions in critically ill postoperative patients. Crit Care Med 1990;8:392–398.

36. Shoemaker WC, Appel PL, Kram HB, et al: Sequence of physiologic patterns in surgical septic shock. Crit Care Med 1993;21:1876–1889.

37. Shoemaker WC, Appel PL, Kram HB, et al: Temporal hemodynamic and oxygen transport patterns in medical patients with sepsis and septic shock. Chest 1993;104:1529–1536.

38. Shoemaker WC, Wo CCJ, Chan L, et al: Outcome prediction of severely injured patients by noninvasive monitoring beginning in the emergency department. Chest 2001; in press.

39. Shoemaker WC, Wo CCJ, Sullivan MJ, et al: Invasive and noninvasive monitoring of acutely ill sepsis and septic shock patients in the Emergency Department. Eur J Emerg Med 2000;7:169–175.

29 Hemodynamic Therapy for Circulatory Dysfunction

William C. Shoemaker

Monitoring and Initial Care of Acute Illnesses

Shock syndromes are affected by age, previous illnesses, comorbid conditions, cardiac reserve capacity, time from onset, and delays in recognition and in fluid resuscitation that affect cardiac, pulmonary, and tissue perfusion to various degrees. An integrated approach to monitoring and therapy that begins in the emergency department is based on continuously monitored patterns obtained with recently available noninvasive monitoring systems. The approach is to identify hemodynamic problems and to titrate therapy to optimal goals as expeditiously as possible. Early or preventative therapy is easier and more effective than waiting until the patient is admitted to the intensive care unit after organ failure has occurred.

Use of a Therapeutic Algorithm

A branched-chain decision tree or clinical algorithm (Fig. 29–1) for high-risk surgical patients has been developed. Priorities were assigned according to decision-making rules based on survivor and nonsurvivor patterns from previous series, outcome predictors, controlled prospective clinical trials of the oxygen delivery/oxygen consumption (DO_2/VO_2) concept, and responses of various therapeutic agents.[1]

The general algorithm (see Fig. 29–1) may be used as an initial starting point for most cases; for future studies, however, better management may be provided by modifying this simplified, general-purpose algorithm to provide physicians and nurses with clearer guidance relevant to the patient's specific circumstances. Modification may be necessary based on the following: age, gender, various diagnostic and high-risk categories, previous preoperative hyperdynamic states (e.g., trauma, stress, sepsis, recent surgery, late-stage cirrhosis), previous hypodynamic states (e.g., hemorrhage, hypovolemia, cardiogenic problems), actual time elapsed postoperatively, terminal states, specific postoperative organ failure (e.g., respiratory, renal, hepatic, cardiac, central nervous system), and postoperative complications (e.g., sepsis, septic shock, disseminated intravascular coagulation, nutritional failure).[2]

Strategies for Therapeutic Decisions Using DO_2 and VO_2 as Criteria

The basic strategy is to optimize hemodynamic and oxygen transport variables in the first 8 hours postoperatively based on the range defined empirically by the survivors' values (as a first approximation). Then, additional therapy may be titrated more gradually to reach the second end point, in which DO_2 is increased (with appropriate safeguards) until there is no further increase in VO_2. The objective is to minimize the degree and the duration of tissue hypoxia by using physiologic goals as proxy outcome measures for gross, rapid titration and by using the concept of "VO_2 independence" for gradual titration to the final end point.[3] The strategy is to attain the mean values of survivors rapidly as a first approximation of therapeutic goals.

DO_2 values before therapy and DO_2 and VO_2 interactions after therapy provide objective criteria for evaluation of therapeutic goals and the relative effects of alternative therapies. As a first approximation, the mean values for survivors of each etiologic category may be used as the therapeutic goal. These goals were developed for the first 8 hours after high-risk surgery and the first 24 hours after trauma. The usefulness of further increases in DO_2, when done early in the postoperative or the post-traumatic course, to maximize VO_2 in the presence of an oxygen debt has been demonstrated repeatedly.[2, 4–11]

The responses to alternative therapy may be a measure of therapeutic efficacy and appropriateness. When suboptimal DO_2 and VO_2 are present, a trial of therapy is indicated. The therapy that is most effective should be given subsequently in a standardized dose and time frame. If that therapy is effective, additional therapy may be given to attain the best values possible. If the therapy is not effective, another agent may be tried and titrated in a similar manner. The agent that

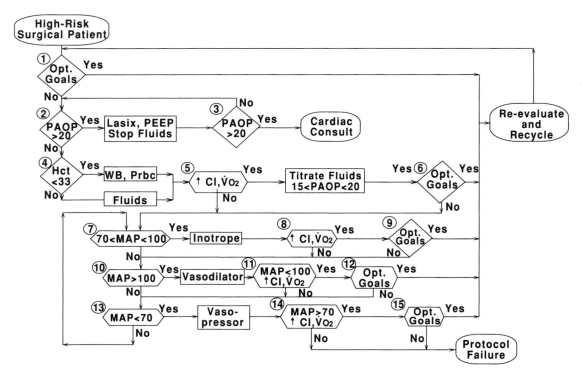

FIGURE 29–1. Revised branched-chain decision tree.

Step 1: Determine whether the patient has reached the optimal goals. Measure cardiac index (CI), oxygen delivery (DO₂), and oxygen consumption (VO₂). If CI is more than 4.5 L/min/m², DO₂ is more than 800 mL/min/m², and VO₂ is more than 170 mL/min/m², the goals are reached, and the first objective of the algorithm has been achieved. Re-evaluate and recycle at intervals to maintain these goals. If any of the preceding optimal values were not reached, proceed to step 2.

Step 2: Take pulmonary artery occlusion pressure (PAOP). If PAOP is greater than 20 mm Hg, proceed to step 3; if PAOP is less than 20 mm Hg, proceed to step 4.

Step 3: If PAOP is greater than 20 mm Hg, and there is clinical or radiographic evidence of salt and water overload or clinical findings of pulmonary congestion, give furosemide intravenously at increasing doses to produce diuresis and to lower PAOP. If not, consider vasodilators, nitroprusside, or nitroglycerin if mean arterial pressure (MAP) is more than 80 mm Hg and systolic arterial pressure (SAP) is greater than 100 mm Hg; titrate the dose needed to maintain PAOP between 15 and 20 mm Hg and MAP at greater than 80 mm Hg. If unsuccessful, obtain cardiology consult and place on cardiac protocol.

Step 4: If hematocrit (Hct) is less than 33%, give 1 U of whole blood (WB) or 2 U of packed red blood cells (Prbc). If Hct is greater than 33%, give a fluid load (volume challenge) consisting of one of the following (depending on clinical indications of plasma volume deficit or hydration): 5% plasma protein factor, 500 mL; 5% albumin, 500 mL; 25% albumin (25 g), 100 mL; 6% hydroxyethyl starch, 500 mL; 6% dextran-60, 500 mL; lactated Ringer's solution (RL), 1000 mL.

Step 5: If the blood or the fluid load improves CI, DO₂, or VO₂, continue to give appropriate fluids to increase these variables; if these are improved with adequate volume, proceed to step 8. Continue to infuse fluids until PAOP is between 15 and 20 mm Hg; if PAOP reaches 20 mm Hg before optimal goals are reached, proceed to step 8.

Step 6: If optimal goals are reached, recycle; if not, proceed to step 8.

Step 7: If MAP is between 70 and 100 mm Hg, give dobutamine by constant intravenous infusion to optimize CI, DO₂, and VO₂.

Step 8: Titrate dobutamine beginning with 2 μg/min/kg and gradually increasing to 20 μg/min/kg, provided there is improvement in CI, DO₂, or VO₂ without further lowering of blood pressure until goals are met.

Step 9: If goals are reached, re-evaluate and recycle. If goals are not reached or it becomes evident that higher drug doses are not more effective or that they produce hypotension, tachycardia, or dysrhythmia, continue dobutamine at its most effective dose range and proceed to step 10.

Step 10: If MAP is greater than 100 mm Hg, give a vasodilator, such as nitroprusside, nitroglycerin, labetalol, or prostaglandin E₁.

Step 11: Titrate vasodilators to decrease MAP and to increase CI, DO₂, and VO₂. If there is no improvement in CI, DO₂, or VO₂ with the vasodilator or if hypotension (MAP of less than 80 mm Hg, SAP of less than 110 mm Hg) occurs, reduce the dose of or discontinue the vasodilator. If there is improvement in CI, DO₂, or VO₂, titrate vasodilator to its maximum CI, DO₂, or VO₂ effects consistent with satisfactory pressures.

Step 12: If optimal goals are reached, re-evaluate and recycle at intervals to maintain optimal goals.

Step 13: If these goals are not reached and MAP is less than 80 mm Hg with an SAP of less than 110 mm Hg, give dopamine or another vasopressor.

Step 14: Titrate vasopressor (dopamine) to the lowest dose that maintains MAP of more than 70 mm Hg and SAP of more than 110 mm Hg and that increases CI, DO₂, and VO₂ to their optimal values. If pressure cannot be maintained or optimal goals cannot be reached, the patient is considered to be a protocol failure; consider re-evaluation and recycling.

Step 15: If optimal goals are reached, re-evaluate and recycle. Opt., optimal; PEEP, positive end-expiratory pressure. (From Shoemaker WC, Appel PL, Kram HB: Oxygen transport measurements to evaluate tissue perfusion and titrate therapy: Dobutamine and dopamine effects. Crit Care Med 1991;19:672–688.)

achieves the most salutary effects for each clinical stratification may be determined by retrospective analysis plus prospective verification.

Proposed Therapeutic Plan

We propose modifications of a therapeutic plan previously guided by invasive thermodilution cardiac index measurements; this and similar concepts were evaluated prospectively in a large number of randomized and nonrandomized clinical trials.[4-11] If cardiac index as measured by means of bioimpedance is not 4.5 L/min/m² or greater, the pulse oximetry is not greater than 94%, the transcutaneous partial pressure of oxygen is not greater than 60 torr, and the central venous pressure is less than 18 mm Hg, administer fluid therapy, principally colloids, and whole blood or packed red blood cells as needed to attain these values and to maintain hematocrit values at 34%. Fluids are continued until the cardiac index increases to 4.5 L/min/m² or the central venous pressure rises to more than 18 mm Hg. When there is no further increase in cardiac index, give inotropic agents (e.g., dobutamine) in increasing doses from 5 to 40 μg/kg/min or give phosphodiesterase inhibitors. When hypertensive episodes are present or when there is an inadequate response to fluids and inotropic agents, give a therapeutic trial of vasodilators (e.g., nitroprusside, nitroglycerin, hydralazine, labetalol). To prevent sudden hypotension, the patient must receive a fluid volume load that is adequate to restore blood volume before administration of vasodilators and inotropic agents with vasodilating actions ("inodilators"). This necessitates blood volume (not total body water) restitution, because a patient may have 4+ pitting edema and still be hypovolemic. Titrate inotropic and vasodilator therapy to bring blood pressure to acceptable levels and cardiac index up to optimal values. If hypotension is not corrected by administration of adequate fluids and inotropes, give vasopressors to maintain diastolic, mean, and systolic pressures of more than 70, 80, and 100 mm Hg, respectively, in patients who were previously normotensive. Vasopressors are used as a last resort because their α-adrenergic effects intensify the uneven metarteriolar vasoconstriction that is a basic underlying hemodynamic mechanism of shock. Persistent hypotension of less than 90/60 mm Hg may limit cerebral and myocardial perfusion, however.

Assessment of Fluid Therapy

For many acute illnesses seen in the emergency department, fluid administration is an integral part of therapy. In the initial resuscitation, most acutely ill patients receive several liters of intravenous crystalloids; those with pulmonary edema or acute myocardial infarction may also receive some colloids when central venous pressure or pulmonary artery wedge pressure is less than 18 mm Hg. The response to transfusions or fluid therapy is conventionally assessed by intermittent recording of vital signs and other indirect markers of hypovolemia (e.g., skin turgor, urinary output, capillary refill); correction of these indirect markers is supposed to signify adequate intravascular expansion. These markers have limited sensitivity and specificity for the adequacy of fluid therapy, however. Improvement in cardiac, pulmonary, and tissue perfusion, as measured noninvasively, reflects appropriate outcome.[12, 13] With immediate feedback on the effects of each fluid, therapy may be titrated to achieve and maintain optimal physiologic goals.

Noninvasive Monitoring to Guide Therapy

The indications for therapy can be defined by diagnostic categories, which include diseases that compromise circulatory function or that produce organ failure or death (Table 29–1). When the diagnosis is known, patients may profit from hemodynamic monitoring, which will enable specific therapy to be titrated to achieve optimal values for that condition. Clinical signs and symptoms reflect unstable hemodynamic states in widely varying conditions. Usually, hypovolemia, low-flow states, and poor tissue perfusion are underlying problems. Noninvasive monitoring may be undertaken in the emergency department in specific diagnostic conditions with suspected deficits, or it may be employed because nonspecific clinical assessment suggests underlying circulatory dysfunction. In either case, monitoring is used to measure the degree of circula-

TABLE 29–1. Diagnostic Categories Prone to Develop Circulatory Dysfunction

Blunt trauma
Gunshot wounds
Stab wounds
Burns
Crushing injuries
Hemorrhage
Acute myocardial infarction
Heart failure with or without pulmonary edema
Dysrhythmias
Pneumonia
Cellulitis
Sepsis
Heat exhaustion
Alcoholic cirrhosis
Hyperemesis gravidarum
Drug overdose
Protracted vomiting or diarrhea
Prolonged diuretic therapy
Seizures

tory impairment and to titrate therapy to achieve these goals as expeditiously as possible.[11-16]

The key to initial resuscitation is earlier warning via noninvasive monitoring systems employed in the emergency department and prompt adequate therapy titrated to achieve optimal physiologic goals. This is in contrast to the situation in chronically ill medical patients, for whom resuscitation is complex and controversial. The crucial problems are the following: What is the nature of the circulatory disorder we are treating? How do we describe and measure it? Beginning in the emergency department, what are the early temporal hemodynamic patterns that determine outcome? How do various fluids, transfusions, blood products, and plasma substitutes affect outcome?

Fluid and Transfusion Therapy

Hypovolemia is the most common cause of low flow and is the most easily correctable. For critically ill high-risk postoperative patients, vigorous fluid therapy that does not cause the pulmonary artery wedge pressure to exceed 20 mm Hg is the first and most important step in achieving the optimal goals. It is appropriate to reach these goals without overexpanding the interstitial space with crystalloids.

In critically ill patients, it is important to correct acute anemia associated with blood loss. Usually, packed red cells are given to maintain hematocrit at 30% to 33%. In healthy ambulatory patients, a hematocrit of 25% to 30% may be readily tolerated, but critically ill patients often require sufficient transfusions to achieve a hematocrit that will optimize the DO_2 value.

Prospective Trials of Lactated Ringer's Solution and Albumin

In a prospective randomized crossover study, invasive hemodynamic monitoring was used to measure the relative effectiveness of 1.0 L of Ringer's lactate (RL) solution and 100 mL of 25% albumin given to postoperative patients in early adult respiratory distress syndrome (Figs. 29–2 and 29–3).[17] (Early was defined as being within 24 to 48 hours of diagnosis.) Each agent was given to each patient; half the patients received RL solution first, then crossed over to the colloid, and the other half received albumin first, then RL solution.

Data are shown for the baseline control, for the infusion period, and for regular intervals for 180 minutes thereafter. These data show that 1000 mL of RL solution increased blood volume by only 200 mL at the end of the infusion, which was the maximum volume effect; this effect lasted less than 1 hour. The administration of 100 mL of 25% albumin increased blood volume an average of 450 mL, which lasted

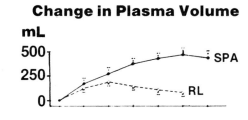

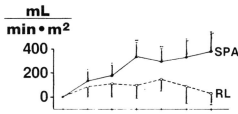

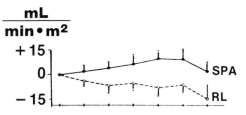

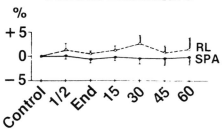

FIGURE 29–2. Comparison of changes in plasma volume, cardiac index, oxygen consumption, and pulmonary venous admixture (shunt) after 25 g of albumin in 100 mL (SPA) and 1000 mL of lactated Ringer's solution (RL) were given in random order to a series of postoperative patients shortly after the onset of adult respiratory distress syndrome. (From Shoemaker WC, Appel PL, Bishop MH: Temporal patterns of blood volume, hemodynamics, and oxygen transport in pathogenesis and therapy of postoperative adult respiratory distress syndrome. New Horiz 1993;1:522–536.)

about 4 hours. The slightly greater response to starch lasted about 6 hours.

In essence, the colloids did not leak in the early stages of acute illness; rather, the 25% albumin dragged 350 mL of interstitial water back into the plasma volume. With this increase in plasma volume,

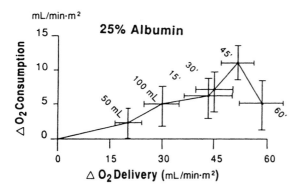

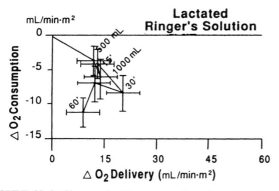

FIGURE 29–3. Changes in O_2 consumption plotted against corresponding changes in O_2 delivery during and 15, 30, 45, and 60 minutes after infusion of 100 mL of 25% albumin *(top)* and 1000 mL of lactated Ringer's solution *(bottom)*; values are mean plus or minus the standard error of the mean. (From Shoemaker WC, Appel PL, Bishop MH: Temporal patterns of blood volume, hemodynamics, and oxygen transport in pathogenesis and therapy of postoperative adult respiratory distress syndrome. New Horiz 1993;1:522–536.)

there was an increase in cardiac index, colloidal osmotic pressure, and VO_2 without worsening of the alveolar-arterial oxygen tension difference—the $P(A–a)O_2$ gradient, or the pulmonary shunt. Albumin significantly improved both DO_2 and VO_2, whereas RL solution transiently increased DO_2 and actually decreased VO_2 because it expanded the amount of interstitial water, which increased the oxygen diffusion pathway and the diffusion time.[18] The data indicate that in early postoperative states and in early adult respiratory distress syndrome, colloids are remarkably effective. This suggests that capillary leak, if present, does not yet limit the therapeutic effectiveness of colloids. In the terminal stage in nonsurvivors, however, neither colloids nor crystalloids are effective and both increase capillary leak.

Blood Volume Effects of Albumin and Starch

In a prospective randomized crossover study, the blood volume response to 500 mL of 6% hydroxyethyl starch was compared with the response to 500 mL of 5% albumin in a series of critically ill patients, with each

agent being given to each patient (Fig. 29–4).[19] Blood volume effects of hydroxyethyl starch persisted 6 to 10 hours; the effects of 500 mL of 5% albumin and of 100 mL of 25% albumin persisted 3.5 to 4.5 hours; and the effects of 1000 mL of RL solution lasted about 45 minutes to 1 hour. In other studies, the hemodynamic effects of dextran 40 and gelatin lasted about 1.5 to 2 hours. Thus, the effects on plasma volume, flow, and oxygen transport were found to be greater and more sustained after colloid administration than after crystalloid administration.

In the initial resuscitation of the hypertensive trauma patient or in a patient who is on a salt-restricted diet preoperatively, 25% albumin may be useful. Similarly, the patient who has been given excessive amounts of crystalloids resulting in massive peripheral or pulmonary edema may do better with concentrated albumin. In many cases, 6% hetastarch or the newly approved pentastarch is appropriate.

Effects of Colloids and Crystalloids

The relative effectiveness of various types of fluid therapy was studied in patients shortly after admission to the emergency department as well as in patients in the operating room and the intensive care unit. The common hemodynamic patterns in nonsurvivors included decreased flow and decreased tissue perfusion, reflected by reduced cardiac index, reduced DO_2, and reduced VO_2 on invasive monitoring and by reduced flow and reduced tissue perfusion on noninvasive monitoring. More important, both invasive and noninvasive monitoring was used to evaluate the earliest phase of shock as well as initial resuscitation and subsequent therapeutic responses to various fluid regimens in the emergency department.

Table 29–2 describes increases in cardiac index, mean arterial pressure, arterial hemoglobin saturation by pulse oximetry ($SapO_2$), transcutaneous oxygen tension/fraction of inspired oxygen ($PtcO_2/FIO_2$), and transcutaneous partial pressure of carbon dioxide ($PtcO_2$) in 65 instances after 2 units of packed red blood cells were given as well as 500 mL of colloids (5% albumin, fresh frozen plasma, and 6% hydroxyethyl starch) and 1000 mL of crystalloids (RL solution) to patients with traumatic injury shortly after admission to the emergency department. These data document improvements in pressure, flow, and tissue perfusion after transfusions of packed red blood cells and colloids. There was a significant increase in cardiac index, mean arterial pressure, and oxygen transport after administration of packed red blood cells and colloids (albumin, starch, and fresh frozen plasma); crystalloids (1000 mL of RL solution) did not significantly improve cardiac index or oxygen metabolism. In these emergency conditions, continuing blood

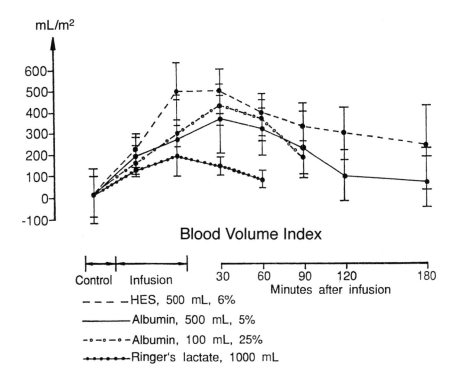

FIGURE 29–4. Changes in blood volume from two prospective randomized crossover studies: 1000 mL of Ringer's lactate solution versus 100 mL of 25% albumin, and 500 mL of 6% hydroxyethyl starch (HES) versus 500 mL of 5% albumin. Measurements are made during a 30-minute control period and a 60-minute infusion period and are then followed for 3 hours after the infusion ends. *Dots* are mean values, *vertical lines* are standard error of the mean.

losses were present in many patients. Nevertheless, whole blood, packed red blood cells, and colloids improved these variables under comparable conditions.[20]

Table 29–3 shows the effects of 172 administrations of 500 mL of 5% albumin, fresh frozen plasma, and 6% hydroxyethyl starch or hetastarch. It demonstrates statistically significant improvements in cardiac index, mean arterial pressure, and tissue perfusion. Table 29–4 summarizes the effects of 132 infusions of 1000 mL of RL solution given to emergency department patients with traumatic injury; no significant changes in the hemodynamic variables were noted.

Inotropic Agents

Inotropic agents may be used after the maximum effects of fluid therapy have been attained. Dobutamine, which is an inotrope and a vasodilator (inodilator), is the agent of choice because it improves cardiac

contractility and also, by its β_2-blocking effect, relaxes previously vasoconstricted metarterioles and thus improves microcirculatory flow and tissue oxygenation.[21] Initially, the drug may be started at 5 μg/kg/minute and may be increased as required to reach optimal goals. Hypotension may occur when hypovolemia has not been corrected. Alternatively, the phosphodiesterase inhibitors (amrinone or milrinone), which also have a β_2-blocking action, may be used to optimize DO_2 and VO_2. They are more difficult to titrate, however, and infrequently produce bleeding problems and dysrhythmias.

Vasopressors

Dopamine, norepinephrine, and epinephrine are often used to correct hypotension. They should be administered after fluid resuscitation of blood flow, because vasoconstriction may worsen tissue perfusion at

TABLE 29–2. Hemodynamic Changes Detected by Noninvasive Monitoring in Emergency Patients

Variable	Prbc, 2 Units (n = 65)	Colloids, 500 mL (n = 15)	RL, 1000 mL (n = 65)
CI, L/min/m^2	0.59 ± .15*	0.59 ± .10*	0.30 ± .21
MAP, mm Hg	6.2 ± 3.7	9.2 ± 4.1†	−0.7 ± 2.1
SaO$_2$, %	−1.8 ± 1.44	−0.9 ± .4	−0.5 ± .4
PtcO$_2$/FIO$_2$	22.6 ± 15.2	40.7 ± 13.9*	9.2 ± 6.2
PtcCO$_2$	−3.1 ± 2.5	0.9 ± 1.6	0.2 ± 1.5

*$P < .01$.
†$P < .05$.
Values are mean ± standard error of the mean.
CI, cardiac index; MAP, mean arterial pressure; Prbc, packed red blood cells; PtcCO$_2$, transcutaneous carbon dioxide tension; PtcO$_2$/FIO$_2$, transcutaneous oxygen tension/fractional inspired oxygen concentration; RL, Ringer's lactate; SaO$_2$, arterial oxygen saturation.

TABLE 29–3. Hemodynamic Changes Detected by Noninvasive Monitoring after Administration of 500 mL of Various Colloids to Emergency Patients

Variable	5% Albumin (n = 15)	FFP (n = 45)	Hydroxyethyl Starch (n = 87)	Total
CI, L/min/m²	0.46 ± .09*	0.50 ± .15*	0.53 ± .05*	0.51 ± 0.04*
MAP, mm Hg	1.73 ± 2.1	3.7 ± 1.3†	5.4 ± 1.5*	4.4 ± 0.92*
SaO₂, %	−0.4 ± 0.4	−0.2 ± 4.5	−0.1 ± 1.5	−0.2 ± 0.19
PtcO₂/FIO₂	10.5 ± 3.4*	14.7 ± 5.1*	19.5 ± 4.8*	17.9 ± 3.2*
PtcCO₂	0.9 ± 1.1	−1.2 ± 0.8	0.0 ± 0.4	−0.4 ± 0.4

*$P < .01$.
†$P < .05$.
Values are in mean ± standard error of the mean.
CI, cardiac index; FFP, fresh frozen plasma; MAP, mean arterial pressure; $PtcCO_2$, transcutaneous carbon dioxide tension; $PtcO_2/FIO_2$, transcutaneous oxygen tension/fractional inspired oxygen concentration; SaO_2, arterial oxygen saturation.

the microcirculatory level as a result of α_1-agonist actions on metarterioles.[21]

Vasodilators

Vasodilators (e.g., nitroprusside, nitroglycerin, hydralazine, labetalol, and prostaglandin E_1) may be used when the pulmonary artery wedge pressure exceeds 20 mm Hg and optimal goals have not been met. Be sure that blood volume has been fully restored and that the arterial pressure is normal before starting vasodilators. β_1-Blockers such as propranolol should be avoided because they decrease the cardiac index and tissue oxygenation.

Crystalloids

Based on experimental and clinical studies, Shires and colleagues used the labeled sulfate ($^{35}SO_4$) method to determine that in both hemorrhagic and traumatic shock, there is a reduction in extracellular water (ECW) in excess of the measured plasma volume losses.[22] They also reported increased intracellular water after shock, which they assumed was due to leaking of salt and water into the body's cells. Both hemorrhagic and traumatic shock were thought to have the same pattern and underlying mechanisms, and no distinction between the two was necessary. Hemorrhagic

shock is associated with reduced ECW from shifts of water within the body, reduced transmembrane potential, and altered intracellular electrolyte concentrations, producing intracellular swelling of skeletal muscle cells. Replacement of the ECW deficit is considered to be of paramount importance for restoration of cellular metabolism and survival.

Critique of the Labeled Sulfate Method

There are several serious flaws in the labeled sulfate method of measuring ECW, including (1) the inappropriate choice of labeled sulfate as an indicator of the amount of ECW, (2) failure to achieve equilibrium of sulfate in shock, (3) failure to distinguish the physiologic effects of hemorrhage from those of trauma, and (4) errors in intracellular water values calculated from spuriously low ECW values.[22]

The crystalloid approach is based on measurement of ECW by the ^{35}S method, which does not measure the same ECW volume as ^{82}Br, ^{38}Cl, ^{22}Na, and ^{24}Na. Results using the latter are consistent with each other and with total body water (measured by use of tritiated water) minus the intracellular water (measured by use of radiopotassium). These isotope studies agree with data obtained from studies of ashed bodies of recently deceased patients. The sulfate method gives an estimation for ECW of about 16% of body weight, whereas the bromide space is normally 24% of body weight, or about 50% more than the sulfate space.

TABLE 29–4. Hemodynamic Changes Detected by Noninvasive Monitoring after Administration of 1000 mL of Ringer's Lactate Solution to Emergency Patients

Variable	ED (n = 65)	OR (n = 45)	ICU (n = 22)	Total (n = 132)
CI, L/min/m²	0.30 ± .21	0.06 ± .09	0.14 ± .15	0.19 ± 0.11
MAP, mm Hg	−0.7 ± 2.1	−2.9 ± 2.1	1.4 ± 3.4	−1.1 ± 1.4
SaO₂, %	−0.5 ± .4	−0.8 ± 1.5	0.1 ± 0.3	−0.5 ± 0.3
PtcO₂/FIO₂	9.2 ± 6.2	−3.0 ± 12.9	16.5 ± 14.4	6.9 ± 6.1
PtcCO₂	0.2 ± 1.5	−1.3 ± 0.7	0.1 ± 2.6	−0.3 ± 0.9

Values are mean ± standard error of the mean.
CI, cardiac index; ED, emergency department; ICU, intensive care unit; MAP, mean arterial pressure; OR, operating room; $PtcCO_2$, transcutaneous CO_2 tension; $PtcO_2/FIO_2$, transcutaneous O_2 tension/fractional inspired oxygen concentration; SaO_2, arterial oxygen saturation.

A major problem is that sulfate is predominantly an intracellular ion, which eventually equilibrates in the intracellular pool. Estimation of ECW via the labeled sulfate method is based on the equilibration of the injected label in the body's extracellular pool before it enters the cells, where it is metabolized. The labeled sulfate begins to enter the cells before it is completely equilibrated in the ECW, however.[22]

Initially, the measurement of ECW was based on values obtained at the arbitrary time of 45 to 60 minutes after injection, but this resulted in very small ECW values because mixing was not yet complete. This problem was solved by selecting arbitrary times on the radioactivity-time curve to calculate ECW, on the assumption that most or all of the injected labeled sulfate was in the ECW at these times and that none had entered the cells.

In addition, there is a slower falloff of the labeled sulfate during non–steady state shock conditions that results in ECW values that are lower than normal. This delay in equilibration is interpreted as reduced extracellular fluid in shock conditions, but the delay is more likely due to impaired circulation resulting from the underlying shock state. It is obvious that if the heart stops before the labeled sulfate leaves the plasma volume, the volume of distribution of the label may closely approximate the plasma volume, which is about one fourth the ECW volume. Similarly, if the impaired circulation in shock delays sulfate equilibration in the ECW, spuriously low ECW values result.[18]

In essence, the sulfate method does not fulfill the two necessary conditions of isotope methodology: (1) that the boundary conditions of the space being measured are known and (2) that there is complete mixing of the injected labeled compound within these boundaries. Incomplete equilibration of the sulfate label results in spuriously low ECW values under normal conditions and even greater disparities in shock, when equilibration takes longer.

Most patients with traumatic injury also have hemorrhage, but these two conditions have different responses. Hemorrhage reduces plasma volume and redistributes the ECW by transcapillary migration of fluid from the interstitium to refill plasma volume in accordance with Starling's law of the capillaries. In contrast, the steroid stress responses of trauma lead to fluid retention with increased ECW but without correction of the hypovolemia. In high-risk postoperative patients, the [82]Br space averaged 8 L in excess of normal values after blood losses were replaced; at that time, blood volumes were still 500 mL deficient.[18] Other investigations have found no reduction in ECW following hemorrhage other than the fluid removed during the production of hemorrhagic shock.[18]

The concept that fluid is sequestered somewhere in the ECW assumes that the sulfate label is normally equilibrated in the ECW in shock. Failure to achieve equilibration of the sulfate label results in spuriously low ECW values. When excessive body water is known to develop with massive fluid infusions, the extra water is thought to be in the third space, which by definition is the transcellular space that includes the peritoneal cavity (ascites), the pleural cavity (effusion), the intraluminal space of the bowel, the synovial membranes, and the anterior chamber of the eye. Failure to find the missing water is best explained by a delay in mixing of the label, not by the disappearance of ECW into a third space.

A widely held concept is that plasma volume is one third of the ECW, but this has not been documented in shock and trauma states. Giving crystalloids in an amount that is three times the estimated blood loss to correct hypovolemia depends on the assumption that fluids will equilibrate with the plasma volume in shock as well as in normal states. In postoperative states, however, only 20% of administered RL solution remains in the plasma volume at the end of infusion, and most of this leaks into the ISW 40 to 60 minutes later.[17]

In essence, a reduction in sulfate space has not been demonstrated to be the cause of shock or death. The decrease in sulfate space after hemorrhagic hypotension and its correction with fluid therapy indicate that these may be associated with shock but are not necessarily its cause. The correction of sulfate-measured ECW volume without correction of blood volume deficits has not been shown to reduce mortality or morbidity in controlled clinical trials. Moreover, there is no direct evidence that ECW reduction is an important pathogenic problem or that it is directly related to outcome. Furthermore, peripheral edema, which occurs in most patients with shock or traumatic injury, indicates expanded, not contracted, ECW. A finding of reduced ECW (calculated via the sulfate method) when there is actually an expanded amount of ECW with hypovolemia may lead to further expansion of body water and adult respiratory distress syndrome without blood volume correction.[18, 21]

Therapy for Acute Low-Flow States

Vasodilators such as nitroprusside, nitroglycerin, hydralazine, labetalol, and prostaglandin E_1 may be used when pulmonary artery wedge pressure exceeds 20 mm Hg and optimal goals are not met. It is necessary to ensure that blood volume has been fully restored and that the arterial pressure is normal before starting vasodilators. β_1-Blockers such as propranolol should be avoided because they decrease cardiac index and tissue oxygenation.

If there are hypertensive episodes or an inadequate response to fluid or inotropes, a therapeutic trial of vasodilators should be given. (See previous discussion, "Proposed Therapeutic Plan," for more details.)

Dopamine, norepinephrine, and epinephrine are often used to correct hypotension. They should be used after fluid resuscitation of blood flow because uneven metarteriolar vasoconstriction worsens tissue oxygenation.

Titration to Optimal Goals

Therapeutic goals were defined empirically as the median or the mean values for survivors of "all comers" for a given disorder. This approach obscures the fact that there is actually a wide range of values.[9] It is not possible to test a range: Prospective trials of therapeutic goals require that a single arbitrary cutoff point be tested. Therefore, the goals described previously should be considered first approximations of optimal values. After the mean survivor values for DO_2 and VO_2 have been attained, it is appropriate to increase circulatory function further to ensure that the VO_2 is at its maximum. For example, if therapy increases DO_2 by 50 to 100 mL/min/m², and VO_2 also increases by 15 to 25 mL/min/m², supply-dependent VO_2 may be assumed, and further therapy should be considered. If, in contrast, no increase in VO_2 resulted from significant increases in DO_2, supply-independent VO_2 may be assumed, suggesting that the oxygen debt has been corrected or the microcirculatory defect is irreversible or has not been corrected with the therapy and the dose used.[18, 22–25]

DO_2 Responses to Therapy as Criteria of Outcome

The capacity of tissues to maintain VO_2 while DO_2 is decreasing represents a compensatory circulatory response. It is important to recognize increased DO_2 as a compensation as well as to understand its limitations. First, there is a wide range of DO_2 and VO_2 values for both survivors and nonsurvivors, but it is not possible to test a range of values, only an arbitrary cutoff point. The prospective clinical trials, therefore, have only tested the hypothesis for all patients in a general overall fashion; they do not provide specific goals for high-risk subgroups (previous cardiac or respiratory conditions, multiple trauma, sepsis, and so forth). When median values were used as therapeutic criteria, 49% of patients in the reference series did not reach the median value but still survived, whereas 50% required more than the median value to survive. Obviously, the criteria can be only a "first approximation" for each individual high-risk patient. Even with these limitations, the optimization of DO_2 and VO_2 values has been shown to be cost effective.[25] Ultimately, with advanced information systems, customized optimal values may be developed for individual patients according to their specific clinical conditions.

Summary

Early Physiologic Responses to Acute Illness

An appropriate basic assumption is that low flow, poor tissue perfusion, shock, and other forms of circulatory dysfunction can be recognized early via objective noninvasive criteria and that more promptly delivered therapy might be more efficacious. Noninvasively monitored data may be used to titrate early fluid and inotropic therapy to achieve optimal physiologic criteria to prevent development of lethal organ failure. To a large extent, circulatory findings in acute illnesses may be explained by well-documented physiologic responses to trauma. Tissue injury, hemorrhage, pain, fear, and hypovolemia activate the sympathoadrenal axis, releasing epinephrine and norepinephrine from the adrenal medulla and the sympathetic effector neurons. The continued stress of hypovolemia, hypotension, and tissue injury and the sympathoadrenal response activate the hypothalamic-hypophyseal-adrenal axis via afferent neural signals. This activation causes corticotropin-releasing hormone to be released by the hypothalamus and elaboration of adrenocorticotropic hormone by the adenohypophysis. Adrenocorticotropic hormone stimulates the adrenals to secrete cortisol, which increases cardiac output and in part mediates the post-traumatic hypermetabolic state. The hypermetabolic state, which requires increased blood flow, makes tissues more susceptible to local ischemic events.

The cardiopulmonary effects of catecholamines immediately after trauma include increases in blood pressure, heart rate, cardiac contractility, minute ventilation, and peripheral vasomotor tone. Although these adaptive effects are often beneficial, especially in minor insults, exaggerated but uneven peripheral vasoconstriction in severe trauma or hemorrhage leads to increased but maldistributed microcirculatory flow with localized areas of hypoperfusion, tissue hypoxia, and intravascular hypovolemia. The hypoxic acidotic endothelium of poorly perfused capillaries activates macrophages and leukocytes and produces cytokines, platelet-activating factor, eicosanoids, intravascular coagulation, and many other known and unknown immunochemical cascades; the activated macrophages and the white blood cells produce oxygen free radicals and local tissue destruction, which mark the systemic inflammatory response syndrome. With resuscitation and reperfusion of hypoxic capillaries, these activated cellular and immunochemical mediators are washed into the venous circulation and lead to the systemic inflammatory response syndrome, end-organ dysfunction, multiple vital organ failures, and death.

The survivors have greater physiologic reserve capacity and the ability to generate the increased flow and tissue perfusion needed to provide adequate tissue oxygenation in the presence of increased metabolic need. Differences in hemodynamic patterns between survivors and nonsurvivors have motivated investigators to suggest aggressive fluid therapy titrated to reach optimal physiologic goals, defined by the patterns in survivors, as a strategy to improve patient outcome. Fluid therapy is titrated to maintain intravascular volume, improve tissue perfusion, and overcome regional circulatory deficiencies caused by uneven, maldistributed vasoconstriction.

Conclusions

We conclude that patients with traumatic injury can be appropriately monitored noninvasively beginning in the emergency department. The changes identified during the first few minutes or hours of hospitalization demonstrate circulatory deficiencies, adequacy of physiologic responses, and effectiveness of therapy. Patients who fail to respond with adequate tissue bed perfusion—as manifested by tissue perfusion and oxygenation—have a higher likelihood of complications and death. Early hemodynamic monitoring leads to better understanding of physiologic patterns in survivors and nonsurvivors, earlier identification of circulatory deficiencies associated with poor outcomes, and more definitive therapeutic protocols that improve outcome.

References

1. Shoemaker WC: Resuscitation algorithms in acute emergency conditions. In Grenvik A, Ayres SM, Holbrook PR, Shoemaker WC (eds): Textbook of Critical Care, 4th ed. Philadelphia, WB Saunders, 2000, pp 47–58.
2. Shoemaker WC, Appel PL, Kram HB: Hemodynamic and oxygen transport responses in survivors and nonsurvivors of high risk surgery. Crit Care Med 1993;21:977–990.
3. Shibutani K, Komatsu T, Kubal K, et al: Critical level of oxygen delivery in anesthetized man. Crit Care Med 1983;11:640–645.
4. Shoemaker WC, Appel PL, Kram HB, et al: Prospective trial of supranormal values of survivors as therapeutic goals in high risk surgical patients. Chest 1988;94:1176–1186.
5. Shoemaker WC, Kram HB, Appel PL, et al: The efficacy of central venous and pulmonary artery catheters and therapy based upon them in reducing mortality and morbidity. Arch Surg 1990;125:1332–1338.
6. Boyd O, Grounds M, Bennett D: Preoperative increase of oxygen delivery reduces mortality in high risk surgical patients. JAMA 1993;270:2699–2704.
7. Berlauk JF, Abrams JH, Gilmour IJ, et al: Preoperative optimization of cardiovascular hemodynamics improves outcome in peripheral vascular surgery. Ann Surg 1991;214:289–297.
8. Yu M, Levy MM, Smith P, et al: Effect of maximizing oxygen delivery on morbidity and mortality rates in critically ill patients: a prospective randomized controlled study. Crit Care Med 1993;21:830–838.
9. Wilson J, Woods I, Fawcett J, et al: Reducing the risk of major elective surgery: Randomized controlled trial of preoperative optimisation of oxygen delivery. BMJ 1999;318:1099–1103.
10. Boyd O, Hayes MA: The oxygen trail: the goals. Br Med Bull 1999;55:125–139.
11. Bishop MW, Shoemaker WC, Kram HB, et al: Prospective randomized trial of survivor values of cardiac output, oxygen delivery, and oxygen consumption as resuscitation endpoints in severe trauma. J Trauma 1995;38:780–787.
12. Shoemaker WC, Belzberg H, Wo CCJ, et al: Multicenter study of noninvasive monitoring as alternatives to invasive monitoring of acutely ill emergency patients. Chest 1998;114:1643–1652.
13. Bishop MH, Shoemaker WC, Shuleshko J, Wo CCJ: Noninvasive cardiac index monitoring in gunshot wound victims. Acad Emerg Med 1996;3:682–688.
14. Shoemaker WC, Wo CCJ, Chan L, et al: Outcome prediction of severely injured patients by noninvasive monitoring beginning in the emergency department. Chest 2001; in press.
15. Shoemaker WC, Wo CCJ, Sullivan MJ, et al: Invasive and noninvasive hemodynamic monitoring of patients with acute myocardial infarction in the emergency department. Ann Emerg Med 2001; in press.
16. Shoemaker WC, Wo CCJ, Sullivan MJ, et al: Invasive and noninvasive hemodynamic monitoring and therapy of patients with heart failure in the emergency department. Eur J Emerg Med 2001; in press.
17. Hauser CJ, Shoemaker WC, Turpin I, Goldberg SJ: Oxygen transport responses to colloids and crystalloids in critically ill surgical patients. Surg Gynecol Obstet 1980;150:811–818.
18. Shoemaker WC, Kram HB: Effects of crystalloids and colloids on hemodynamics, oxygen transport, and outcome in high risk surgical patients. In Simmonds RS, Udekuo AE (eds): Debates in Clinical Surgery. Chicago, Year Book, 1990, pp 263–315.
19. Lazarove S, Waxman K, Shoemaker WC: Hemodynamic, blood volume, and oxygen transport responses to albumin and hydroxyethyl starch infusions in critically ill postoperative patients. Crit Care Med 1980;8:254–260.
20. Shoemaker WC, Wo CCJ: Circulatory effects of whole blood, packed red cells, albumin, starch, and crystalloids in resuscitation of shock and critical illness. Vox Sang 1998;74(suppl 2):69–74.
21. Shoemaker WC, Appel PL, Kram HB, et al: Hemodynamic and oxygen transport monitoring to titrate therapy in septic shock. New Horiz 1993;1:145–159.
22. Ford HR, Shires GT III, Shires GT: Colloids should not be used in the resuscitation of the patient in hemorrhagic shock. In Simmonds RS, Udekuo AE (eds): Debates in Clinical Surgery. Chicago, Year Book, 1990, pp 250–262.
23. Shoemaker WC, Appel PL, Kram HB, et al: Comparison of hemodynamic and oxygen transport effects of dopamine and dobutamine in critically ill patients. Chest 1989;96:102–106.
24. Shoemaker WC, Appel PL, Kram HB: Role of oxygen debt in the development of organ failure, sepsis, and death in high-risk surgical patients. Chest 1992;102:208–215.
25. Boyd O, Grounds RM, Bennett ED: The cost implications of reducing mortality by perioperatively increasing oxygen delivery. Clin Intensive Care 1994;5:21–27.

INDEX

Note: Page numbers followed by the letter f refer to figures and those followed by t refer to tables.